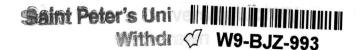
W9-BJZ-993

The Medical Cost-Containment Crisis

Fears, Opinions, and Facts

Edited by
Jack D. McCue

The Medical Cost-Containment Crisis

Fears, Opinions, and Facts

Health Administration Press Perspectives
Ann Arbor, Michigan 1989

94 93 92 91 90   5 4 3 2

Library of Congress Cataloging-in-Publication Data
The Medical cost-containment crisis.
    Includes bibliographies and index.
    1. Medical care, Cost of—United States. I. McCue, Jack D.
[DNLM: 1. Cost Control. 2. Economics, Medical—United States.
W 74 M4889]
RA410.53.M39 1989   338.4'33621'0973   88-34784
ISBN 0-910701-43-1 (soft)

Health Administration Press
A division of the Foundation of the
    American College of Healthcare Executives
1021 East Huron Street
Ann Arbor, Michigan 48104-9990
(313) 764-1380

Contents

**VIEWPOINTS OF BUSINESS, ORGANIZED
MEDICINE, GOVERNMENT, AND THE MEDICAL-
INDUSTRIAL COMPLEX**

IV **COST-CONTAINMENT EFFORTS: MIXED
RESULTS OF CONTROLS ON TECHNOLOGY USE,
EDUCATION, RATIONING, AND INFORMATION
SYSTEMS**

List of Figures

List of Tables

Acknowledgments

The Kate B. Reynolds Health Care Trust provided generous support for the symposium that was the starting point for this book. Dennis Hoban, Ed.D., James Leist, Ed.D., Charles J. Hansen, M.A., and Richard Janeway, M.D. provided encouragement, support, and advice. Secretarial help provided by Linda Griffin made it possible to keep this complicated project organized.

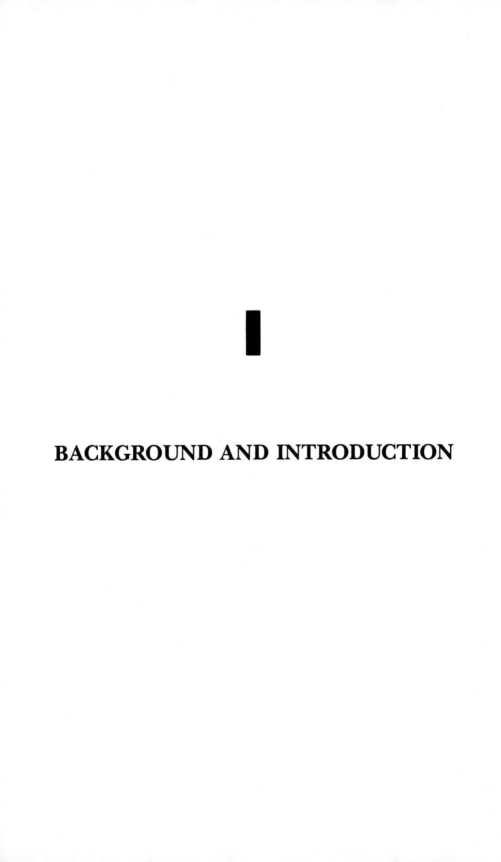

BACKGROUND AND INTRODUCTION

Introduction

*The High Cost of Medical Care:
An Introduction to the
Cost-Containment Debate*

Jack D. McCue

Americans believe that the United States is in a medical
care cost crisis. Since the early 1980s, the federal government and the
private insurers who finance much of the cost of medical care have
advocated and implemented crisis-oriented, radical changes in the health
care system to reduce the rate of rise in medical costs. So pervasive are
the changes that, as Duffy credibly asserts in Chapter 4 of this book, the
physician and the third-party payer (Medicare, Medicaid, or a private
insurer) now form the primary decision-making relationship in complicated medical and surgical problems. The patient, who can rarely afford
the expense of high-technology care out-of-pocket, serves in an advisory
capacity, ultimately receiving the care that his insurer decides is worth
the expense.

Despite our increasingly energetic moves over the last decade, the
true dimensions and nature of the medical cost crisis are still hard to
grasp. Americans do not want less medical care—every public poll has
concluded that an overwhelming majority wants more. As the population continues to age, and the healthy, affluent, middle-aged population
retires, it is certain that first class medical care will become an even
greater national priority. Nor are Americans especially unhappy with
the quality of their medical care. It is difficult for anyone to be uncrit-
ically complimentary about a service such as medical care. In Chapter 3,

Mechanic describes a few reasons why we can never be wholly pleased with our experiences during the dependency and peril of a serious illness.

Nor are we disenchanted with expensive medical technology. We crave the nostalgic warmth and security of our family doctor of the 1950s (who retired in southern Florida 15 years ago), but we are really more impressed by expensive medical technology. Every frugal primary care physician will ruefully admit that the reassurance value of a $750 CT brain scan (better yet, a $1,200 MRI scan!) for a patient with headaches exceeds the value of the physician's empathy and interpersonal skills. The fact is that both patients and physicians want the certainty that technology promises, and we think it is worth the cost. We and our employers pay expensive medical insurance premiums—one of the very first concerns of laid-off workers is medical insurance for their families (and appropriately so)—and we expect our insurance to pay for sophisticated medical care, without excessive concern for expense.

Still, while we want the best for ourselves and our families, Americans also believe that medical care is too expensive. Our concern for the cost of care seems directed mostly at our out-of-pocket expenses and public expenditures through taxation or the support of Medicare. Our feelings about modern medical care are similar to the vague belief that, in general, life has become too complicated, impersonal, and expensive. Ironically, it seems that many of our attempts to contain costs have actually resulted in increased complexity and bureaucracy—to an extent that would have seemed unbelievable only a decade ago—without resulting in dramatic decreases in the costs of medical care.

The popular support for medical cost-containment programs seems to come from the general concern that we are not getting our money's worth. And there is a basis for this concern. If I go to my physician with complaints of dyspepsia, he will tell me to take better care of myself and not to work so much; but he might also order an abdominal ultrasound to be sure that I do not have gallstones. If gallstones are found (giving me an excuse to return to my self-abusive life-style), they may or may not be responsible for my symptoms; it is impossible for my physician to be certain. So, we decide that I should undergo elective cholecystectomy. When all is said and done, the total cost for evaluation and treatment will be approximately the same as the cost of my basic family car.

Did I get my money's worth? My dyspepsia might still bother me because the gallstones might actually have been asymptomatic (or I might subsequently develop stress-related non-ulcer dyspepsia as I attempt to deal with the insurance paperwork), but two things are certain: my gallstones were indeed removed, and nearly every item charged to my account during hospitalization is defensible. (Whether each expense was *necessary* is a far more difficult question, and it might be worth a little thought to the difference between a defensible, justifiable service and a necessary medical service.) Furthermore, I can assure the reader that there was less waste in my elective cholecystectomy than in the manufacturing of my family car: the hospital president did not receive a multimillion dollar bonus last year; my hospital is not unionized and has never dealt with feather-bedding; every syringe or piece of suture is as competitively bid as any component of my car; and my surgeon is no better paid than many automobile company executives who have had far less education and training (my general surgeon has had nine expensive, arduous years of post-college education and training). But I still have a disquieting belief that it should not cost as much to remove my gallstones as to purchase a car—am I not entitled, as a hard-working, tax-paying American, to the right to be free of the pain of an easily correctable disease such as cholelithiasis? Does my belief that good medical care should be a fundamental right interfere with an objective assessment of how expensive medical care should be?

It is helpful to look at what Americans spend on medical care in comparison with other nations (Figure 1). Our expenses per capita are average; in comparison to those of Canada or West Germany, they are rather modest; and they are surprisingly little more than in Great Britain, where one must wait months to years for elective surgery in decaying facilities which are understaffed by underpaid health care workers (*New York Times*, 7 August 1988, 1). As one might predict, the share paid by the U.S. government is much less than in nationalized health systems; we pay a much larger amount out-of-pocket and through private insurance than other industrialized nations (Figures 1 and 2—the methodologies for these data are different, yielding different numbers for per capita expenditures). Another major difference is that we clearly spend a greater percentage of our gross national product (GNP) on health care than do other nations (Figures 1 and 3).

Each reader must decide independently whether it is proper for a wealthy nation with a rapidly aging population to spend a large proportion of its GNP on medical care. The vigorous interdisciplinary debate in this book may contribute to that decision; it will certainly convince the reader that there are no simple answers to the questions posed by consumers, health economists, politicians, ethicists, and industry. Do we pay too much for medical care, and if so, whose fault is it? Is there excessive wastefulness? Are our solutions to the problems of rising costs of medical care worse than the problems? Do we have the ethical courage and honesty to face the consequences of rationing medical care?

The majority of the contributors to this book are physicians, but they write with knowledge of the many facets of the medical cost-containment debate and not necessarily from the perspective of medical practitioners. Business, organized medicine, for-profit hospitals, edu-

FIGURE 1

Health Care Expenditures, 1985

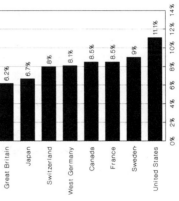

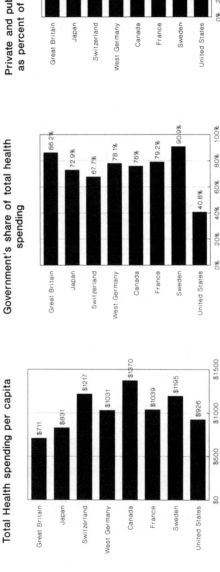

Sources: The Organization for Economic Cooperation and Development and U.S. Department of Human Services.

FIGURE 2

Who Paid Our Medical Bills of $2,130 per Person in 1987

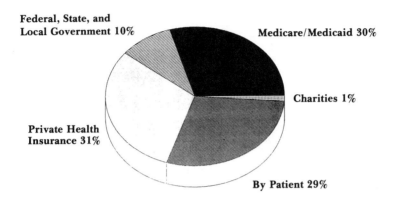

Source: Health Care Financing Administration.

cators, health policy researchers, charitable foundations, ethicists, and sociologists are also engaged in the debate in this book. Nevertheless, the orientation of this book is most in keeping with the interests of the medical care industry and its practitioners.

While many of the chapters are written by scholars and are indeed scholarly in their analysis, the book is not intended to be a comprehensive description of medical economics. It is intended, instead, to serve as a forum for debate among representatives of the major groups involved in cost containment.

BACKGROUND

The initial chapters attempt to give an overview of the medical cost-containment debate: Janeway looks to the past and asks how we got to the point where about 11 percent of our entire gross national product is directed to providing medical care; Freymann looks forward, asking what we want medical care to be like in 20 years, and describing what it will probably be like.

As Janeway indicates, medical care costs have risen dramatically. Each American spent $82 per year for medical care in 1950, and 23 years later spent $1,459; the total expenditures for health-related

FIGURE 3

Medical Costs as a Percentage of GNP

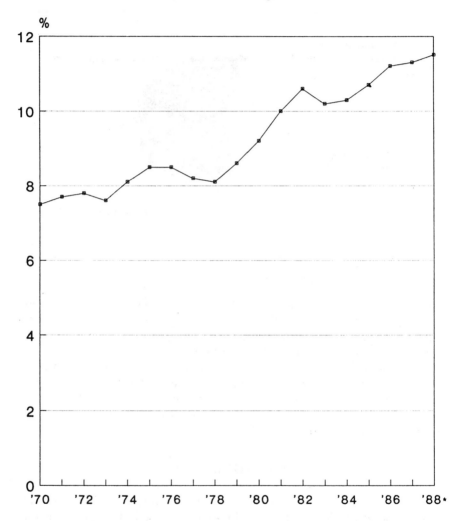

Source: Health Care Financing Administration.
*Estimate.

services and goods rose from $12.7 billion in 1950 to $423.8 billion in 1985.[1] Such statistics are surely breathtaking and perhaps alarming, but Janeway insists that we consider what we have bought with that money as we demand an analytic account of why we spend so much on medical care. Medical costs have been driven up by general inflation, population growth, demographic changes, increased voluntary usage by consumers, and increased willingness of government to spend larger amounts of money derived from our increasing affluence, much as government has been willing to spend more on military weaponry.

But the nature and cost of both military weaponry and medical care have been irreversibly changed by technology and scientific research. We must remember that, when we compare the cost of medical care in 1950 with that in 1990, we are comparing two demonstrably different items. To cite an example, an automobile bought in 1990 will be many times more expensive than one bought in 1950, but it will also be safer, more comfortable, and more efficient; hence, such cost comparisons of either automobiles or medical care will be interesting but not necessarily fair.

In his former role as the president of the National Fund for Medical Education, Freymann was concerned with encouraging research and projects that would help prepare medical education for the future. His forward-looking view of the medical cost crisis is provocative in its breadth. Cost containment, he predicts, will be so pervasive that it becomes part of the fabric of medical care—and we will be as poorly prepared—educationally, technologically, and ethically—for the problems of future medical care as we are for the problems created by changes in medicine over the past two decades.

DOCTORS AND THEIR PATIENTS

Mechanic, a prominent medical sociologist who is especially interested in medical economics, draws a disquieting picture of the complex human ramifications of the simplistic responses of bureaucrats and government to the demands for reduced cost of medical care. His chapter deserves careful reading and rereading. The differences between the social disruptions created by a reduction of funds devoted to research in and production of widgets, and decreasing the availability of expensive medical technology or cutting funds available for medical research, are rarely appreciated.

One small but extensively analyzed part of sociology is the doctor-patient relationship. It is a relationship in which nearly everyone participates at some point in life, and during a serious illness it can become our most important personal relationship. Duffy examines the potentially pernicious effect of cost-containment interventions which threaten to make the patient's relationship to his physician less important than the relationship with the government or an insurer in determining the care that can be provided.

Veatch postulates, and many of the contributors to this book agree, that technologic developments and economic changes have outstripped our ethical understanding of those changes. The hypocrisy of rationing medical care while claiming that all can have equal access to the best medical care is uncomfortably apparent; rationing is inevitable, and the ethical dimensions of limiting medical care should be addressed openly.

BUSINESS, ORGANIZED MEDICINE, GOVERNMENT, AND THE MEDICAL-INDUSTRIAL COMPLEX

The contributions of businesses to the financing of medical care, indirectly through employee health insurance benefits and directly through employee health clinics, probably equal the amount of government spending for Medicaid and Medicare; yet they have received little attention in discussions of cost containment. In 1987, 40 percent of the nation's health care bill was paid by government, 31 percent by private insurers whose premiums were paid at least in part by business, and 29 percent by individual patients (1988 HCFA data). Hayes presents original data that document the size of business contributions and provide a basis for understanding why further increases directly raise the cost of their products and reduce the competitiveness of American businesses in the international market.

The other influence of business on health care costs is, of course, the growth of for-profit medical care businesses. Two opposing views are presented: Frist and Howard describe how investor-owned hospitals have demonstrated that medical care can be delivered more efficiently and less expensively, and have, therefore, taught not-for-profit hospitals how good business practices could be adapted in their operations. Wohl disagrees: Businesses, whether manufacturing or medical, seek to increase their numbers of customers and their profits, and to control their market. Their goals are, therefore, inimical to cost-effective medical care. Perhaps the truth lies between these two views.

The impetus for medical cost-containment programs came primarily from the growth in government expenditures for the Medicare and Medicaid programs. Approximately 20 percent of the U.S. population has their medical care paid for by one of these programs: Medicaid serves mostly children, and Medicare serves the elderly. Even physicians, who must deal with these programs daily, do not fully understand who these programs serve and how they serve their target populations. Sorkin's historical description of Medicare and Medicaid thus makes it possible to better understand how cost-containment interventions will affect the medical care of two vulnerable groups of the population.

Finally, organized medicine, and the American Medical Association (AMA) in particular, has been blamed for vigorously opposing government programs such as Medicare, and then standing by passively as hospitals and physicians eagerly reach in the deep pockets of government programs. The view from inside the AMA is different, of course, and Schwarz describes its attempts to encourage cost containment. It is doubtful that other unions or lobbyist groups have made similar attempts to encourage reduced consumption of government funds by their members (we should remember that a majority of physicians are not AMA members).

COST-CONTAINMENT EFFORTS

Some of the varied attempts to control medical costs are described in this section. McPhee, Showstack, and Schroeder describe the complicated issues involved in reducing the use of medical technology by physicians, and why efforts to change clinical decision making to reduce costs without diminishing the quality of care have rarely succeeded. Hoban, Hansen, and McCue similarly describe the variable results, at best, of attempts to encourage cost-consciousness through medical education; and Lyle et al. describe the frustration and confusion experienced by medical school faculty when they tried to discourage the unnecessary use of expensive medical resources at their university hospital.

The experiences with rationing of medical care described in Great Britain lurk uncomfortably behind the platitude that claims we must "get more for less." Merrill and Cohen give a clear-sighted description of what rationing medical care means, where it leads us, and how it might be avoided.

Komaroff and Lee describe how the continuing information revolution predicted for the future by Freymann can influence the costs of medical care now. Useful, timely information provided to those who make cost-related decisions can lead to more efficient use of resources in medicine as well as in business.

AT THE MARGINS OF COST CONTAINMENT

Three issues (many more could have been chosen) are explored to illustrate the complexity and multidimensionality of medical cost containment. The elderly are the major consumers of medical resources per capita. Yet, as Hazzard points out, since their medical care is not shaped to meet their needs, they often receive inappropriate and unnecessary treatment and do not receive the (often less expensive) care that could best meet their needs. We all agree that we must strive to maintain the quality of care as we attempt to cut costs—but how? Dans describes what quality assurance means, and how quality is measured and monitored. Neuhauser, the editor of a major health care services research journal, examines research issues such as ethics and liability that must be addressed to permit public policy to *shape* our system of medical care, rather than to *respond* with piecemeal solutions, as in the past.

Two participants in the national debate are missing from this book: First, consumers (or patients, as we once called them) are only indirectly represented. A single chapter on the patient's perspective could not do justice to the economic viewpoints of healthy, acutely ill, disabled, young, and old patients. Second, there is no comprehensive description—either in this book or in the medical-legal literature—of the economic impact of the malpractice liability disaster that now confronts medicine. Liability problems do not belong to medicine alone, but they are surely most disruptive there. Every practitioner, every day, makes decisions based on the fear of litigation that have cost consequences. Before the medical liability problem can be solved, however, our society must face ethical issues such as the right to die, the right to live a meaningless life, or whether maloccurrence ("bad luck") is compensable and by whom. Although these topics are not covered in the chapters of this book, pertinent discussions of the issues are provided in the reference list which follows.

Another issue, costs related to paying physicians, is not explored in detail in this book. Physician reimbursement is a relatively small part of medical care expenditures which is often exaggerated in importance in the minds of the lay press and the public. It is not addressed here because it is nearly impossible to determine objectively what anyone should be paid for a service or what a person's services are truly worth. The sociology and psychology of the debate on paying doctors may be far more interesting and important than the relevant economics. Again, the references listed on the following pages discuss physician reimbursement.

This book is intended to give readers insight into how terribly complex medical cost containment is—the consequences of changes are not just economic, they are human. We must not forget that pain, death, disability, and injustice may result from mistakes in our attempts to correct the problems we find in our often wasteful medical care system, the system which many people consider the world's best.

NOTE

1. The figures for 1987 (the most recently reported year as of the date of publication) are: $500 billion total spending, with $541 billion estimated for 1988 and $590 billion estimated for 1989.

RECENT REFERENCES AND SUGGESTED READINGS

Journal Articles

Abraham, K. S. "Medical Liability Reform: A Conceptual Framework." *Journal of the American Medical Association* 260 (1988): 68–72.

Blendon, R. J.; Aiken, L. H.; Freeman, H. E.; et al. "Access to Medical Care for Black and White Americans. A Matter of Continuing Concern." *Journal of the American Medical Association* 261 (1989): 278–81.

Bloom, B. S., and Jacobs, J. "Cost Effects of Restricting Cost Effective Therapy." *Medical Care* 23 (1985): 872–80.

Brook, R. H. "Does Free Care Improve Adults' Health? Results for a Randomized Controlled Trial." *New England Journal of Medicine* 309 (1983): 1426–34.

Brook, R. H., and Lohr, K. N. "Monitoring Quality of Care in the Medicare Program: Two Proposed Systems." *Journal of the American Medical Association* 258 (1987): 3138–41.

Chassin, M. R.; Kosecoff, J.; Park, R. E.; et al. "Does Inappropriate Use Explain Geographic Variations in the Use of Health Care Services? A Study of Three Procedures." *Journal of the American Medical Association* 258 (1987): 2533–37.

Donabedian, A. "The Quality of Care. How Can It Be Assessed?" *Journal of the American Medical Association* 260 (1988): 1743–48.

Drummond, M.; Stoddart, G.; Labelle, R.; et al. "Health Economics: An Introduction for Clinicians." *Annals of Internal Medicine* 107 (1987): 88–92.

Evans, R. G.; Lomas, J.; Barer, M. L.; et al. "Controlling Health Expenditures— The Canadian Reality." *New England Journal of Medicine* 320 (1989): 571–77.

Feldstein, P. J.; Wickizer, T. M.; and Wheeler, J. R. C. "Private Cost Containment: The Effects of Utilization Review Programs on Health Care Use and Expenditures." *New England Journal of Medicine* 318 (1988): 1310–14.

Ginzberg, E. "A Hard Look at Cost Containment." *New England Journal of Medicine* 316 (1987): 1151–54.

Hadley, J., and Berenson, R. A. "Seeking the Just Price: Constructing Relative Value Scales and Fee Schedules." *Annals of Internal Medicine* 106 (1987): 461–66.

Health and Public Policy Committee, American College of Physicians. "Medicare Payment for Physician Services." *Annals of Internal Medicine* 106 (1987): 151–63.

Himmelstein, D. U., and Woolhandler, S. "Cost without Benefit: Administrative Waste in U.S. Health Care." *New England Journal of Medicine* 314 (1986): 441–45.

————. "The Corporate Compromise: A Marxist View of Health Maintenance Organizations and Prospective Payment." *Annals of Internal Medicine* 109 (1988): 494–501.

Hsiao, W. C.; Braun, P.; and Yntema, D. "Estimating Physicians' Work for a Resource-Based Relative-Value Scale." *New England Journal of Medicine* 319 (1988): 835–41.

Hulka, B. S., and Wheat, J. R. "Patterns of Utilization: The Patient Perspective." *Medical Care* 23 (1985): 438–60.

Iglehart, J. K. "Canada's Health Care System" (3 parts). *New England Journal of Medicine* 315 (1986): 202–8.

Luft, H. S. "Competition and Regulation." *Medical Care* 23 (1985): 283–300.

Reynolds, R. A.; Rizzo, J. A.; and Gonzales, M. L. "The Cost of Medical Professional Liability." *Journal of the American Medical Association* 257 (1987): 2776–81.

Robinson, J. C., and Luft, H. S. "Competition and the Cost of Hospital Care, 1972 to 1982." *Journal of the American Medical Association* 257 (1987): 3241–45.

Robinson, J. C.; Luft, H. S.; McPhee, S. J.; and Hunt, S. S. "Hospital Competition and Surgical Length of Stay." *Journal of the American Medical Association* 259 (1988): 696–700.

Roper, W. L. "Perspectives on Physician-Payment Reform: The Resource-Based Relative-Value Scale in Context." *Health Care Financing Administration* 319 (1988): 865–67.

Russell, L. B., and Manning, C. L. "The Effect of Prospective Payment on Medicare Expenditures." *New England Journal of Medicine* 320 (1989): 439–44.

Sager, M. A.; Easterling, D. V.; Kindig, D. A.; et al. "Changes in the Location of Death After Passage of Medicare's Prospective Payment System." *New England Journal of Medicine* 320 (1989): 433–39.

Schwartz, W. B. "The Inevitable Failure of Current Cost-Containment Strategies: Why They Can Provide Only Temporary Relief." *Journal of the American Medical Association* 257 (1987): 220–24.

Selker, H. P., and Griffith, J. L. "How Do Physicians Adapt When the Coronary Care Unit Is Full? A Prospective Multicenter Study." *Journal of the American Medical Association* 257 (1987): 1181–85.

Shapiro, M. F.; Ware, J. E.; and Sherbourne, C. D. "Effects of Cost Sharing on Seeking for Serious and Minor Symptoms." *Annals of Internal Medicine* 104 (1986): 246–51.

Shortell, S. M., and Hughes, E. F. X. "The Effects of Regulation, Competition, and Ownership on Mortality Rates among Hospital Inpatients." *New England Journal of Medicine* 318 (1988): 1100–6.

Siu, A. L.; Sonnenberg, F. A.; Manning, W. G.; et al. "Inappropriate Use of Hospitals in a Randomized Trial of Health Insurance Plans." *New England Journal of Medicine* 315 (1986): 1259–66.

Watt, J. M.; et al. "The Comparative Economic Performance of Investor-Owned Chain and Not-for-Profit Hospitals." *New England Journal of Medicine* 314 (1986): 89–96.

Books

Danzon, P. M. *Medical Malpractice.* Cambridge, MA: Harvard University Press, 1985.

Eisenberg, J. M. *Doctors' Decisions and the Cost of Medical Care.* Ann Arbor, MI: Health Administration Press, 1986.

Glaser, W. A. *Paying the Doctor: Systems of Remuneration and Their Effects.* Baltimore, MD: Johns Hopkins University Press, 1970.

———. *Paying the Hospital: Foreign Lessons for the U.S.* New York: Columbia University Center for the Social Sciences, 1982.

Chapter 1

*The Costs of Medical Care in a
Society with Changing Goals:
A Longitudinal View*

Richard Janeway

Editor's Note—From 1950 to 1985, expenditures for medical care increased more than 35-fold, and currently they constitute about 11 percent of the U.S. gross national product (GNP). The causes of the increase are multiple: inflation in the economy in general, real growth, and inefficiency. Inefficiency and waste are relatively small components of costs and are, therefore, a negligible cause of increasing costs. General inflation is the major reason for increased costs, and the medical care industry may well have endured a higher rate of inflation than other major segments of the economy because of pressures to raise health care worker salaries to competitive levels.

Real growth is a smaller, but important part of increasing costs. Among the causes of real growth—that is, a growth in the quantity of medical services (not just the price, which would be inflation)—are growth of the population, the dramatic increase in the number of elderly Americans who are the major consumers of medical services, improved access to medical care for the poor and disadvantaged, and technologic advances. Real growth has brought benefits, Janeway reminds us, and some of those benefits will have to be sacrificed if we decide to reduce expenditures for medical services.

Viewing our perceived cost crisis historically, we are reminded that we arrived in the current circumstances by design, not by accident. Government and private funding of medical research and the goals of the Great Society, which include equal access to medical care for all Americans, are part of the foundation of our medical care system. If we decide to institute radical changes in the economics of the medical care system, we should honestly examine how those past goals may be undercut by attempts to economize, and whether we should choose to continue to pursue those goals which have been accomplished, to a large degree, by the modern medical care system.

The increasing costs of medical care in the years leading up to 1987 are best viewed through a historical context that recognizes our passage first through what has been called "the age of scientific awakening" in the 1950s and then through the social and medical expansionist goals of the Great Society of the 1960s. Before costs are considered, however, benefits should also be taken into account. What has happened to the health of the nation in the last 3½ decades?

To cite a few examples of changes in our nation's health, the age-adjusted overall death rate per 100,000 people has declined precipitously from 841.5 in 1950 to 540 in 1986 (see Figure 1.1). A 36 percent decrease in the death rate over 36 years cannot be a chance occurrence. Similarly, the age-adjusted death rate for diseases of the heart has been reduced by 41 percent, and the death rate from cerebrovascular disease has been cut by a remarkable 64 percent (see Figures 1.2 and 1.3).

Although medicine cannot be credited for all of this good news, dramatic decreases in these selected death rates began about 1965 when the federal government initiated its massive intervention in research and demonstration programs related to heart disease, cancer, and stroke.

FIGURE 1.1

U.S. Age-Adjusted Overall Death Rate:
Selected Years 1950–86

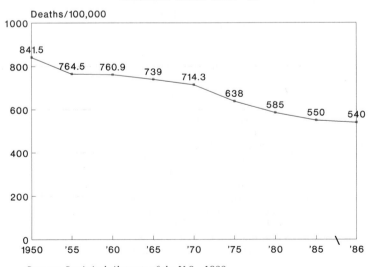

Source: *Statistical Abstracts of the U.S.*, 1988.

FIGURE 1.2

U.S. Adjusted Death Rate for Diseases of the Heart: Selected Years 1950–85

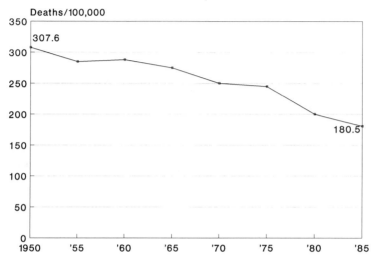

Source: *Statistical Abstracts of the U.S.*, 1988.

FIGURE 1.3

U.S. Adjusted Death Rate for Cerebrovascular Disease: Selected Years 1950–85

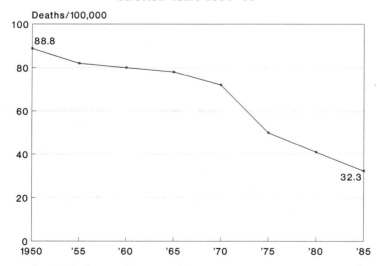

Source: *Statistical Abstracts of the U.S.*, 1988.

FIGURE 1.4

Infant Mortality in the United States:
Selected Years 1950–86

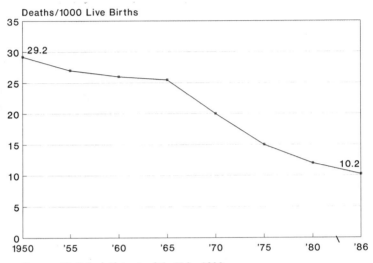

Source: *Statistical Abstracts of the U.S.*, 1988.

Similarly, infant mortality declined from 29.2 to 10.2 per 1,000 live births, related to the combined impact of the institution of social programs designed to guarantee access to high-quality medical care and other supportive services (see Figure 1.4).

Of the three major causes of adult death, only cancer has shown an increase, and at least part of this increase can be explained by the increasing longevity of the population, and another part by intemperate personal life-style decisions and other environmental factors (Figure 1.5).

COSTS

Benefits do not come without costs. Indeed, the cost of health care in the United States rose from $12.7 billion in 1950 to an estimated $423.8 billion for 1985 (see Figure 1.6). The projected expenditures for 1986 total $466 billion. Although it is an oversimplification, we are spending, in nominal dollars, approximately 36.6 times as much as we were spending 35 years ago, and major segments of our society are seriously questioning whether the benefits we produce are worth the costs we incur.

Another way of examining this increase is the rise in per capita costs of approximately 21-fold in the last 35 years; but this is a mislead-

FIGURE 1.5

U.S. Adjusted Death Rate for Cancer: Selected Years 1950–85

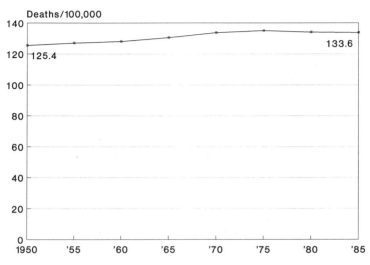

Source: *Statistical Abstracts of the U.S.*, 1988.

FIGURE 1.6

Total National Health Expenditures: Selected Years 1950–85

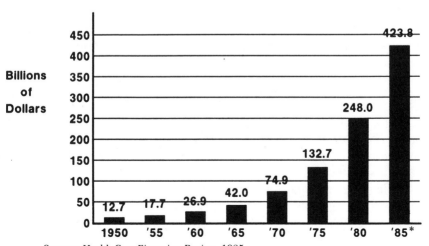

Source: *Health Care Financing Review*, 1985.

*Estimate.

FIGURE 1.7

National Health Expenditures per Capita:
Selected Years 1950–83

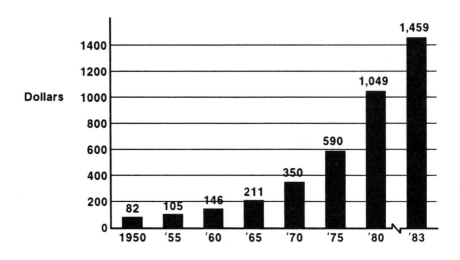

Source: *Statistical Abstracts of the U.S.*, 1985.

ing statistic (see Figure 1.7). Expenditures are very unevenly distributed among age groups and, within the elderly population, expenditures are unevenly distributed between survivors and decedents, and by timing of expense. Quoting per capita expense thus distorts the actual low cost figures for health care for the huge majority of working Americans.

COMPONENTS OF COST

A longitudinal look at the distribution of national health expenditures from 1950 to 1983 shows that the largest portion of the increase in expense can be accounted for by the costs of hospitalization and physician services (see Figure 1.8).

When the percentage distribution of expense is used to compare components of cost in 1950 and 1983, it becomes apparent that the hospital cost component has risen from 30.4 percent of total expenditures to 41.4 percent in 1983, while payments to physicians have fallen from 21.7 percent to 19.4 percent of total health care expenditures (see Figure 1.9). The most rapidly increasing cost on a percentage basis is nursing home care, which was 1.5 percent of total expense in 1950 and

FIGURE 1.8

Growth in Major Components of National Health Care Expenditures:
Selected Years 1950–83

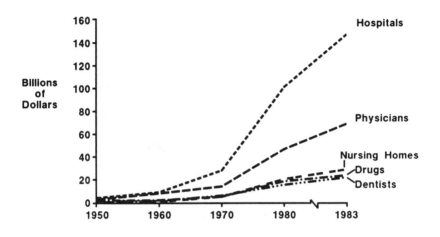

Source: *Statistical Abstracts of the U.S.*, 1985.

FIGURE 1.9

Percent Distribution of Total National Health Expenditures:
Selected Years 1950–83

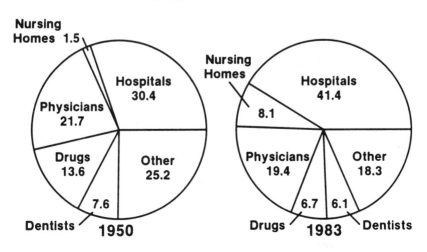

Source: *Statistical Abstracts of the U.S.*, 1985.

FIGURE 1.10

Source of Growth in National Health Expenditures:
Selected Years 1950–85

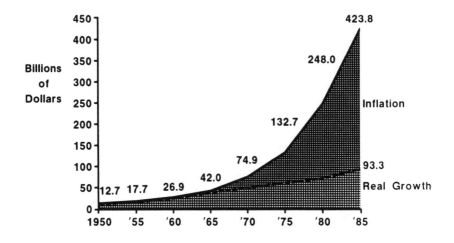

Source: *Health Care Financing Review*, 1985.

had risen to 8.1 percent in 1983. Nursing home care costs will continue to be the most rapidly increasing percentage component of cost for the foreseeable future because of the increasing longevity of the population.

CAUSES OF COST INCREASES

There are three elements that can be aggregated to account for almost all of the increase in the cost of health care in the United States. These elements are *inflation, real growth,* and *inefficiency.* Fraud and abuse receive major rhetorical attention, but can be subsumed within inefficiency without causing major numerical distortion.

Inflation

The major cause of the increase in national health expenditures is attributable to inflation within our economy as a whole (see Figure 1.10). If one considers 1950 dollars to be "real dollars" (dollars for which the deflating effect of inflation has been arithmetically corrected), only $93.3 billion of our total health expenditures in 1985 represented "real

FIGURE 1.11

Cumulative Percent Increase in Inflation:
Selected Years 1950–85

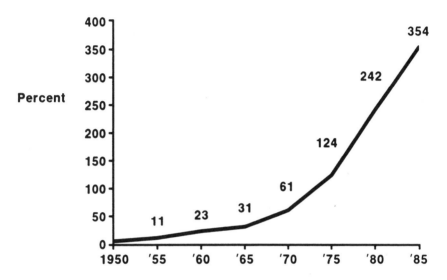

Source: *Statistical Abstracts of the U.S.*, 1988.

growth" (growth in quantity of services) in system costs, including any inherent inefficiency, fraud, and abuse. One need only note the 354 percent cumulative increase in the consumer price index (CPI) from 1950 to 1985 to validate this assertion (see Figure 1.11).

The cost of running a hospital has undergone inflation out of proportion to the general CPI, however, and was 4.33 times the 1967 base in 1986, approximately 32 percent higher than the all-items CPI (see Figure 1.12). Part of the increment is due to wage increases that were deemed essential by our society to redress the economic imbalance borne by historically underpaid personnel in nursing services and other support positions. A significant portion, however, is related to cost-based reimbursement policies which gave no incentive for hospitals to be prudent buyers. Finally, part is related to the real growth of utilized available services.

Real Growth

Real growth within the system can be accounted for by growth and aging of the population, by improvements in access to care, and by

FIGURE 1.12

Growth of Hospital Market Basket and CPI All Items
(base 1967 = 1.00): 1966–86

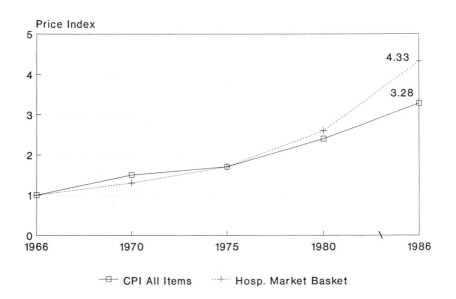

Source: *Statistical Abstracts of the U.S.*, 1988.

scientific and technical advances. The population of the United States increased by 63 percent from 1950 to 1988 (see Figure 1.13). But even more significant is the dramatic change in the age distribution of the population (see Figure 1.14).

Increased life expectancy has a cost. On a per capita basis, people 65 years of age or older averaged $3,593 of personal health care expenditures in 1983, while those under age 65 incurred costs of only $995. Personal health care expenditures in the age group from one to 18 years are negligible in comparison to any other age grouping (see Figure 1.15). The distribution of expenditures among the elderly is not only uneven between decedents and survivors, it is unevenly distributed over time. These disparate expenditure distributions will become the focus of one of the most difficult ethical and policy disputes ever encountered by our society.

It is predicted that by the year 2000 there will be 35 million people in this country over the age of 65, and almost 16 million people over

FIGURE 1.13

U.S. Total Population by Age: Selected Years 1950–88

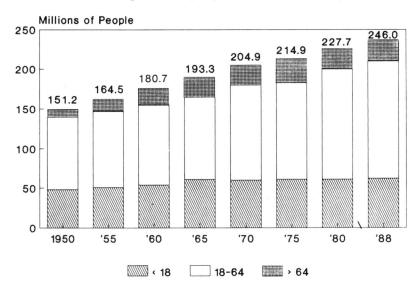

Source: *Statistical Abstracts of the U.S.*, 1988.

FIGURE 1.14

Percent Increases of Population by Age Group: 1950–83

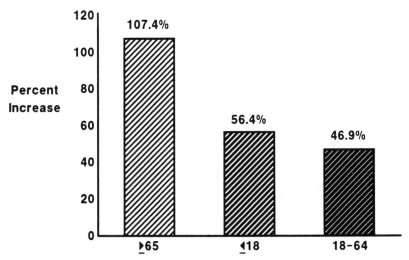

Source: *Statistical Abstracts of the U.S.*, 1985.

FIGURE 1.15

Per Capita Personal Health Care Expenditures by Age: 1983

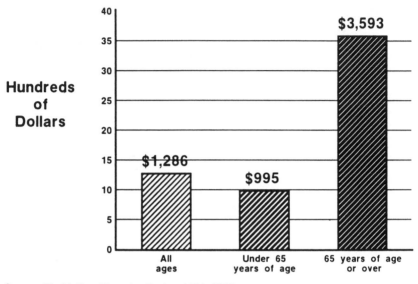

Source: *Health Care Financing Review,* 1984, 1985.

FIGURE 1.16

Growth of Elderly Population: Selected Years 1950–2000

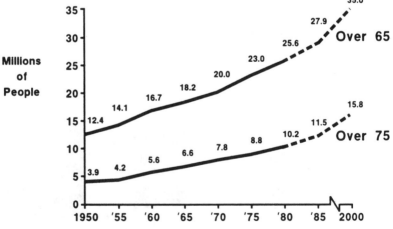

Source: *Statistical Abstracts of the U.S.,* 1985.

FIGURE 1.17

Percentage of Whites and Nonwhites Seeing a Physician
in a 12-Month Period

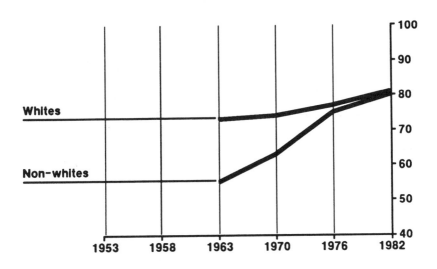

Source: Center for Health Administration Studies, University of Chicago.

the age of 75 (see Figure 1.16). This age group happens to be the most
rapidly growing segment of the United States population in percentage
terms. By the year 2040 it is projected that there will be 68.8 million
people (plus or minus about a million) age 65 and over in the United
States, and there will be almost 12 million people over the age of 85.
This so-called demographic imperative will have to be considered as we
plan for future medical care expenditures.

Access to medical care was dramatically changed when Medicare
and Medicaid were begun in 1965. The data in Figure 1.17 demonstrate
that the difference between the percentage of whites and nonwhites who
saw a physician in this country in a 12-month period in 1982 is statistically insignificant. When high-, medium-, and low-income groups are
compared, only statistically insignificant differences among the groups
are seen (see Figure 1.18). The most dramatic change in access-to-care
statistics is seen in the number of physician visits per person per year
(see Figure 1.19).

The frequency with which low-income patients visit physicians is
now higher per year than is the frequency within the middle- and high-
income groups, perhaps a result of the association between poverty and

FIGURE 1.18

Percentage of High-, Medium-, and Low-Income People Seeing a
Physician in a 12-Month Period

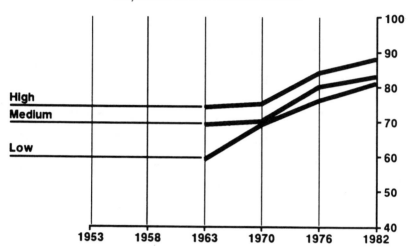

Source: Center for Health Administration Studies, University of Chicago.

FIGURE 1.19

Average Number of Physician Visits per Person per Year
(Excludes Phone Calls)

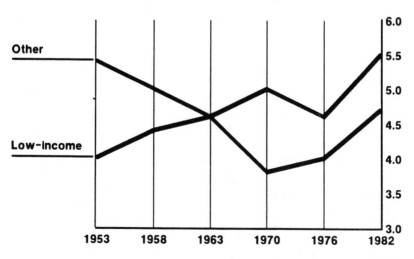

Source: Center for Health Administration Studies, University of Chicago.

poor health. Equality of access to care, it appears, has nearly been achieved.

Scientific Advances. Scientific advances such as kidney dialysis, coronary care, coronary artery bypass surgery and balloon angioplasty, cancer chemotherapy, intensive care units, stroke rehabilitation, neonatal intensive care units, and organ transplantation were not available in 1950. Our society voted its approval of these scientific developments through taxation and philanthropy and now must decide whether it wants to pay for continuing use of those advances.

Inefficiency

There is inefficiency, overutilization, waste, fraud, and abuse within the medical care system, as there is in all institutions. One of the major causes of inefficiency and overutilization is the direct and indirect costs of malpractice insurance. The direct cost of this insurance expense quadrupled from $700 million in 1975 (remember, we thought we had a crisis that year) to $3 billion in 1982, an interval of only seven years. In the three years leading to 1985, the cost of malpractice insurance expense increased 2.4 times to an estimated $7.2 billion (see Figure 1.20). It is probable that costs will rise another 35 percent in 1986 to approximately $10 billion. The cost is largely passed on directly to patients through higher hospital charges and physician fees. The perceived need of professionals to practice defensive medicine, lest they get sued for an act of omission rather than one of commission, also results in medical costs that are directly passed on to patients.

In 1980, each of the 100 counties in North Carolina had at least one physician delivering babies. In January 1986, there were eight counties without a physician provider, and by 1987 an estimated 29 counties in North Carolina will be without a physician who would deliver babies. Family physicians in each of those 29 counties deliver an average of 25 babies yearly. Their malpractice insurance cost rose to $22,000 in 1986, which will make it economically impossible for them to practice obstetrics at any kind of reasonable charge to their patients.

Overutilization. Overutilization of inpatient services has been an important determinant of increased cost during the past 35 years. What are some of the reasons? In 1950, 83 percent of all payments made by patients to doctors were out-of-pocket payments. By 1983, out-of-pocket personal payment for services was down to 28 percent of expenditures (see Figure 1.21).

Similarly, direct personal payment for hospital care has decreased from 30 percent to 7.5 percent in the same number of years. How does

FIGURE 1.20

Total National Malpractice Insurance Expenditures

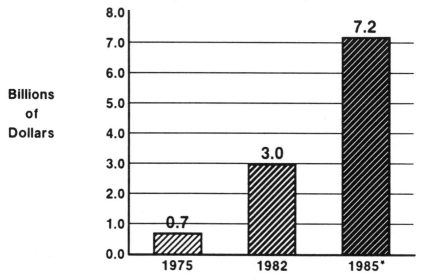

Source: American Medical Assurance Co., 1984.
*Estimate.

FIGURE 1.21

Percent of Self-Payment for Personal Health Care Expenses

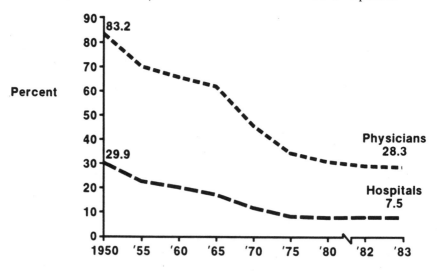

Source: *Health Care Financing Review*, 1984.

FIGURE 1.22

Estimated Sources for Real Growth
in the Cost of Medical Care
($93.3 Billion), 1950–85

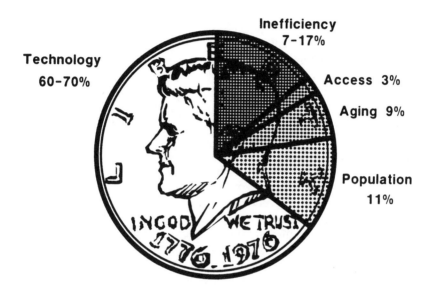

this relate to the causes of overutilization? Simply stated, there is far less pain associated with payment when the payment source is one step removed from your pocketbook, and therefore little reluctance to consume medical services. The removal of pocketbook cost also influences the decision to admit to the hospital or to provide less expensive ambulatory care. Notably, there has been no significant change in the percentage of third-party payment for personal health care since 1980, a result of the changing policies of government, industry, and insurance companies in their attempts to control the rise in the costs of medical care.

If approximately 78 percent of the costs of health care since 1950 can be accounted for by systemic general inflation, then real growth accounts for only $93.3 billion of the $423.8 billion expended on health care in 1985 (see Figure 1.22). Within that real growth category, technology accounts for 60 to 70 percent of the increase. Inefficiency, according to experts, accounts for 7 to 17 percent. The size of the population and the aging of the population account for about 20 percent of the overall increase in health care cost. Access to care, which has improved so dramatically, has not been considered a major element in the cost increase.

A HISTORICAL VIEW OF THE COST OF SOCIAL LEGISLATION

The 1940s

When Old Age Survivor's Insurance was fully implemented during the presidency of Franklin D. Roosevelt, it was envisioned as a relatively inexpensive program that would encourage people to retire at age 65. This statement must be placed in appropriate temporal and political context to be fully understood. At the time of implementation of the Social Security Act, we were still in the Great Depression, and this new "safety net" was designed to create jobs. It is important to remember that the average life expectancy at that time was 64 years! Social Security payments were legislated to begin at age 65.

The cost of a "relatively inexpensive," socially responsible Social Security program, independent of any costs associated with Medicare, has risen from $800 million in 1950 to about $179.2 billion in 1984 (see Figure 1.23). This 224-fold increase exceeds the 31-fold increase in national health care expenditures in the same interval by a multiple of 7.3. Inflation, indexing, and twice-a-year cost-of-living adjustments have taken their toll, but one of the major reasons for the cost increase is simply that people are living longer than anyone in Washington ever dreamed possible in the late 1930s. With 26 million potential voters aged 65 and over, we must assume that this component of federal expenditures will not be measurably restrained.

The 1960s

In the mid-1960s, we adopted the goals of the Great Society. One of the components of that Great Society was that all members of our society were to have access to quality health care at some reasonable cost. Medicare, Medicaid, the Food Stamp program, and Aid to Families with Dependent Children (AFDC) were created, and in fact, the entire welfare system (both federal and state) was altered to reflect the goals of the Great Society. As a result, combined federal and state welfare expenditures, exclusive of any health programs, were about $555 billion in 1985, the latest year for which there are reliable statistics (see Figure 1.24). Combined federal and state welfare expenditures in 1985 were about the same as national health expenditures that year.

FIGURE 1.23

Social Security Costs Less Medicare

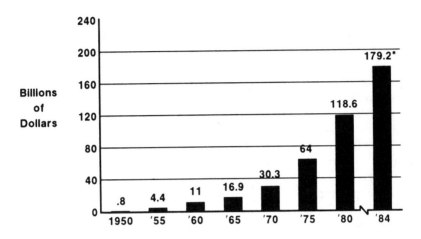

Source: *Statistical Abstracts of the U.S.*, 1985.
*Estimate.

FIGURE 1.24

Federal and State Welfare Expenditures (Excluding Health):
Selected Years 1950–85

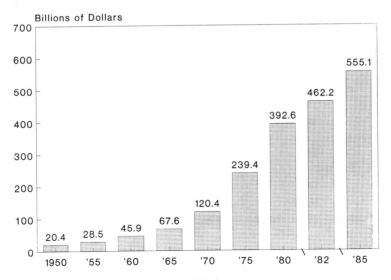

Source: *Statistical Abstracts of the U.S.*, 1988.

The 1980s

So where do the policy decisions of past decades leave us? In the more conservative environment of the 1980s, many groups in our society have been calling for fundamental change in our social, financial, and political infrastructure. The health care sector of the economy is only one among the many sectors that have come under scrutiny. Viewed in the context of the emergence of our health care system over the last four decades, we must remember that it is only recently that serious and concerted attention has been given to the need to change course. Changes in such a massive economic and social system cannot be made rapidly without major disruptions.

The five major interest groups (consumers, insurers, government, industry, and providers) address health care cost containment with different perspectives, different degrees of willingness to make changes, and different agendas. The only similarities are that each wants to get the benefits and each wants to avoid the costs. Have the combined agendas of business, government, insurers, and consumers and the responses of providers had significant effect? Hospital admissions have declined remarkably in spite of the increased age and size of the population (see Figure 1.25). The average length of a hospital stay has declined precipitously both in anticipation of and because of the implementation of prospective hospital reimbursement by diagnosis-related group (DRG). Average length-of-stay fell to 6.65 days in 1984, and in most cases has continued to fall, from the relative plateau of 7.2 days that had been the average from 1979 through 1982 (see Figure 1.26).

The burden of medical costs is being shifted to employees, as is depicted in Figure 1.27. The percentage of companies requiring employees to pay a deductible expense tripled from 17 percent in 1982 to 52 percent in 1984, and will exceed 60 percent in 1985. Similarly, the provider community has responded to these strategies by moving more surgery to the ambulatory setting (see Figure 1.28).

THE DEBATE GOES ON

The cost-benefit debate will focus on the following issues: whether we are going to concentrate on public health or personal care, prevention versus treatment; whether we are going to enhance the quality of life or merely extend it; and what the role of personal responsibility for payment versus public entitlement to cost reimbursement is to be. Are we going to take care of our old, or are we going to take care of the young? Are we going to continue to accomplish technical miracles (albeit that some of them are what Lewis Thomas has called "half-way

FIGURE 1.25

Estimated U.S. Hospital Admissions in Millions

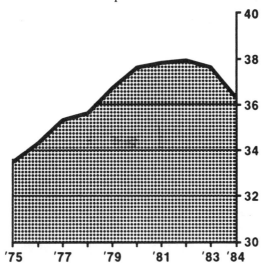

Source: American Hospital Association.

FIGURE 1.26

Average Length-of-Stay at U.S. Hospitals in Number of Days

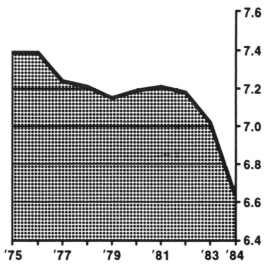

Source: American Hospital Association.

FIGURE 1.27

Shifting the Burden of Medical Costs:
Percentage of 250 Large Corporations Surveyed That Require
Employees to Pay a Deductible for Medical Expenses

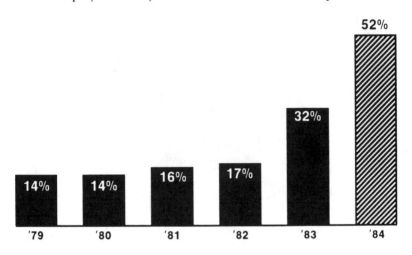

Source: Hewitt Associates.

FIGURE 1.28

Ambulatory Surgery as Percent of Total Surgeries

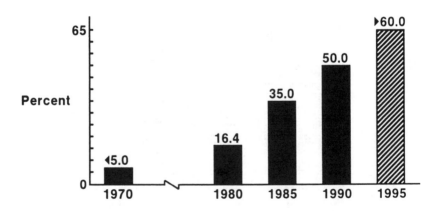

Source: J. Goldsmith.

technologic" treatment improvements rather than true cures), or are we going to have cost limitations that prohibit technological and scientific advances within the system?

Taking an important example to explore the differing standpoints of the federal policymaker and the ethical medical practitioner, perhaps the most vexing issue our society must openly debate involves the costs and the distribution of costs within the Medicare program. Lubitz and Prihoda (1984) pointed out in *Health Care Financing Review* some remarkable facts about the distribution of Medicare expenditures between decedents and survivors, and about the timing of those expenditures in relation to date of death (see Table 1.1).

There were 18,342,000 survivor enrollees in Medicare in 1978: 7,679,000 (almost 42 percent) of those people did not utilize *any* of the resources of the Medicare system. Less than $100 per person was expended on another 3,597,000 people. In other words, over 60 percent of the covered population accounted for only 1.2 percent of total reimbursements to survivors. Recognizing that 77 percent of the expenditures were made on behalf of 10.6 percent of the recipients (dead and alive), the question must be asked: "Where should we be spending our money in the Medicare program?"

The number of people covered by Medicare who died in 1978 was 1,142,000 (see Table 1.2). The costs associated with decedents were $4.97 billion. For 89,000 of those people who died there were no Medicare funds expended. Another 86,000 people had reimbursable expenses of less than $100 per person. Medicare costs were less than

TABLE 1.1
1978 Medicare Reimbursements for Survivors

	Survivors	
Reimbursement Interval	*Number of Enrollees (thousands)*	*Amount of Reimbursements (millions)*
Total	18,342	$13,365
No reimbursement	7,679 ⎱ 61%	0 ⎱ 1.2%
Less than $100	3,597 ⎰	159 ⎰
$100 to $1,999	5,111	2,917
$2,000 to $4,999	1,252	3,984
$5,000 to $9,999	516	3,540
$10,000 to $14,999	124	1,485
$15,000 to $19,999	37	627
$20,000 to $29,999	20	479
$30,000 and over	5	173

Source: *Health Care Financing Review*, Spring 1984.

$2,000 per person for 44 percent of the decedents. Seventy-six percent of the costs were concentrated on 31 percent of the decedent recipients, and that tells only part of the story (see Figure 1.29). For the combined expenditures of survivors and decedents, almost 80 percent of the funds expended through Medicare were expended on 8 percent of the patients solely within the hospital setting. These statistics focus on only one of the cost-benefit trade-offs that will have to be addressed broadly by all segments of our society, if cost alone continues to be the major focus for decision making.

Cost cannot be allowed to be the only important factor in decision making. It is true that national health expenditures represented an estimated 10.8 percent of the GNP in 1985. Why is this percentage perceived to be so important? Health care costs as a percentage of GNP were at a relative plateau from 1983 to 1986, and could decrease if the economy shows robust growth and restrained inflationary pressure (see Figure 1.30). The important question to ask and to answer is, of course, whether any given percentage of the GNP is an appropriate expenditure for health care, for welfare, or for that matter, for automobiles. The other important question is whether economists should determine the answer to the first question. Cost is one of the major medical care issues that must be addressed by our society; but it has to be considered broadly, from ethical, scientific, social, and medical viewpoints, and not just from an economic perspective. Medical caregivers must be actively involved in this decision-making process.

TABLE 1.2

1978 Medicare Reimbursements for Decedents

Reimbursement Interval	Decedents	
	Number of Enrollees (thousands)	Amount of Reimbursements (millions)
Total	$1,142	$4,969
No reimbursement	89 ⎫	0 ⎫
Less than $100	86 ⎬ 44%	4 ⎬ 5.1%
$100 to $1,999	336 ⎭	279 ⎭
$2,000 to $4,999	274	919
$5,000 to $9,999	217	1,546
$10,000 to $14,999	84	1,024
$15,000 to $19,999	32	552
$20,000 to $29,999	19	439
$30,000 and over	5	205

Source: *Health Care Financing Review,* Spring 1984.

FIGURE 1.29

Percent of Medicare Expenses in the Last Year of Life,
According to Selected Time Intervals before Death:
United States, 1976 (time before death in days)

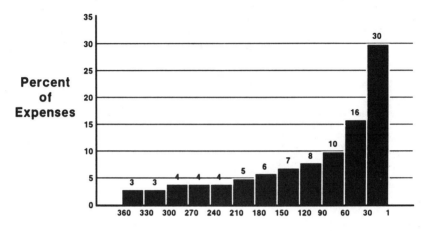

Source: *Health Care Financing Review*, Spring 1984.

FIGURE 1.30

National Health Expenditures as a Percentage of
Gross National Product: Selected Years 1950–85

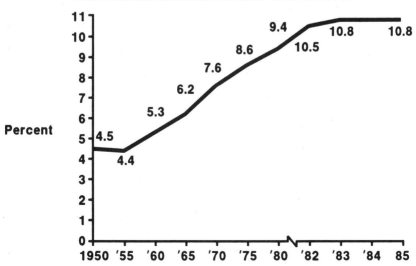

Source: *Statistical Abstracts of the U.S.*, 1985.

ACKNOWLEDGMENT

The author acknowledges the valuable contributions to this manuscript by William Luginbuhl, Vice President for Health Affairs and Dean, University of Vermont, whose ideas generated the original framework for the cost analysis, and Dennis Durden, Vice President, RJR Nabisco for providing a corporate perspective. The data used in the figures in this chapter come from uncopy-righted publications of the Health Care Financing Administration and the Bureau of Census, and were the most recent data available at the time of publication.

REFERENCE

Lubitz, J., and Prihoda, R. (1984). "The Use and Costs of Medicare Services in the Last Two Years of Life." *Health Care Financing Review* 3:117–31.

Chapter 2

Medical Cost Containment: Preparing for the Year 2010

John Gordon Freymann

Editor's Note—Medical cost containment may no longer be an issue after the year 2010. Freymann predicts that allocation of scarce resources will be so much a part of the fabric of medical care that physicians will no longer remember the 1970s and 1980s when health care resources were used with profligacy. Our "cost problem" will have been solved.

The problems underlying the management of scarce medical resources—access to care for the poor, the rights of patients and physicians to determine the care that will or will not be given, and the ineffectual and destructive medical-legal liability system—that must be addressed now are fundamentally ethical and legal problems, not just economic questions.

The other research that we must work on now to prepare us for a radically changed future includes: how doctors can use computer-video technology to help handle the medical information explosion; developing better ways to teach in the outpatient setting, where most acute medical care will be delivered; the quantification of quality of medical care; achieving better understanding of the reasoning and decision making that lead good clinicians to cost-conscious medical judgments; developing in or selecting for medical students the values and personal qualities of physicians that lead to better care; and most important, a forthright examination of the ethics of medical care in a new age characterized by high technology and the coexistence of affluence and poverty.

To prepare for the year 2010, we must first project an image of what our world will be like in that year. What will we encounter in the economy, in the social concerns of the American people, in the health care system, and in the physician population?

First, the political economy. In 2010, the nation will still be suffering from a hangover after the wildest spending binge in our history. Looking back, we will see that we spent trillions in pursuit of the will-o'-the-wisp of military security, only to find less security than we had before. We blew most of what was left on personal consumption, and we saved very little. We did all this by running up an astronomical national debt which we financed by selling off many of our national assets to foreigners. This left us a debtor nation—a status we thought we had left behind forever in 1914.

In a nation reduced to near penury by this spree, cost-consciousness will have become a way of life. The reflex answer to every improvement—even upkeep on our national infrastructure, which includes the health care system—will be, "We can't afford it." Thus in 2010 we will find ourselves in a position similar to that of our British counterparts today—short on everything and getting grim satisfaction out of a philosophy of "make do, wear it out, do without."

At the same time, however, it is likely that the concerns of society will have changed dramatically (and paradoxically, considering the state of the economy). We will witness a reversal of the hedonism of the '80s, in which selfishness was elevated to such heights that the concept of "two-tiered" health care was accepted with hardly a murmur of disagreement. This forecast is reasonably reliable because the political philosophy of Americans has historically been one of fairness, a concern that all citizens have at least a minimum share of the nation's goods.

Once before in this century we saw an anomaly comparable to today's hedonism: the "return to normalcy" heralded by Warren Gamaliel Harding and fostered by Calvin Coolidge. It lasted just 12 years, which is about how long this one will last. At some point around 1992, people will no longer be able to ignore what the slashing of social services has wrought: one American in seven living below the poverty line, perinatal mortality on the rise, and our cities beginning to rival Cairo and Calcutta with their hosts of homeless people. Furthermore, the middle class will feel the bite, too. The most likely trigger for political action will be the erosion of Medicare, which will cause the elderly to coalesce into a single block of nearly 30 million voters. Once the realities sink in, Americans will reaffirm their traditional social standards. Thus, in 2010, we will find in the body politic a greater willingness to share than seems possible today. A two-tiered health care system will be inconceivable.

The health care system is but one component of the total national system, and it is therefore subject to the multiple pressures on the latter as well as its own intrinsic pressures. These pressures will have transformed health care by 2010. The system will be dominated by vertically integrated organizations that encompass the full spectrum of health care facilities from tertiary hospitals to home care. It will be staffed by salaried health care professionals, including many doctors. Most of these expanded hospitals will be divisions of regional and a few national health care corporations, both for-profit and not-for-profit, financed through their own insurance systems. Therapies now barely visible on the horizon will have been deployed. Pharmacologic agents will bridge the mind-body gap. Immunologic tools may have conquered cancer and other degenerative diseases such as arthritis. The genetic keys to blights such as insulin-dependent diabetes, atherosclerosis, and alcoholism will be found and preventive measures may have begun. And, since 2010 will be the year when the first "baby boomers" retire, the system will be caring for a population in which the proportion of elderly is soaring. The problems we now face with acquired immunodeficiency syndrome (AIDS) will have been solved or played out, but new diseases, as we have now learned, are always a threat. Perhaps our willingness to pollute or drastically alter our natural environment will have brought on new health problems.

By 2010, the physician population will have changed drastically, too. Many of its 600,000 members will be salaried. Most will have graduated from medical school since 1980. To them, the "golden age" in which cost was no object will only be history that is hard to believe. They will never have known a time when cost was not a consideration in every clinical decision. The older members of that cohort will be in their forties and fifties and will have taken over many positions of professional leadership.

If these predictions are accurate, cost will no longer be an issue by 2010. The "cost problem" as we know it today—profligate use of health resources—will have been solved. We will have done again what Americans have done so many times before: we will have created a new problem by oversolving an old one. (For example, we solved the doctor shortage of the 1950s so thoroughly that we created a doctor glut.) By 2010, we will have controlled costs so tightly that we will have created another problem: how to maintain quality of care when cost control is second nature to all health professionals.

Thus, in order to prepare for the year 2010, we must embark immediately on a research agenda designed to maintain and enhance the quality of health care. In rough order of *ascending* importance, research to maintain and enhance quality should focus on the following areas.

MEDICOLEGAL RESEARCH

The most pernicious effect of "malpractice madness" on the health care system is not increased costs but crippled services (obstetrics and midwifery are stark examples) and hobbled innovation. Studies are needed to quantify the burden malpractice suits (and fear of such suits) place on the system. These data could then be used to craft legislative reforms which still guard the rights of those with legitimate claims, without dragging the whole system down into expensive mediocrity.

ECONOMIC RESEARCH

Economic research covers many areas. How is the nation going to finance long-term care so that all who need it can get it without reducing themselves and their families to penury? How can this be done without drawing off resources that will still be needed for acute care? How will the assessment of new technologies be organized, by whom will it be controlled, and how will the responsible agency make decisions for or against release of effective but expensive technologies? In the tightened circumstances of 2010, the nation will no longer be able to afford the luxury of haphazard development and dissemination of technologies such as the artificial heart. The ultimate question in economic research will be how much of the gross national product (GNP) society is willing to set aside for health care. Can this be determined rationally, or will the nation continue to grapple with this vital question in an emotional political debate?

RESEARCH IN APPLICATIONS OF COMPUTERS AND TELEVISION

Research in applications of computers and television in health care and education evokes a parallel to the impact that printing made on medieval society after it was invented in the middle of the fifteenth century. Today we collect the products of the first 50 years of that innovation (books published before 1500) as curious "incunabula." Computers and television came on the scene midway through the twentieth century, and it is likely that future centuries will view developments in these areas between 1950 and 2010 as incunabula, too. We haven't seen anything yet! Computer-video technology will flower in the early years of the twenty-first century, so our research efforts between now and then should focus on the applications of these technologies *in* health care and the effect of these technologies *on* health care.

Interactive computer-video systems will become prime educational tools by 2010, invading the territory of textbooks and journals and quite possibly replacing them entirely. Educators should start preparing for this now by trying to anticipate how this revolution will affect the relation of teachers to students. Moreover, computer-video systems will place the information resources of the world at the fingertips of any doctor seeking a consultation. This will enhance the effectiveness of primary physicians and reduce the power and influence of specialists.

We need to learn how doctors can use this vast information pool effectively and efficiently without going on wild goose chases after every obscure diagnostic possibility, and how primary physicians can know when a clinical situation calls for intervention by specialists. It is just a step from this electronic consultative role to artificial intelligence and the emergence of computers as clinical decision makers. Will artificial intelligence ever completely displace physicians' acumen? Research will be needed to establish the optimal balance between man and machine to provide the best patient care.

RESEARCH IN EDUCATIONAL METHODS

Research is also needed in the area of educational methods that do not involve electronic media. One of the problems to be solved involves a long-overdue adjustment: the coordination of medical education with the delivery system that uses the products of that education. With the decline of hospital inpatient care and the rise of ambulatory care, this need can no longer be ignored. Educators must develop ways to teach the coming generation of doctors how to practice in ambulatory settings without abandoning the valuable aspects of bedside teaching.

Further research is also needed on improving the thinking processes of physicians. Top priority should go to transforming decision analysis from an arcane mathematical exercise to a practical tool doctors can apply in everyday clinical management. This will be crucial in the world of tight resources. Doctors will be able to use this tool to *reason* how to use resources with maximum effectiveness and minimum cost and risk. Without it, the probable recourse will be to constrain clinical options by having gimlet-eyed accountants prepare lists of things which doctors can not order.

RESEARCH ON WAYS TO QUANTIFY QUALITY

Research on ways to quantify quality is essential, since maintaining and enhancing quality will be the main challenge to medicine in the cost-conscious world of 2010. One research challenge is the objective measurement of the clinical abilities of medical students, residents, and practicing physicians. While it is commonly acknowledged that tests of factual recall do not measure clinical skills, such tests are still the mainstay of evaluation, from application for admission to medical school to licensure and specialty certification. There are still no valid and reliable objective measures that can be inexpensively applied to large numbers of practitioners to test how well they care for patients. Measuring quality of care itself is still primitive. We once naively believed that the structure and process of health care would predict quality; that is, if the proper resources were available and the doctor went through the proper rituals (e.g., careful history, complete physical examination), the care would automatically be of high quality. Now we know that structure and process are important but that they are only part of the equation. The outcome of care is another part, but assessing outcome is harder than it looks. An outcome may be good in the near range (i.e., when a patient survives) but not in the long range, where function and quality of life are concerned. We have no way at all to measure the value of the "samaritan" functions of medicine such as counseling and reassurance. Regional variations in medical practice are another problem. Research is needed to establish whether the care is really sufficient in regions where doctors use resources most frugally, and what level of use is optimal.

RESEARCH ON EDUCATION FOR DOCTORS

Research should also address the intellectual equipment doctors must carry to function in the health care system of the twenty-first century. Since many doctors will be salaried employees, how will they be able to temper the organizations in which they work, be they for-profit or not-for-profit, with the humanism that is essential to quality care? Ways must be found to teach doctors how to work as salaried employees while remembering that the welfare of the patient, rather than the fiscal welfare of their employees, is the primary concern of their profession. This can be done, for the key to the primacy of the patient's interests lies not in how a doctor is paid but in the values that distinguish the doctor from the businessman. How can these values be instilled and maintained? Educators must find a way and, at the same time, they must find ways to teach the principles of organizational behavior. Only with this knowledge will physicians be able to function effectively within organizations as advocates for their patients and to parry confrontations with management which threaten to compromise the quality of care.

Some managers should be physicians. This will require special training that combines in one person the knowledge and skills of both a businessman and a healer. These attributes may seem contradictory, but they can be reconciled if educators select students with qualities that enable them to combine these skills. Because other health professionals, particularly nurses, will have more important and responsible roles in the new health care system, doctors must also learn how to work as colleagues with their fellow professionals. Doctors will no longer be "captains of the ship" in 2010, and any residue of this attitude must be exorcised from their education. Finally, since health policy in 2010 will be set in the political arena (even more than it is now), all doctors should learn about forms of political action, and a few should be prepared to assume political leadership roles while still maintaining the traditional medical values that place public welfare first.

RESEARCH ON PERSONAL QUALITIES OF PHYSICIANS

There is a pressing need for research into the personal qualities that enable physicians to maintain the traditional values of their profession while at the same time functioning in organizations and political systems. Doctors who cannot work in collegial fashion with other health professionals and who cannot sustain their values when interacting with administrators will not give good care. But how will those who select the novitiates of the profession be able to predict which ones will and which ones will not be able to do this 20 years down the line? Lacking research instruments, admissions committees are flying blind. All we know now is that past academic achievement, the current gauge for selection, predicts only future academic achievement. Research must first establish the personal characteristics desired in twenty-first century physicians and then develop instruments that will measure these qualities. The entire selection process must be revamped. Since those being selected today are the very doctors who will bear the full brunt of the revolution in health care, there is no time to waste.

RESEARCH ON ETHICS

Research on the ethics of health care is most important of all. Traditional medical ethics have centered on prevention of death. The technologic advances of the last 30 years, and those that will come between now and 2010, call for refocusing medical ethics on enhancing function and quality of life. This would be true even if cost were no object. However, the economic strictures we will face, at the same time that society is demanding that all Americans have access to quality care, make a new ethic mandatory. Such a revolutionary change cannot be made by medicine alone—it will represent a societal consensus and will be implemented at the national political level—but doctors should be among the leaders in starting it. They will inevitably be instrumental in applying a new ethic. The medical profession cannot escape responsibility for decisions in the management of individual patients, even though they may share more of this responsibility with patients and families than ever before. Without a consensus on the ethics of the new world of health care, American doctors will be forced to use vague rationalizations to justify their clinical decisions, as their confreres in Britain's National Health Service are already doing (Aaron and Schwartz 1984). It will be far better for American doctors to confront the dilemmas of this new world and to make decisions on the basis of a new ethic they fully understand.

CONCLUSION

To those of us who grew up in the world of twentieth-century medicine, the new millenium so close at hand is strange and frightening. Yet it is our responsibility to prepare the new generation of physicians to carry on the values that must be retained if medicine is to continue as a profession. Without values that put the welfare of patients first, medicine will degenerate into another high-tech business in which *caveat emptor* is the guiding philosophy. We must cast aside both our nostalgia and our fears. We must face economic reality. We must accept the fact that much of the revolution in health care is a consequence of advances medicine made on our watch. We must prepare those who follow us to maintain and enhance the caring function of our profession under circumstances more trying than we and our forebears ever knew.

Medicine has always found answers to the unknown through research. The research agenda outlined here may provide many of the answers to the problems of tomorrow, which are already pressing in on us today.

REFERENCE

Aaron, H. J., and Schwartz, W. B. (1984). *The Painful Prescription: Rationing Hospital Care.* Washington, DC: The Brookings Institution.

DOCTORS AND THEIR PATIENTS: THE PERSONAL DIMENSION OF MEDICAL COST CONTAINMENT

Chapter 3

Cost Containment, Patient Expectations, and Doctor-Patient Relationships: A Sociologist's Point of View

David Mechanic

Editor's Note—It is sobering to compare the crudeness of medical cost-containment interventions with the complicated human behaviors and motivations that result in increasing use of medical care. While it seems clear that the public desires reduced expenditures for medical care, there seems to be little support for reduction in availability of medical services or in access to medical care. In fact, as Mechanic asserts, the public favors paying more for better, useful, and more technologically sophisticated medical services; people are understandably distressed by wastefulness, the provision of unnecessary or unwanted services, and profit-seeking behavior in health care providers.

Cost-containment interventions may have negative effects on the focal point of medical care, the patient-physician relationship. Initial government efforts have eroded coverage and access to care for minorities, the poor, and the near poor. Implicit rationing shifts the physician's role from patient advocate to resource allocator; explicit rationing shifts power from physicians to bureaucrats and dilutes the roles of cultural values, subtlety, personal choice, and nuance—important aspects of personalized medical decision making. Giving physicians a stake in the results of cost-containment efforts means that patients may not be informed of some of their medical care options because of their expense. Mechanic points out that patients cannot judge whether a treatment about which they are ignorant might be worthwhile, but that even the unfounded fear that treatment options are being withheld can seriously undermine the trust that must be present between doctor and patient.

Physicians and the general public believe that costs can be constrained without impairing the quality of medical care. In a 1984 American Medical Association (AMA) survey, 71 percent of doctors and 86 percent of the general public questioned agreed that "medical care costs can be reduced without reductions in the quality of care" (Freshnock 1984). The challenges, of course, are to implement constraints so as to eliminate marginal and unnecessary care, to substitute less expensive for more costly services without harming quality, and to do this in an equitable and acceptable way.

WAYS OF CONSTRAINING COSTS

The costs of medical care, and the resulting burden on state and federal budgets, have encouraged forceful efforts to constrain expenditures. The large federal deficit, and growing potential for continuing cost escalation resulting from new technologies, an aging population, an increased supply of doctors, and aggressive for-profit marketing, make continuing pressures inevitable. Cost-conscious bureaucrats are not necessarily sensitive to the needs or preferences of patients and doctors; they are inclined to use crude regulatory devices that provide control over budgets. If we are to minimize the dislocations that flow from such regulatory efforts, both patients and doctors will need to consider how they might cooperate in patterns of practice that are more consistent with the known benefits and costs of alternative medical interventions. Costs of care can be contained by reducing the consumption of services or changing their mix or price, by making the production of services more efficient, or by legitimizing functional alternatives.

Consumption of Services

It is generally agreed that preventing or delaying illness is not only a valuable goal in itself but is also likely to reduce the demand for care. Additional gains are also possible by limiting patients' psychological dependence, by changing conceptions of the value of varying types of care, and by making patients more aware of the costs of service relative to benefits received. The large improvements in longevity in the United States in the past two decades are difficult to account for specifically, but there is much circumstantial evidence to suggest that a significant component of the change is attributable to reduced risk resulting from earlier identification and control of hypertension, changes in smoking patterns, and other factors related to standards of living and improved health behavior. There is significant potential for health advantages in further reducing smoking or preventing it among the young, identifying medical risk early and treating it appropriately, and minimizing alcohol and drug abuse, inactivity, obesity, and high levels of risk taking and violence. These are, however, complex behavioral patterns that often reflect social and cultural tensions and do not simply yield to exhortation or even sophisticated educational approaches. While gains have been made, it is prudent to be realistic about the difficulty of the task, the intractable social problems that encourage poor health behavior, and the limits of our knowledge and ability to intervene. Much of the solution to changing behaviors associated with poor health involves broad social policies which are not readily under the control of doctors.

Changing patients' conceptions of medical care and what is appropriate, in contrast, involves changing the culture of medical care. The growth and impressive potential of medical technology produces its own imperatives, and patterns of services are more technically oriented than patients' needs or prudent expenditure patterns would justify. While traditional modes of insurance and physician payment have exacerbated this problem, it stems from the public's admiration of technologic advances and aspirations for new "technologic fixes." Patients today are better educated and more sophisticated about medical matters, and health and medicine are popular and dominant media themes. Consumers not only follow biomedical and technological developments but, as repeated surveys show, are their most avid champions. While the public favors cost-containment efforts, it also supports continued and even larger expenditures for new biomedical technologies. These views have been skillfully shaped and reinforced by the biomedical science establishment, scientifically sophisticated physicians, and medical technology industries. Cultural redefinitions would encourage patients to demand different ways of dealing with many problems, but this is no easy challenge in the context of public conceptions and existing economic incentives.

At a simple level, a better-educated public, more aware of the risks and limitations of seemingly impressive medical procedures and of the large variations in medical practice, may be less likely to demand dangerous and unnecessary interventions. Moreover, as patients become better informed, some physicians who have a strong bias toward action and toward the use of radical interventions in marginal instances may be more aggressively questioned or even resisted. Despite much discussion about informed patients and a partnership in care, most patients are exceedingly docile and reluctant to challenge physicians' authority and decisions (Haug and Lavin 1981; Gray 1975, 195), and most physicians remain unaccustomed to such relationships. The challenge here is fairly subtle, requiring that patients learn to question constructively and meaningfully, and that physicians learn to respond in a way that supports perceptions of the doctor's competence and good intentions.

Factors Affecting Production of Services

Methods of production refer to the way in which problems are handled, the time devoted to each case, the routine procedures performed, and the apportionment of tasks among personnel. For example, nurse practitioners or physician assistants can substitute for physicians in carrying out some functions. Moreover, clinicians and clinics may vary in the amount of time that they schedule for new and routine visits, the routine procedures performed with new patients, and modes of dealing with common problems. Production of services may be affected in four ways: by changing the mix of personnel, by changing technologic inputs, by changing the content of the encounter, or by changing the auspices of care.

While just a decade or two ago there were incentives for identifying ways of substituting less expensive personnel for physicians to increase productivity, the increasing numbers of physicians and competition for patients has changed this agenda markedly. Yet, as medical care plans compete in a context of constrained expenditures, and as reimbursement is transformed from fee-for-service to capitation and other prospective forms of payment, incentives for new types of substitution will become apparent. Already some hospitals are replacing house staff with physician assistants, and prepaid health plans may experiment much more than they did earlier in the use of nurse clinicians, nurse practitioners, physician assistants, psychologists, and other personnel. While such plans could not be innovative in a hostile medical environment or where recruitment of physicians was difficult, the changing context and physician surplus altered power relationships and opportunities.

There is great potential to conserve resources by changing the unnecessary use of new and old technology and treatments. Wennberg (1984) and his colleagues have demonstrated the extraordinary variable use rates among hospital markets in diagnostic tests, surgery, and treatments. As Wennberg explains:

> The procedures exhibiting the most variation are often for conditions that are part of the aging process. The controversies arise because for such conditions the natural history of the untreated or conservatively treated case is often poorly understood, and well-designed clinical trials are notably absent. Examples include hysterectomy for non-cancerous conditions, prostatectomy for benign hyperplasia of the prostate, tonsillectomy for hypertrophy of the tonsil, and coronary bypass surgery for mild angina. Well-defined scientific norms simply do not exist to limit the practice

options physicians select to treat these maladies. As a consequence, the opinions of individual doctors can vary substantially, based on subjective experience. Because many of the conditions are associated with the aging process, the number of candidates that could qualify for operative intervention is sometimes upwardly limited only by the size of the population.

Wennberg attributed these fluctuations to practice variations that become most apparent as uncertainty increases. For example, variation is relatively modest in inguinal and femoral hernia repair, hip repair except for joint replacement, and the treatment of specific cerebrovascular disorders and gastro-intestinal hemorrhage. In contrast, variations among areas is very large in knee operations, transurethral operations, tonsillectomy, the treatment of chest pain, kidney and urinary tract infections, adult bronchitis and asthma, and peptic ulcer, among others. He reports that sharing information with medical societies and physician groups helps moderate these very large and expensive variations.

The concept of practice variation, however, is exceedingly vague, and the difficulty is in knowing what the proper standard should be. Schroeder (1984) has noted eight factors that in no way exhaust alternative hypotheses for these variations: (1) the belief that more services will improve quality of care, (2) patient demand, (3) defensive medicine, (4) fiscal incentives, (5) medical practice variables, (6) educational background of the physician, (7) knowledge of costs of medical services, and (8) participation in medical teaching. The assumption typically made is that it is prudent to reduce variations to a lower average level in the absence of evidence demonstrating better outcomes from a more generous style of practice. This is a reasonable assumption only if linked with careful monitoring of outcomes and continuing study of the natural history of disease processes and the efficacy of varying interventions.

There is inconsistent evidence that knowledge of variation has an impact on subsequent behavior. A successful program would not only have to monitor variation but also communicate results to physicians in a simple and understandable way and induce them to take such information seriously. Behavior change is more likely to occur and to be more enduring if (1) monitoring practice variations has medical society sponsorship, (2) it is endorsed by prominent physicians in the community, and (3) face-to-face discussions of practice differences occur among physician groups. The analysis of variations is motivated to reduce those on the high side, but careful analysis might justify increases in areas where service levels are lower than physician consensus would support. The program of review is likely to have more credibility if it addresses issues of underservice as well. Enduring changes are also more likely to occur when consistent with economic incentives.

Little thought has been given to how data on practice variations could be shared with consumers so as to influence the demands they make on physicians. Second-opinion programs have been widely implemented, but few efforts have been made to communicate to patients the extent of variation that typifies ordinary medical practice. Physicians are understandably hesitant to advertise such information since patients' awareness of disagreement can contribute to erosion of trust, patient insecurity, and the diminution of physician authority. But an awareness of variations in patterns of practice, if sensibly and meaningfully communicated to the patient, could increase the patient's role in decisions about selecting a more conservative or aggressive pattern of care for a particular problem. If skillfully done, it could also contribute to confidence in medical credibility. As the population becomes better educated and more sophisticated, new bases for physician authority will be necessary in any case.

Communicating such information meaningfully to 240 million patients is a formidable task, but new power configurations in health care make this more feasible. Employers and consumer organizations increasingly show a more vital interest in health care decisions and could play an indispensable role in analyzing such information and providing guidance to employees and clients. Some are already aggressively doing so. Few patients seek hospitalization and surgical intervention and many would like to avoid painful and inconvenient procedures. Patients undergo these interventions because they believe them to be necessary and unavoidable. Making patients more aware of variations and alternatives will probably contribute only modestly to cost containment, but it could assist them in making more thoughtful and prudent purchases of medical services.

Reducing technical interventions, of course, also changes the content of encounters, but incentives for increasing cognitive services, counseling, education, and behavioral modification have been exceedingly weak. Physicians earn far more for technical procedures than for these other functions. One analysis found that average office-based physicians could earn 50 to 60 percent more per hour spent in hospital care than in their offices, and the types of inputs used in hospitals per hour of physician time may cost twice as much as those used in office-based practice (Blumberg 1979). In the absence of altered reimbursement incentives, performing cognitive and behavioral tasks works against the physician's interest. Even when the specialties espouse a philosophical orientation consistent with behavioral care, such as among family practitioners, the dominant pattern is a short encounter time which is antithetical to the requirements of serious counseling, education, or behavioral modification. Many of these services can be provided effectively by nurses, educators, psychologists, and others whose remuneration levels allow longer patient encounters. As competition for patients increases, however, physicians may be more resistant to such substitution. The essential point is that whatever the physician's education or medical philosophy, it is unlikely to be translated into practice if the context or constraints work against it.

Finally, services can be provided more economically in some settings than in others. This is a deceptively simple issue, and whether a particular setting is more or less expensive depends on the nature of the problem and the necessary course of care. Moreover, it is essential to differentiate between the price of a service and the aggregate costs of care, since changing the auspices of service also affects the population of potential clients. The National Hospice Study found, for example, that hospice care, particularly in home-based hospices, was less expensive than cancer care in clinical centers, without significantly diminishing pain control or the patients' quality of life. However, the extent of savings depended on when patients first entered a hospice and how long they survived (Mor and Kidder 1985). Many studies show that home-based long-term care can sustain patients' functioning at a lower cost per patient than institutional care, but the extension of home care benefits attracts many new clients who managed to avoid institutionalization by using informal supports. Many patients attracted to home care benefits are not those most at risk for institutionalization, yet targeting and screening those at highest risk is very difficult (Weissert 1985).

In recent years we have seen a transformation in the auspices of surgical care with many procedures performed in doctors' offices or surgi-centers in contrast to hospitals. New technologies make it increasingly feasible to provide a wide range of services in doctors' offices and homes, and medical supply firms are investing significant research and development efforts in technologies that can be used in these settings. While this shift clearly accounts for part of the reduction in hospital admissions, we know less about the implications for aggregate costs. Experience suggests that reduced length of hospital stay, and a shift of care from hospital to other auspices, can be achieved without demonstrable adverse consequences. It remains unclear, however, how far these trends can be pushed without diminishing quality.

There is a compelling need for a better understanding of the relationships between production methods, the changing pool of clients seeking service, and treatment outcomes. There is an implicit bias among many physicians that more is better and that the marginal expenditure for small increments of further information is justified. Alternative investments of these resources in knowing the patient better, and communicating more effectively, may yield more valuable results than increasing the intensity of technical inquiry or intervention. It may also be desirable to shift services to other sectors, where they can be provided equally well and at less cost by nonmedical personnel. The boundaries of medical care have expanded enormously in recent decades, forcing many common problems of living into the medical arena. With physicians and health care plans searching for new clients in an increasingly competitive context, we would do well to try to prevent the expansion of that context to include social problems and aging.

THEORIES ABOUT RECRUITING AND TRAINING PHYSICIANS

The hope of every sector is to attract outstanding individuals, and to have them properly socialized so that they behave in an exemplary way. We want health care professionals who are technically competent and can provide high-quality care, who respond to their clients with interest and compassion, and who use medical resources intelligently and in a cost-effective way. There are basically three theories about how these objectives can be achieved, all of which are correct to some degree. The first argues that the quality of personnel depends on the types of persons who are attracted to or recruited for an endeavor. The second notion is that quality viewed broadly is largely determined by adequate professional training. The third argues that professional behavior is affected by the opportunities and constraints of the practice situation, including group structures, peer influences, work load, controls, and types of remuneration. Each theory has implications for the changing health care context.

The first theory suggests that the quality of care is a product of selection criteria used in recruiting members of a profession. The most appropriate prospects are drawn to the medical arena when the screening process is consistent with the qualities desired. It is commonly argued that changing the character of medical care requires changing the selection process. It is maintained that current selection processes reinforce a technical perspective (in contrast to a broader one), and give preference to those valuing prestige and remuneration in contrast to public service. By selecting students differently, it is argued, we will produce physicians who are more humane, more devoted to public service, and more willing to practice in minority and poverty areas and in specialties where they are most needed. Although such beliefs are widely shared, there is little evidence that they are correct. We can reliably screen for aptitude and knowledge, but have no adequate screening instruments for measuring humaneness or desire to serve the public. It is unlikely that we can improve professional quality by changing existing criteria for admission. Students attracted to a medical career, for whatever reason, will learn to present the attitudes necessary to gain admission. Modifying the nature of medical activities, and their rewards, is more likely to change the type of person recruited.

A second approach to insuring quality is through the educational process itself and the types of professional socialization that accompany it. During medical school and residency training, the student not only acquires knowledge and technical skills but also a wide range of attitudes, perspectives, and orientations to medical care. While there is considerable evidence to suggest that the content of medical education encourages and reinforces concern with technical and highly specialized endeavors, the long-term impact of medical training on attitudes, values, and modes of behavior is less clear.

There are many who believe that the key to change is modification of curricula. Although there is little evidence that changing educational content alone has much impact on future behavior, when such content is reinforced by appropriate faculty models and clinical experience, there is greater promise for altering behavior. In recent years, efforts have been made to go beyond curricular changes by bringing new types of faculty into medical education and developing clinical experiences in a variety of new care settings. However, the core values of medicine do not appear to have altered appreciably. A major change has been the rapid growth of family practice and primary care residency training programs. Such programs have been broader in scope than traditional programs, and they give attention to health promotion, prevention, and social and behavioral factors. The graduates of these residency programs practice in ways that are more consistent with perceived public need than graduates from more traditional programs. The comparative quality of their practice is difficult to assess because the criteria for quality in ambulatory care are vague.

An argument frequently made for self-regulation among professionals proposes that the processes of recruitment and socialization during medical school and residency are so rigorous that they insure a high level of professional behavior. Once admitted into medical school, however, few students are dropped for either academic or moral deviations, and medical education has much lower rates of attrition than almost any other professional educational endeavor. Medical education may require some testing of commitment and perseverance, but it does not require proof of moral standards beyond what is expected in the culture more generally.

While medical students must impress their mentors to obtain attractive residency positions, medical graduates are rarely excluded from residency training, and usually only for extreme deviance. There are enough residencies to accommodate even the dullest prospects, and what little research there is suggests that sorting of medical personnel between high- and low-quality hospitals goes on, but almost no one is excluded.

The third view of shaping professional behavior focuses on the opportunities and constraints of the practice setting. This view considers such issues as the hierarchical structure of practice, modes of remuneration, the organization of work, the management of patient demands, and the checks and controls exercised over physician discretion. Physicians exercise a great deal of discretion and autonomy in even the most organized medical settings, and it is in this context that the behavior of physicians is most likely to be influenced by social policy, and particularly by payment incentives.

There are three basic ways in which providers can be paid: (1) on a fee-for-service basis, (2) on a capitation or salary basis, and (3) on a case-episode basis. These techniques can be combined in many ways, producing a range of incentives affecting productivity, efficiency, responsiveness, and quality. Each mode of payment may encourage either over- or underutilization, but lacking any broad consensus on appropriate care, allegations about under- and overutilization are difficult to assess.

Fee-for-service systems, in theory at least, can promote any practice goals desired if they can be explicitly defined. One can manipulate reimbursement rates to encourage or discourage any procedure, test, intervention, or assessment process. In practice, such systems almost always reinforce the provision of definable technical procedures in contrast to less tangible aspects of medical care. The reluctance to change the schedules for fee-for-service payment reflects not only dominant values in the medical arena but also the difficulty of monitoring the provision of less tangible preventive, educative, and counseling services. Patients also tend to share the value put on technical assessment and interventions, and are more questioning of large fees for simply talking with a physician.

While the combination of fee-for-service and third-party payment encourages procedures, capitation and case-episode payment are more restrictive. If such payments are sufficiently high, they may result in patterns of service comparable to fee-for-service. The logic of moving to these alternative modes of payment, however, is to ration care. But changes in the structure of remuneration also have implications for the source of authority and the ethics of medical decision making.

TYPES OF RATIONING

There are three major approaches to rationing care (Mechanic 1979). Most prevalent is cost sharing, as exemplified by coinsurance and deductibles, which serves to inhibit the purchase of some types of medical services. Although cost sharing relieves the burden on the taxpayer or on insurance programs, it differentially affects the poor as compared with the affluent, inhibits necessary as well as "trivial" care, is burdensome and costly to administer, is unpopular, and encourages evasion and deception. Although cost sharing is increasing, other approaches are gaining ascendancy as well.

An alternative is for administrators to decide the types of care that will be covered. This is typically done by insurance companies when they exclude or limit payment for certain services such as psychotherapy, dentistry, and optometry. Although such exclusions have usually applied to entire areas of service, there is no logical requirement that explicit rationing be restricted in this way. In theory, explicit decisions can be made about payment for selected diagnostic, therapeutic, or rehabilitative services and the circumstances under which they can be provided. Peer review groups have become more active in this area, particularly in respect to hospital admission and surgery. Such decisions represent direct efforts to limit physician autonomy and discretion.

The alternative is to ask physicians to make rationing choices by imposing restraints on the resources available to them. Implicit rationing refers to limitations on resources (as in capitation or prospective payment), and limitations on numbers of beds, available specialist positions, residency slots, and so on. In such cases, policymakers do not specify the decisions that physicians should make, but rather put them in a position where they must consider their choices more carefully. Inefficiencies in the care of some patients affect what the physician will be able to do for others. Implicit rationing is the cost-containment device most typically used by health maintenance organizations (HMOs) and by the British National Health Service. There is no attempt to specify how physicians should practice, nor are there limitations on their professional discretion. There is insistence, however, that they work within economic constraints. A political dialogue will be needed to define what these constraints will be.

RATIONING AND DOCTOR-PATIENT RELATIONSHIPS

Aggressive efforts are being made to increase both patient and physician awareness of the costs of medical care. With respect to patients, there have been extensive increases in copayment both to encourage cost-consciousness and, especially, to shift a larger proportion of the costs from insurers to the insured. With respect to physicians, initiatives are still being debated, but the introduction of diagnosis-related groups (DRGs) for hospital payment, the freezing of medical fees under Medicare, and the increasing efforts to extend capitation arrangements all affect how they view practice and consider options.

The economic incentives affect both doctors and patients, but often in different ways. Here it is essential to make distinctions between how patients pay for their care, how health programs are reimbursed, and how the physician is paid. Many other factors, such as patient need, attitudes and values, and the way in which a health care plan is organized, affect utilization of services and cost as well; but the financial structure is crucial.

Most insured patients pay for care on a fee-for-service basis, but utilization is affected primarily by the degree of cost sharing required. In the Rand Health Insurance Experiment, persons in the free care condition had expenditures that were about 50 percent higher than those with income-related catastrophic insurance. Patients are more likely to be cautious in using care when they are substantially at risk for out-of-pocket costs. In contrast, patients who are comprehensively insured or who pay for care on a capitation basis, as in an HMO, have less incentive to reduce their demands for services, unless there are other barriers to care (e.g., difficulty getting an appointment, long waiting times, greater travel distance, or bureaucratic resistance). Physicians, in contrast, have greater incentive to provide services when paid on a fee-for-service basis and least incentive when they are capitated and share the risk associated with high expenditures.

Theory suggests that the economic incentives affecting the physician in a fee-for-service context should be moderated by the counterincentive among patients to limit out-of-pocket costs. Moreover, physicians are believed to be somewhat sensitive to the burden of medical care costs on the patient. The extensive growth of comprehensive insurance, however, has undermined patients' cost-consciousness, contributing to a high level of medical care consumption at the margins where neither patients nor doctors have strong incentive to limit expenditures. Potential insurance premium increases may, in theory, affect consumption patterns, but any individual's behavior has so little effect on aggregate costs that any link between individual behavior and future premiums is tenuous. Moreover, employers typically pay most of the premium, diluting any incentive that might exist.

In HMOs, physicians have little incentive to use services at the margin, but pressures to limit costs are weaker than generally appreciated. There may be administrative pressure on HMO physicians to be frugal, but such influences are not seen as fully legitimate and physicians practice much as they do in other contexts, justifying their actions in terms of medical necessity and quality (Freidson 1975). Patients have little incentive to seek frugality under the prepayment mechanism and their contractual right to all necessary services. Utilization of ambulatory and preventive services is higher in HMOs than in typical fee-for-service practice as a result, although some HMOs reduce utilization by making access difficult.

It is well understood that HMOs, particularly the closed-panel pre-paid practices, save resources by their lower rates of hospitalization and surgical intervention, and these savings are sufficiently large to more than offset other effects. Patients typically do not insist on surgery or hospitalization unless physicians encourage it, and thus these matters are almost exclusively under physician control. But the fact that the HMOs do not conserve resources in respect to all dimensions of care, and provide few incentives for physicians or patients to do so, explains some important facts about HMO savings. The reduction in hospital use in HMOs, while substantial and important, has an upper limit as defined by prudent standards for hospitalization and surgery. The fact that costs in HMOs increase in a way comparable to those in other settings (Newhouse et al. 1985) suggests that HMOs have yet to make significant progress in altering styles of medical care more generally or in limiting variabilities in most aspects of medical practice.

Physicians in most HMOs are not truly at financial risk, although serious efforts are being made to change that situation. The physicians' employment may depend on the financial viability of the plan, but since the standard for pricing is the fee-for-service sector, financial failure is not a salient concern. While some HMOs offer physicians bonuses when savings are achieved, these are relatively small compared to total remuneration and the impact of any single physician's behavior on the magnitude of savings also appears to be too small to be significant.

Constraints can be substantially increased in HMOs as well as in other settings, but the desirability of doing so is not clear. Perhaps most useful within such plans is to have an informed medical authority that discourages procedures of little value (or those that are unnecessarily risky), that monitors performance and provides appropriate feedback, and that works with doctors in an educative forum to modify practices through peer influence. While such efforts have had limited success, the changing balance of influence between individual physicians and medical care organizations, and growing consciousness among doctors as to the importance of these issues, make the potential of such efforts more promising.

A powerful incentive is offered by placing the individual physician at serious financial risk. However, this alternative raises profound ethical issues since it clearly induces conflict between the interests of doctor and patient. Few patients want their physician to have a salient financial stake in doing less than they could in critical situations, and even if all physicians behaved ethically, the recognized conflict of interest would result in heightened uncertainty and suspicion. While some argue that a comparable situation already exists in fee-for-service medicine, with the physicians' bias toward diagnostic and surgical procedures consistent with their economic advantage, patients are probably more suspicious of services withheld. In the case of bias toward care, patients know they have the option of another opinion or refusing the procedure. It is more difficult to protect oneself against unknown possibilities.

The implications of the ethical conflict inherent in putting the physician at financial risk have encouraged some observers to favor explicit rationing in which external authorities place limits on procedures (Fried 1975). In such situations the physician has less room for decision but can remain the patient's advocate. While this approach may offer some emotional satisfaction, it allows power to shift from the service to the regulatory level, so that decision making becomes less sensitive to the nuances of situation, taste, and culture. Physicians must not yield this authority.

Implicit rationing, involving macro budgetary constraints but with physicians responsible for micro decision making, shifts the physician role, however subtly, from advocacy to allocation (Mechanic 1986a). It is not clear how much conflict the relationship can tolerate without negative consequences for quality, nor have we adequately explored mechanisms that help preserve trust. There is a fundamental difference between putting a system of care at risk, which may affect the remuneration of the individual physician, and making that risk specific and salient to the individual physician. In the former case, the risks are spread sufficiently to leave a forceful place for professionalism and ethical purpose, while the latter alternative presses both.

One technique for maintaining budgetary control but encouraging physician advocacy is to finance care through capitation but reimburse physicians by fee-for-service. Capitation establishes the total pool for physician payment, but should fees in the aggregate exceed the pool, they are only reimbursed on a pro rata basis. Such a system encourages a general tendency toward frugality, but in any individual case the link between behavior and personal interest is too limited to erode professional and ethical orientations. In theory, such a system should eliminate waste without undermining the physician's commitment to the individual patient or to high-quality care. It may create, however, greater tensions among physicians who, under such payment arrangements, are more inclined to resent those who reduce their payment per service.

THE FUNCTION OF FEEDBACK

There are those both within and outside medicine who are skeptical that variations in practice can be contained, given the uncertainty about appropriate standards. Nor do they believe that physicians will cooperate sufficiently to avoid forceful intrusion from regulators. The public is the physician's strongest ally in resisting the excessive intrusion of private and public administrative authority. But the public must believe that physicians are making the necessary efforts to deal with waste and abuse. The increasing supply of physicians, and the realities of an emerging consensus among employers, government, and much of the educated public about the need to control costs, suggest that public pressures and the threat of administrative interventions will introduce stronger inducements for physician self-regulation than ever before.

The evidence on efforts to change practice is mixed, suggesting that the task is a difficult one. Programs to contain variation seem to be more effective when there is a general consensus that particular procedures are overused, as in the case of tonsillectomy and hysterectomy. Myers and Schroeder (1981), in a review of the efforts to reduce hospital services, found limited evidence that a sustained reduction could be achieved through educational efforts, and this view was supported in a prospective study by Schroeder and his colleagues. However, evidence in many fields of behavior change suggests that education combined with other incentives can be forceful where education alone is limited in effectiveness.

We tend to underestimate the deterrent value of feedback and of making physicians aware that their practice patterns depart markedly from those of their peers. Well-organized comparative information, appropriately combined with carefully structured standards established by the physician's peers, contributes to the restraint of questionable practices. More important, such efforts can encourage physicians to look more critically at the marginal value of procedures and services. Myers and Schroeder found that audit with feedback and education was most successful in reducing physician ordering (Myers and Schroeder 1981), although systematic auditing in this manner could be costly.

FUTURE UNCERTAINTY

The practice of medicine is undergoing great ferment and, as incentives change, they are likely to alter how physicians and patients behave. More physicians will work in complex organizational contexts and under capitated arrangements or other financial constraints. While underservice becomes a risk, patients are sufficiently demanding and public media sufficiently vigilant to limit this threat.

The evolution of public expectations is an important aspect of the political process. The public recognizes cost problems but is less concerned than are policymakers. The public continues to put high value on the potentialities and contributions of the doctor, wants the best available technologies, and supports research efforts on major disease problems. It wants more rather than less medical care coverage, welcomes the growth of supply, and values immediate and responsive access. One implication is that the public will not actively support efforts to cut back significantly on services it sees as valuable, and efforts to reduce cost will have to be coordinated carefully with public education and understanding. Thus far, cost-containment efforts have not reduced options for most people, so tensions have remained at acceptable levels.

The largest challenge in the years ahead will be to our notions of equity in access to needed services. While the average person will be responsible for more cost sharing and out-of-pocket costs, such requirements are unlikely to erect major barriers to care. In contrast, minorities who are dependent on public programs, and particularly the poor and near poor, face an erosion of coverage and access to needed care (Mechanic 1986b). The changing configuration of health care providers, and the financial pressure they face, make it unclear who will take responsibility for the uninsured and underinsured, often populations with high levels of need for medical care.

There is much concern at present with the excess capacity that characterizes our health care system. Studies repeatedly indicate the excess of hospitals, beds, physicians, and varied ancillary services. It is ironic that we seem unable to tap this capacity to insure that those most in need receive care, and that the most vulnerable segments of our population are maintained in the mainstream of care.

Under financial pressure, government has found it easier to disenfranchise the poor and powerless than to impose greater discipline on providers and patients. Perhaps it is inevitable that the many groups that benefit from the existing organization and financing of health care seek to preserve their advantages; and it is extraordinarily difficult to achieve equity when budgets are no longer expanding. The fact is, however, that our system of care, despite cutbacks, is generously financed and should be sufficient to provide an adequate level of care for the entire population. We need a more coherent framework that reorders existing incentives so as to guarantee health insurance coverage for the entire population, and that allocates existing resources in a clear relationship to apparent need.

In this time of deficits and budget cutbacks it may appear naively idealistic to anticipate that equity will be high on the nation's agenda. Whatever the immediate constraints and difficulties, we would do well to keep this important goal in mind. While it would be foolish to expect those who are more fortunate to give up their advantages, there exists a strong and continuing belief among the public that access to health care should be universal and not dependent on financial resources. If people perceive that this value can be achieved without foregoing necessary services for themselves and their families, a resolution will be possible.

REFERENCES

Blumberg, M. S. (1979). "Physician Fees as Incentives." In *Proceedings of the 21st Annual Symposium on Hospital Affairs*, 20–32. Chicago: University of Chicago, Graduate Program in Hospital Administration and Center for Health Administration Studies.

Freidson, E. (1975). *Doctoring Together: A Study of Professional Social Control*. New York: Elsevier.

Freshnock, L. (1984). "Physicians and Public Opinion on Health Care Issues. Survey and Opinion Research." Paper presented to the American Medical Association, Chicago, September.

Fried, C. (1975). "Rights and Health Care: Beyond Equity and Efficiency." *New England Journal of Medicine* 293: 241–45.

Gray, B. (1975). *Human Subjects in Medical Experimentation*. New York: Wiley–Interscience.

Haug, M., and Lavin, S. (1981). "Practitioner or Patient—Who's in Charge?" *Journal of Health and Social Behavior* 22: 212–19.

Mechanic, D. (1979). *Future Issues in Health Care: Social Policy and the Rationing of Medical Services*. New York: The Free Press.

———— (1986a). *From Advocacy to Allocation: The Evolving American Health Care System*. New York: The Free Press.

———— (1986b). "Health Care for the Poor: Some Policy Alternatives." *Journal of Family Practice* 22: 283–89.

Mor, V., and Kidder, D. (1985). "Cost Savings in Hospice: Final Results of the National Hospice Study." *Health Services Research* 20: 407–22.

Myers, L. P., and Schroeder, S. (1981). "Physician Use of Services for the Hospitalized Patient: A Review, with Implications for Cost Containment." *Milbank Memorial Fund Quarterly* 59: 481–507.

Newhouse, J. P.; Schwartz, W. B.; Williams, A. P.; and Witsberger, C. (1985). "Are Fee-for-Service Costs Increasing Faster than HMO Costs?" *Medical Care* 23: 960–66.

Schroeder, S. A. (1984). "Reviews: A Medical Educator." *Health Affairs* 3: 55–62.

Weissert, W. G. (1985). "Seven Reasons Why It Is So Difficult to Make Community-Based Long-Term Care Cost-Effective." *Health Services Research* 4: 423–33.

Wennberg, J. E. (1984). "Dealing with Medical Practice Variations: A Proposal for Action." *Health Affairs* 3: 6–32.

Chapter 4

Influences of Doctor-Patient Relationships on the Cost of Medical Care

F. Daniel Duffy

Editor's Note—A caring, successful patient-physician relationship can promote cost-effective medical care through efficient use of medical resources and avoidance of unnecessary testing. Since the physician controls most of the ordering of medical resources, however, the effects of patient demand and self-indulgence on costs are rarely given the attention afforded to physician self-indulgence.

As third-party payers have become more intrusive in directing medical care delivery, the patient-physician relationship may become attenuated and distracted by nonmedical matters. Likewise, limiting free choice of physicians by patients, and vice versa, can undermine the commitment of patients and physicians to cost-effective medical care. Both of these efforts, often undertaken in the interest of cost containment, may thus have paradoxical, unanticipated effects on the costs of medical care through the changes they cause in the traditional, "private" relationship between a patient and physician.

Among the important sociological factors that influence decisions to use medical services are the doctor-patient relationship, the physician's and the patient's personal characteristics, and the physician's interaction with the medical profession (Eisenberg 1979). Hulka has reviewed in detail how patient characteristics can influence the cost of medical care (Hulka and Wheat 1985), and the way the physician's relationship to the medical profession influences decisions to use medical services has been reviewed by Eisenberg (1985). This chapter will explore the first of these three influences on the costs of medical care: the doctor-patient relationship.

THE TRADITIONAL DOCTOR-PATIENT RELATIONSHIP

Leaf described the doctor-patient relationship as a ". . . contract between the physician and patient . . . a private affair and no one else's business. The physician makes the diagnosis and, with the informed consent of the patient, manages the treatment. The patient subsequently pays the physician's fee, and that fulfills the contract. At least the physician is the better for the transaction, and with increasing frequency so is the patient" (Leaf 1984). Three levels to the relationship emerge from this description: a private, personal level; a business level; and a legal contract level.

The doctor-patient relationship is usually examined for its humanistic and communication aspects (Reiser and Rosen 1984). The relationship involves a personal commitment of one human being to another, with the physician giving and the patient receiving. The needs of the physician are secondary to the needs of the patient (McDermott 1982). From the commitment to put the patient's needs first springs the principle of sparing no cost for the good of the patient. Levinsky writes, ". . . physicians are required to do everything that they believe may benefit each patient without regard to costs or other societal considerations. In caring for an individual patient, the doctor must act solely as the patient's advocate, against the apparent interests of society as a whole, if necessary" (Levinsky 1984). The Ethics Manual of the American College of Physicians charges the physician to expend all effort for the individual patient and to avoid considering society's interest in containing the costs of medicine when making decisions regarding the individual patient (Ad Hoc Committee on Medical Ethics 1984). As for the physician's personal needs, expectations, and desires in the relationship, little has been written except for some advice on dealing with difficult psychosocial situations and the stress of medical practice (Enelow and Swisher 1986; Groves 1978; Leaf 1984; McCue 1982).

In the legal contract, the physician agrees to be available to the patient and to provide accurate and timely diagnosis and treatment. The patient agrees to try to get well and to pay the fees incurred. The physician is obliged to continue treating the patient who is unable to pay, until the patient is well or has been transferred to the care of another physician (Ad Hoc Committee on Medical Ethics 1984). The escalating numbers of malpractice claims and the increases in liability insurance premiums have heightened awareness of the legal aspects of the relationship, and the quality of human interactions has been diminished by a more legal-minded approach to medical care.

The business aspects of the relationship have generally been neglected in medical education and in scientific research. Although *Medical Economics* and similar periodicals provide advice and direction for the physician, money issues have been treated as the "last taboo" in medicine (DiBella 1980). A failure to deal directly with the money issues during residency, linked with training experiences in which neither the indigent patient nor the salaried resident is concerned with cost or payment, has produced physicians who have unrealistic attitudes about the business contract in the doctor-patient relationship. But the development of expensive new medical technology and pressures for cost containment are now emphasizing the business relationships of medicine, often at the expense of the human interactions.

THE COMPLEX DOCTOR-PATIENT RELATIONSHIP

Before World War II, the most one might expect from an interaction when consulting a physician for a medical illness was a caring relationship. During the past 40 years, science and medical technology have empowered the doctor-patient relationship with the capacity to prevent some diseases and cure others, compensate for disability, and effectively delay progression of incurable disease. Social changes have removed the financial barrier to medical care for most Americans. The aged have gained access through Medicare, the poor and needy through Medicaid, the veteran through the Veterans Administration, and the employed through increasingly comprehensive health insurance benefits at the workplace. Doubling the output of American medical schools has guaranteed adequate physician manpower. The Hill-Burton Act has enabled nearly every community to have its own hospital.

Although these scientific and social advances have reduced disease and increased life expectancy for many, they have also carried a high price in increased cost of medical care. As costs have increased at alarming rates, both business and government have begun looking for ways to reduce spending. Alternative payment plans suggest that traditional medical care is inefficient, and some health maintenance organizations (HMOs) have demonstrated effectiveness in delivering fine medical care at reduced cost (Manning et al. 1984). The need to reduce costs of medical care and the development of cost-effective insurance alternatives have forced an examination of medical care financing and the very process of doctoring.

Today's patient and physician enter into a more complex relationship than the simple "private affair" described by Leaf. The physician brings hospitals, pharmacies, laboratories, ancillary services, and consulting physicians into the doctor-patient relationship. Health insurance and government entitlements now join the relationship as the "third party." The family, socioeconomic status, and subcultural behaviors regarding the sick role profoundly influence the patient's behavior (Hulka and Wheat 1985).

Each of the elements in the expanded doctor-patient relationship provides an opportunity to increase or to reduce the cost of medical care. The physician's attitudes toward expensive medical technology and toward the elite medical profession divert attention from the personal needs of the patient to the possibilities available through modern medicine. The powerful "third party," which was once just an insurance plan, is now transformed into a negotiator of services. Instead of being the patient's agent for financial protection, the third party now pretends to be an advocate for the patient's welfare, while actively intervening between the patient and physician, and actually restricting or directing medical care. At times the patient seems like the third party, with the insurance company and the physician forming the primary relationship. This new relationship with the third party risks distracting the physician from service to the patient, giving primary importance to the economics of medical care (Manning et al. 1984; Levinsky 1984). The power of medical technology and the medical profession adds value and cost to medical care; the equally powerful third party demands economy in providing that care. The individual physician and the individual patient are simultaneously the targets of and the participants in this battle.

THE VALUE OF THE DOCTOR-PATIENT RELATIONSHIP

Studies attempting to determine the value of the doctor-patient relationship have measured the expressed patient satisfaction or expressed physician satisfaction by encounter (Putnam et al. 1985; Bartlett et al. 1984; Ley 1982), by payment of fees, by return for subsequent care (Wartman et al. 1983), and by changing physicians (Young et al. 1985). Most studies have measured satisfaction as a function of the content and style of communication (Wasserman and Inui 1983). Some studies have explored the impact of practice arrangements on patient satisfaction and compliance (Weisman and Nathanson 1985; Dutton, Gomby, and Fowles 1985; Linn et al. 1985; Tessler and Mechanic 1975). In each of these studies the relationship between the patient and the physician differed, but the impact of the relationship on the outcome was not specifically studied and may have had a potent and confounding influence on the findings.

Along with satisfaction, effectiveness of the diagnosis and treatment contributes to the value of the medical care. The success or failure of the doctor-patient encounter rests largely with the skills of the physician. The technical skill in performing surgery or other procedures obviously affects the outcome. The cognitive skills involved in disease recognition, hypothesis generation, and problem solving influence the physician's decisions. Less obvious, but equally important, are the physician's communication skills and the style of communication used in the doctor-patient relationship (Wasserman and Inui 1983).

Szasz and Hollender (1956) classified three communication styles in the doctor-patient relationship: the active-passive, the guidance-cooperation, and the mutual participation relationship. The active-passive relationship exists in the intensive care unit or operating room when the physician controls the patient's life and the patient has little control over his existence. The guidance-cooperation style describes the way a physician provides advice which the patient follows, as in the treatment of an acute illness. The mutual participation relationship works best in the nonacute phase of chronic illnesses in which the physician supervises while the patient performs the daily activities of the treatment. Skills in negotiating plans and forming contracts enable physicians to relate through mutual participation (Anstett 1981; Heaton 1981; Quill 1983). No single style can be mastered exclusive of the others. The ability to use each style and to move flexibly from one style to another with the same patient, during progressive stages of the illness, marks the effective clinician. Tenacious adherence to one style as the right one dooms many relationships to failure.

TYPES OF RELATIONSHIPS

With both satisfaction and medical effectiveness creating the value of medical services, and thus determining the appropriateness of the costs, it is useful to examine how the failure of the doctor-patient relationship to achieve either or both outcomes influences costs. A matrix of satisfaction and medical effectiveness produces four outcomes: mutually satisfying and effective (*ideal*), mutually satisfying but ineffective (*quackery*), unsatisfying to at least one party but effective (*frustrating*), and unsatisfying to at least one party and ineffective (*dangerous*). In applying values to these outcomes, we see that the patient places a premium on satisfaction and effectiveness, while the third party and, at times, the medical technology place the premium on medical effectiveness at the expense of satisfaction.

In the *ideal* relationship one might consider that all costs are justified and that medical care delivery should be manipulated to assure only ideal relationships, ones that are mutually satisfying and effective. However, at times, neither the patient nor the physician may have a choice in the selection of the other. In some clinics or group practices, the initial appointment is determined by the call schedule at the time of the patient's emergency or by the availability of a physician at the time of the scheduled appointment. Although the initial interaction between humans sets the stage for the relationship, there may not be enough time committed to establish the kind of therapeutic relationship that would explore goals, expectations, desires, or preferences of the patient for the interaction. In addition, physicians rarely explicate their own goals, expectations, desires, and preferences (Uhlmann, Inui, and Carter 1984). For most physicians, the primary purpose of the first interaction is to learn enough about the patient to make a diagnosis and effect a satisfactory treatment, relegating interpersonal tensions or conflicts to the category of "best left unsaid." Such avoidance sets in motion the making of a potentially unsatisfactory relationship, yet a relationship which is medically effective. As we will see, dissatisfaction carries a price, a needless cost.

In *quackery*, the satisfying-ineffective relationship may have great value to the patient for whom there is no unnecessary cost. For the third party and for the profession, this relationship is considered wasteful and an embarrassment. However, the relationship will be maintained as long as the diagnosis and treatment remain unimportant to the patient, the patient's family, the physician, or the patient's third party. The nurturing aspects of the relationship may be valued by the patient as much as better medical results. In some instances, neither the patient nor the physician realizes that the relationship results in ineffective medical care. An outsider, frequently a family member or another physician, strains the relationship by suggesting the possibility that a different physician might be able to effect an alternate outcome. Quality assurance measures aim to reduce costs in these relationships.

A relationship resulting in *frustration* becomes excessively costly. Even with an effective medical outcome, an unpleasant relationship provides an environment for excessive testing and treating directed at satisfying needs of either the patient or the physician. If either the patient or the physician believes he has a choice, the unsatisfying relationship will usually end. However, some patients and most physicians will tolerate an unsatisfying relationship for a while if the medical outcome is effective. For the patient, the durability of an unsatisfying relationship depends on the frequency of the encounters, inconvenience, out-of-pocket cost, and availability of an alternative relationship. Some patients may endure an unsatisfying doctor-patient relationship, confirming their belief that all aspects of illness and medical care are unpleasant, including the physician. The physician may endure the unsatisfying relationship with the patient, either out of a sense of duty or a fear of losing income.

Dreaded by both patient and physician is the *dangerous* or unsatisfying-ineffective relationship, which is characterized by frustration (for both parties) and lawsuits. Litigation may well be the most costly aspect of a poor doctor-patient relationship. The fees become a focus of anger and control. When neither party can confront the impossible relationship directly, avoidance or overt hostility intervene and the "firing" of either patient or physician puts an end to the unsuccessful interaction.

SPECIFIC INFLUENCES ON THE COST OF MEDICAL CARE

The utilization of medical services varies greatly from one geographic region to another (Barnes et al. 1985; Roos, Roos, and Henteleff 1977), among different practice organizations (Manning et al. 1984), and among practitioners within a given organization (Daniels and Schroeder 1977; White et al. 1984). Many studies have attempted, with little success, to dissect the factors influencing the variability of costs among physicians and practices. Yet the influence of the doctor-patient relationship on variations in cost is often overlooked.

Dissatisfaction prompts some patients to seek another physician, and the "doctor shopping" will increase costs through duplication of services. One reason for changing physicians is unsatisfactory communications (Wasserman and Inui 1983). A dissatisfied patient may disregard a physician's instructions, allowing the illness to progress to a more costly stage. Relationships that have previously been poor may divert a patient from seeking early medical care, thus precluding treatment at a less costly stage of the illness.

Lack of trust can increase medical care costs. The patient may demand unnecessary tests or unneeded consultations to compensate for the lack of trust in the physician's physical diagnosis and opinion. The physician's failure to trust the patient also provokes the ordering of unnecessary tests, and marginally beneficial hospitalization or expensive treatments, to insure control over the patient's illness.

Ambiguity of diagnosis threatens the physician's need to be the expert and drives the physician to increased testing and consultation (Eddy 1984; Pineault 1977). The insecurity over missing a diagnosis may prompt needless workups. When initiating a risky or unfamiliar therapy, the physician may insist on more frequent follow-up examinations and testing (Bennett et al. 1983). The insecurity with the diagnosis and management of psychosocial problems, which confound or masquerade as physical illness, prompts unnecessary testing, consultations, and treatment (Mechanic 1978).

The beliefs of the patient regarding the doctor-patient relationship influence the cost of medical care. Some patients believe doctors are to be avoided and thus miss the opportunity for preventive care. Persons with a strong internal locus of control may employ self-treatment, consulting the physician only after other measures have been exhausted.

To insure the continuation of a meaningful patient-physician relationship, both parties may alter their use of medical services in an attempt to please the other. At this point, the dispensing of medical services is no longer directed toward curing an illness or providing medical care, and such practices become a needless medical cost. Patients may avoid telling the physician about disturbing symptoms or the lack of progress under treatment, fearing the physician will be disappointed. Some patients believe their failure to improve may be a criticism of the physician's skills. Similarly, the patient may lie about following instructions so that the physician will be pleased with the patient and think that it was the medication or treatment that failed. The false reports provoke the physician to perform additional tests, change treatments, and insist upon additional follow-up visits. Patients may silently submit to testing or treatments they do not understand, because they fear offending the physician and being rejected from the relationship. Some patients attempt to hide frustration and missed expectations to avoid displeasing the physician. Each deception causes the physician to test and treat needlessly, escalating medical costs.

Just as well-meaning deception by the patient provokes needless expenses, so can physicians' attempts to please patients increase costs. Patients often request medication, appliances, home or hospital services, or consultations that the physician knows are not required for optimal medical care. The physician also knows, however, that failing to provide access to the services will jeopardize the relationship. Likewise, the physician must certify even routine medical services as necessary in order for the patient's insurance to pay the fee. The conflict in choosing optimum services for the patient places a tension on the doctor-patient relationship (Ginzberg 1981). Some patients expect a barium enema, treadmill, chest x-ray and other studies on an annual basis. Since most of the tests are not harmful, and since the insurance plan will pay the bill if the tests are certified as medically necessary, the physician earns more from the visit, and the relationship will be enhanced. The physician may avoid criticizing the patient's unhealthy life-style to preserve the relationship. Some physicians avoid insisting that the patient stop smoking or drinking, for example, replacing the interdiction with frequent office visits, testing, and medications.

At times during any relationship, each of the partners indulges his own needs at the expense of the other. The doctor-patient relationship is no different, but when such self-indulgence occurs in the medical setting, the cost of care increases. For example, patients are self-indulgent when they seek care from more than one physician at the same time. Multiplication of services, inadequate follow-up, and duplication of treatment may result from self-selection of specialists, the use of more than one primary care physician, or the use of emergency rooms or minor emergency centers for convenient primary care.

Patients who are alone or elderly may use the doctor-patient relationship as a source of social support (Barsky, 1981) and as an escape from loneliness. The physical examination affords a legitimate, and for some the only, opportunity to be touched by another human being. These spin-offs of the doctor-patient relationship may, for some patients, become the reason for frequent but medically unnecessary care. The physician who fails to realize the true reason for the visit may test and treat with needless additional cost.

Other patients indulgently benefit from the sick role (Ries et al. 1981). They control the environment, obtain exemptions from duties, and receive disability payments. For these patients, the doctor-patient relationship becomes part of their livelihood—they must keep the relationship going or lose their benefits. When the disability is fraudulent, the expenses are obviously unnecessary. However, the physician's failure to recognize the maintenance of the sick role as the manifestation of a psychiatric illness might prompt erroneous testing and treatment. Some self-indulgent patients use the relationship to obtain mind-altering drugs. Others scheme to convince the physician to claim medical necessity so that medical insurance will pay for cosmetic surgery.

Physicians are not immune from self-indulgence in the doctor-patient relationship (Hardison 1979). Some physicians encourage frequent, simple office visits to maintain a pleasant relationship with patients and generate fees with a minimum of effort. The advising of costly procedures with marginal indications, particularly if those procedures are performed by that physician, is a form of self-indulgence to generate additional income. In order to organize a busy schedule, some physicians unnecessarily admit patients to the hospital for convenience of the workup or treatment because the hospital provides all the ancillary personnel at no cost to the physician, and more patients can be seen during brief hospital rounds than in the office (Ginzberg 1981). Some physicians demand that the patient make an office visit when a telephone call could solve the problem, again raising the cost of medical care.

Excessive testing as a safeguard against missing a rare diagnosis or as a defense against malpractice claims can be viewed as an indulgent diversion of medical care dollars to meet a physician's need. Excessive consultation in lieu of sound, fundamental knowledge is certainly a dishonest self-indulgence, as are laboratory tests ordered merely to satisfy the doctor's curiosity.

For some physicians, the primary doctor-patient relationship may exist to enhance a valued professional relationship with one's peers. Physicians who practice consultative medicine must nurture the relationship with the referring physician and avoid too close a relationship with the primary physician's patient. When a consultant is called into a case, the primary physician may defer to the consultant's decisions rather than integrate the advice into the total plan for the patient. When more than one consultant is active in decision making, the primary physician's failure to coordinate the order writing may allow duplication of services and increase costs. Most physicians respond to the suggestions, recommendations, and practice patterns of the strong clinical leaders. Should that leader have a cost-expansive attitude toward medical care, the practice of the influenced physicians will be the same. The secondary professional relationships may have as much impact on the decisions to utilize services as do the factors in the primary doctor-patient relationship (Eisenberg and Williams 1981).

CONCLUSIONS

Although the physician makes most of the decisions regarding the services that will be used for the patient's care, the patient decides when to initiate medical care by contacting a physician. Once the two meet, a relationship is established. The relationship may be of trivial value to each member, as exemplified by episodic minor illness care, or the relationship may be highly valued by one or both. The patient with chronic illness, for example, needs a long-term, reliable, and continuous relationship. The primary care physician needs a stable practice of patients who continually seek his services. As the services available to the physician increase, secondary relationships between the physician and the hospital, peers, and consultants influence the doctor-patient relationship. Likewise, the third party, the patient's insurance plan, exerts an influence on the doctor-patient relationship.

Honest, ideal relationships increase the chance of cost-effective care. Faulty relationships stimulate increased utilization of medical resources through doctor shopping and duplication of services. The need to please the other in the relationship may prompt cost-escalating decisions. Self-indulgent behaviors in both patients and physicians, enabled by a long-term relationship, may divert medical care payments to meet nonmedical needs. Hence, improving the doctor-patient relationship is an important focus for cost containment.

ACKNOWLEDGMENT

The help of Barbara McCoy and Carol Butler in the preparation of this manuscript is greatly appreciated.

REFERENCES

Ad Hoc Committee on Medical Ethics (1984). "American College of Physicians, American College of Physicians Ethics Manual: Part I." *Annals of Internal Medicine* 101: 129–37.

Anstett, R. (1981). "Teaching Negotiating Skills in the Family Medicine Center." *Journal of Family Practice* 12: 503–6.

Barnes, B. A.; O'Brien, E.; Comstock, C.; D'Arpa, D. G.; and Donahue, C. L. (1985). "Report on Variation in Rates of Utilization of Surgical Services in the Commonwealth of Massachusetts." *Journal of the American Medical Association* 254: 371–75.

Barsky, A. J. (1981). "Hidden Reasons Some Patients Visit Doctors." *Annals of Internal Medicine* 94: 492–98.

Bartlett, E. E.; Grayson, M.; Barker, R.; Levine, D. M.; Golden, A.; and Libber, S. (1984). "The Effects of Physician Communications Skills on Patient Satisfaction, Recall and Adherence." *Journal of Chronic Diseases* 37: 755–64.

Bennett, M. D.; Applegate, W. B.; Chilton, L. A.; Skipper, B. J.; and White, R. E. (1983). "Comparison of Family Medicine and Internal Medicine: Charges for Continuing Ambulatory Care." *Medical Care* 21: 830–39.

Daniels, M., and Schroeder, S. A. (1977). "Variation among Physicians in Use of Laboratory Tests II. Relation to Clinical Productivity and Outcomes of Care." *Medical Care* 15: 482–87.

DiBella, G. (1980). "Mastering Money Issues that Complicate Treatment: The Last Taboo." *American Journal of Psychotherapy* 24: 510–22.

Dutton, D. B.; Gomby, D.; and Fowles, J. (1985). "Satisfaction with Children's Medical Care in Six Different Ambulatory Settings." *Medical Care* 23: 894–912.

Eddy, D. M. (1984). "Variations in Physician Practice: The Role of Uncertainty." *Health Affairs* 3: 74–89.

Eisenberg, J. M. (1979). "Sociologic Influences on Decision-making by Clinicians." *Annals of Internal Medicine* 90: 957–64.

——— (1985). "Physician Utilization: The State of Research about Physicians' Practice Patterns." *Medical Care* 23: 461–83.

Eisenberg, J. M., and Williams, S. V. (1981). "Cost Containment and Changing Physicians' Practice Behavior." *Journal of the American Medical Association* 246: 2195–2201.

Enelow, A. J., and Swisher, S. N. (1986). *Interviewing and Patient Care,* 3rd ed. New York: Oxford University Press.

Ginzberg, E. (1981). "Economic Changes and Physician-Patient Relations." *Bulletin of the New York Academy of Medicine* 57: 29–35.

Groves, J. E. (1978). "Taking Care of the Hateful Patient." *New England Journal of Medicine* 298: 883–87.

Hardison, J. E. (1979). "To Be Complete." *New England Journal of Medicine* 300: 193–94.

Heaton, P. B. (1981). "Negotiation as an Integral Part of the Physician's Clinical Reasoning." *Journal of Family Practice* 13: 845–48.

Hulka, B. S., and Wheat, J. R. (1985). "Patterns of Utilization: The Patient Perspective." *Medical Care* 23: 438–60.

Leaf, A. (1984). "The Doctor's Dilemma—And Society's Too." *New England Journal of Medicine* 310: 718–21.

Levinsky, N. G. (1984). "The Doctor's Master." *New England Journal of Medicine* 311: 1573–75.

Ley, P. (1982). "Satisfaction, Compliance and Communication." *British Journal of Clinical Psychology* 21: 241.

Linn, L. S.; Brook, R. H.; Clark, V. A.; Davies, A. R.; Fink, A.; and Kosecoff, J. (1985). "Physician and Patient Satisfaction as Factors Related to Organization of Internal Medicine Group Practices." *Medical Care* 23: 1171–78.

Manning, W. G.; Leibowitz, A.; Goldberg, G. A.; Rogers, W. H.; and Newhouse, J. P. (1984). "A Controlled Trial of the Effect of a Prepaid Group Practice on Use of Services." *New England Journal of Medicine* 310: 1505–10.

McCue, J. (1982). "The Effects of Stress on the Physician and Their Medical Practice." *New England Journal of Medicine* 306: 458–63.

McDermott, W. (1982). "Education and General Medical Care." *Annals of Internal Medicine* 96: 512–17.

Mechanic, D. (1978). "Approaches to Controlling the Costs of Medical Care: Short-Range and Long-Range Alternatives." *New England Journal of Medicine* 298: 249–54.

Pineault, R. (1977). "The Effect of Medical Training Factors on Physician Utilization Behavior." *Medical Care* 15: 51–67.

Putnam, S. M.; Stiles, W. B.; Jacob, M. C.; and James, S. A. (1985). "Patient Exposition and Physician Explanation in Initial Medical Interviews and Outcomes of Clinic Visits." *Medical Care* 23: 74–83.

Quill, T. E. (1983). "Partnerships in Patient Care: A Contractual Approach." *Annals of Internal Medicine* 98: 228–34.

Reiser, D. E., and Rosen, D. H. (1984). *Medicine as a Human Experience.* Baltimore, MD: University Park Press.

Ries, R. K.; Bokan, J. A.; Katon, W. J.; and Kleinman, A. (1981). "The Medical Care Abuser: Differential Diagnosis and Management." *Journal of Family Practice* 13: 257–65.

Roos, N. P.; Roos, L. L.; and Henteleff, P. D. (1977). "Elective Surgical Rates— Do High Rates Mean Lower Standards?" *New England Journal of Medicine* 297: 360–65.

Szasz, T. S., and Hollender, M. H. (1956). "A Contribution to the Philosophy of Medicine: The Basic Models of the Doctor-Patient Relationship." *Archives of Internal Medicine* 97: 585–92.

Tessler, R., and Mechanic, D. (1975). "Consumer Satisfaction with Prepaid Group Practice: A Comparative Study." *Journal of Health and Social Behavior* 16: 95–113.

Uhlmann, R. F.; Inui, T. S.; and Carter, W. B. (1984). "Patient Requests and Expectations: Definitions and Clinical Applications." *Medical Care* 22: 681–85.

Wartman, S. A.; Morlock, L. L.; Maltiz, F. E.; and Palm, E. A. (1983). "Patient Understanding and Satisfaction as Predictors of Compliance." *Medical Care* 21: 886–91.

Wasserman, R. C.; and Inui, T. S. (1983). "Systematic Analysis of Clinician-Patient Interactions: A Critique of Recent Approaches with Suggestions for Further Research." *Medical Care* 21: 279–93.

Weisman, C. S.; and Nathanson, C. A. (1985). "Professional Satisfaction and Client Outcomes." *Medical Care* 23: 1179–92.

White, R. E.; Skipper, B. J.; Applegate, W. B.; Bennett, M. D.; and Chilton, L. A. (1984). "Ordering Decision and Clinic Cost Variation among Resident Physicians." *Western Journal of Medicine* 141: 117–22.

Young, P. C.; Wasserman, R. C.; McAulife, T.; Long, J.; Hagan, J. F.; and Heath, B. (1985). "Why Families Change Pediatricians: Factors Causing Dissatisfaction with Pediatric Care." *American Journal of Diseases of Children* 139: 683–86.

Chapter 5

Finite Resources in a World of Infinite Needs

Robert M. Veatch

Editor's Note—The amount that could be spent on health care is, in theory, unlimited: we could, for example, have a daily physical examination and a monthly total body computerized tomography (CT) scan. The imposition of limits is thus inevitable, and these limitations occur in an ethical or philosophical context, as well as in an economic context. The three major philosophical positions on the allocation of health resources are: libertarianism, in which personal autonomy is primary, and everyone may purchase all services that are desired and can be afforded; utilitarianism, in which we attempt to maximize aggregate good, usually through cost-benefit or cost-effectiveness analyses; and egalitarianism, in which resources are allocated to those with the greatest need, regardless of marginal benefit or cost. All positions face serious objections and all have enthusiastic proponents.

The egalitarian position requires that people indicate where medical needs are greatest. It is possible, Veatch argues, for rational, altruistic persons to do so—both for themselves and for others. Clinicians, moreover, should not be asked to be society's cost-containment agents. Their values are not necessarily those of rational, altruistic citizens, and being held responsible for allocating medical resources forces them into a fundamental conflict with their moral obligation to serve their patients, first and foremost.

It is increasingly clear that there is no limit to the amount of the world's resources that could be spent on health care. In the United States alone the current expenditure is greater than a billion dollars per day (Levit et al. 1985). Using just a few of the most recently developed medical interventions to treat relatively small numbers of people could by itself absorb the entire gross national product (GNP). Just supplying transplantation of hearts and kidneys, hemodialysis, coronary bypass surgery, and artificial hearts to all who could plausibly use them would place a drain on national resources that would probably be intolerable. If similar levels of service were extended to all in the world who could benefit from these procedures, the international economy would collapse. It is a given that not everyone in the world can have all the health care that he or she desires. Our resources are finite. Our needs, or at least our desires, are infinite. The ethics of health resource allocation have become a problem of deciding who has ethical claims on scarce resources. Some containment of health care costs is inevitable. The only question is how cost containment ought to take place.

THE COST-CONTAINMENT PROBLEM

Separating Needs and Desires

One approach to this question is to attempt to differentiate needed care from desired care (Bayer, Caplan, and Daniels 1983; Avorn 1983; Daniels 1983). It seems obvious that some people have desires for health care services that are not really needed. That approach, however, raises serious problems. First, efforts to distinguish between needs and desires have been mired in conceptual and normative controversy. While there may be some rough agreement that certain health care interventions are needed more than others, it is not clear that any hard and fast line can be drawn between needs and desires. Different cultures with different resources and different values would probably draw the line differently. Some scholars have attempted to relate needs to typical functioning of the species (Daniels 1983), but it is not clear that people need care when, and only when, it is necessary for typical functioning.

Second, it is not clear that people should have a claim on health care services on the basis of need. Some societies believe it is legitimate for persons to command the attention of physicians and other health care personnel only on the basis of ability to pay. Others believe that persons are entitled to care only when that care would efficiently improve the health statistics of the community. In either case, even if one could establish who has the greatest need, it would not establish who has the right to care.

Macroallocation: Diverting from One Sphere to Another

It is sometimes argued that cost containment in health care is being driven by unjustified greed on the part of those representing other sectors of the economy. It is believed that cost containment permits diversion of health care dollars to other uses such as national defense, highways, tobacco price supports, or whatever one's favorite target may be. To the extent that this is the source of the problem, we cannot avoid recognizing that ethical as well as political decisions are being made. Such diversion of resources requires an ethical judgment that these other spheres have a greater claim on our resources than does health care.

At the same time we cannot escape recognizing that the percentage of GNP devoted to health care has been growing throughout this century. The diversion of resources from other spheres to health care is also an ethical as well as a political decision. If the benefits from these extra health care expenditures were dramatic in terms of reductions of mortality or morbidity, probably no one would question the resource diversion. It is apparent, however, that some of these expenditures produce very little benefit. In fact, in many cases the patients themselves are actively trying to refuse the treatments being rendered.

It has been reported that 22 percent of all Medicare dollars went to patients who died within the calendar year of treatment (Bayer, Callahan, Fletcher, et al. 1983). While some of those treatments were plausibly considered wise at the time they were provided (because there was hope of significant benefit), others were clearly last-ditch, heroic efforts with little possibility of benefit and no desire on the part of the patient. Other treatments were provided not because either patient or physician desired them, but because they were thought necessary to comply with professional standards or to defend against malpractice. Still others (often, but not always, high-tech treatments) were desired by individual patients and providers, but with very little expected benefit per unit of resources invested. Deciding to provide these services because physicians want them, patients want them, or lawyers want them requires an ethical judgment.

The Societal Obligation

Given the enormous financial commitments and the enormous demands on the system, we must determine the extent of our societal obligation. At one extreme, some would argue that costs could be contained efficiently by simply placing all services on a free-market pay-as-you-go basis, with the society taking no responsibility. To be effective, insurance mechanisms would have to be prohibited so that each consumer of health care would pay in full the costs of the services delivered. This would maximize the cost-consciousness of the consumer and probably be quite effective in controlling costs.

Such a scheme, of course, would be devastating for the poor, who would not be able to afford even the basics of care. It would contain costs by jeopardizing the medical welfare of many persons. Even the middle class would not be able to afford many expensive medical interventions. While costs would be contained, reasonable persons would consider the social and ethical price too high.

It is widely recognized that some cost-shifting is appropriate. Persons should at least be permitted to buy insurance, thus pooling risks. Most would also acknowledge that justice requires that society provide some basic care for those who have medical needs, but no resources to provide for themselves. Thus we have national Medicare and Medicaid programs as well as many other health care funding mechanisms funded by governmental and private agencies. Once costs are shifted to third parties, however, the direct financial incentive for consumers to control costs diminishes or disappears. We must face the question of what is fair or just allocation of our limited resources.

The President's Commission for the Study of Ethical Problems in Medicine and Biomedical and Behavioral Research, in its report on *Securing Access to Health Care,* proposed as national policy that, "Equitable access to health care requires that all citizens be able to secure an adequate level of care without excessive burdens" (President's Commission 1983, 4). In doing so they acknowledged that there is a floor below which no one ought to fall, and that the burdens ought not be excessive or fall disproportionately on particular individuals. They also suggested that the government must bear the ultimate responsibility for providing such care when the private sectors are unable to meet this obligation.

This makes it clear that third parties will necessarily be involved and that problems will necessarily arise in a world of finite resources. The right of access is not unlimited. Some restrictions are inevitable, and those restrictions will necessarily be linked to the limits on resources.

A JUST BASIS OF ALLOCATION

In order to determine when care can justifiably be limited in order to control costs, it will be necessary to answer the question of what constitutes a fair or just basis for allocating our scarce resources. Three major positions have emerged in the philosophical and public policy debate. Each has its proponents and emerges to some extent in the interpretation of the notion of an "adequate level of care without excessive burdens."

Libertarianism

The first alternative is one that would eliminate the cost-containment problem by permitting persons to buy whatever they wanted (provided they were able). It is based on the philosophical primacy of liberty or autonomy and is thus linked to the philosophical position referred to as libertarianism (Nozick 1974). Its primary tenet is that people are entitled to those things they possess provided they acquire them justly; that is, by appropriating them from the state of nature or through gift or exchange. Holders of this position support the idea that persons should be able to get any health care that they obtain by free exchange from persons willing to supply them with care. This could be based either on consideration offered or on the charity of the provider (Engelhardt 1986; Sade 1971). Costs would be constrained only by free-market mechanisms.

If everyone started with a fair share of the resources, had similar skills for acquiring resources, and had comparable medical needs, then presumably no problems would result and costs would be easily contained.

The problem, of course, is that initial resources are not distributed equally, nor are the skills for acquiring resources or the needs for health services. Moreover, many people needing health resources—infants, children, the retarded—are never in a position to acquire resources and buy health services. Often they are desperately ill before they ever become autonomous consumers. Some libertarians consistently maintain that the inability of some persons to buy the services they need is unfortunate, but it is not unfair (Engelhardt 1981). It is just the way life is.

While that response has the advantage of being logically consistent, it is not a feasible answer for most people. They feel that society bears some obligation to provide at least the basics of care for those who are desperately ill and who cannot afford to buy the care they need through their own resources. For those who acknowledge some societal obligation, such as the President's Commission, the problem of setting limits on access to third-party provided care becomes a critical part of the cost-containment problem. Two major alternatives remain for grounding cost containment. Each provides its own framework for limiting care and controlling costs.

Utilitarianism

The most popular approach, at least in the past decade, has been to attempt to figure out which health care services are the most efficient, which services provide the most health benefit per dollar invested. The goal is to maximize the total or aggregate amount of good that can be done with the limited resources available. Aggregate social indicators, such as mortality and morbidity rates for the population, are the most important social statistics.

This philosophical commitment is the instinctive inclination of economists and health planners, no matter how alien it might be for physicians and clinicians who are trained ethically to focus on the welfare of the individual patient. The most popular planning tools of these people are cost-benefit and cost-effectiveness analysis (Weinstein and Stason 1977; Shepard and Thompson 1979; Klarman 1973; United States Congress 1980). Both are sophisticated devices for calculating how to maximize the good that is done per unit of investment. Under such approaches the care that is least efficient, that contributes least to aggregate social indicators, is to be eliminated. Countless studies have been funded which deal with interventions ranging from hypertension screening (Stason and Weinstein 1977) to asymptomatic bacteriuria (Rich, Glass, and Selkon 1976). In fact, efficient delivery of care has become so popular in the era of cost containment that it is widely assumed that it is an uncontroversial definitive criterion for deciding what care ought to be eliminated in order for costs to be contained.

Nevertheless, cost-benefit and cost-effectiveness analysis are ethically controversial (Mooney 1980; MacIntyre 1977; Beauchamp 1979; Fein 1971; Baram 1980). One criticism centers on the difficulties in quantification of the benefits and harms. The earliest cost-benefit analyses were based on calculations of the additions to the GNP of investments that resulted from the alternative forms of health care under consideration (Rice and Cooper 1967). They self-consciously limited attention to the economic value of life with controversial implications. Because of inequities and long-standing social patterns of income differentials, health care investments for males tended to be valued more highly than those for females, and those for whites more highly than those for nonwhites. For example, the future contribution to the GNP of a white male age 30 was $129,623 while that of a nonwhite female of the same age was $51,884 (both in 1967 dollars). Moreover, since future earnings decrease with age, the economic value of older persons was less than younger ones, and at retirement the value dropped to near zero.

Although the authors cautioned against drawing policy conclusions directly from the calculations, the temptation was irresistible. Nevertheless, the movement toward more sophisticated strategies of calculating the net benefit of alternative interventions was underway. Some proponents favored adding factors for nonmonetary benefits, such as happiness and other psychological benefits, and nonmonetary harms, such as pain and suffering. Others advocated simply calculating what various people were willing to pay on average for health care interventions (Schelling 1968). A significant controversy over strategies for valuing life emerged (Rhoads 1980; Landefeld and Seskin 1982; Acton 1976). Some reached the pessimistic conclusion that the entire enterprise was inherently biased in favor of quantifiable benefits and harms to the exclusion of unquantifiables such as the sacredness of life, the joy of seeing a grandchild, or the relief of pain. Some have even argued that the approach of cost-benefit analysis and "valuing lives" discriminates against those who prefer a more intuitive life-style.

Although the quantification problems of cost-benefit analysis have been serious, scholars defending the approach have argued that some intuitive comparisons of the benefits of alternative investments of our scarce resources are inevitable and essential. They argue that it is wiser to attempt to be systematic and reflective about these judgments than to guess blindly which of two alternative interventions will do more good (Beauchamp 1979).

If the only objection to cost-benefit analysis were the problems of quantification, the defenders of these efforts would probably win the day; but the second major objection to cost-benefit approaches lies in determining where costs should be cut. The approach rests, in principle, on aggregate net benefits. As such it does not take into account how the benefits and harms are to be distributed. This has led to many criticisms of the entire approach of choosing where to cut costs based on efficiency in maximizing net benefits (United States Congress 1980; Veatch 1980). They argue that efforts to cut costs by eliminating the least efficient care can unintentionally also eliminate care for those with the greatest need. For example, it is widely recognized that treating the poorest socioeconomic classes is more difficult than treating higher classes. If an emergency room adopted a policy of only treating the relatively well-to-do, it is quite possible that the hospital would do more good per unit of investment.

Critics of health planning measures that emphasize aggregate measures such as cost-benefit analysis argue that such an approach can be inequitable. It fails to deliver care where it is needed. They argue that efficiency cannot be the only goal of health care. The consideration of fairness or justice must be included.

As a way of circumventing these problems, some have suggested that the goal of the health care intervention should be chosen prior to the analysis for efficiency. Thus, equity can be taken into account by planners in choosing the end. Cost effectiveness, which is a technique closely related to cost-benefit analysis, can be used to choose which of two techniques most efficiently achieves a predetermined end. Even here, however, similar problems of equity emerge. Insofar as there are differences in two approaches for achieving a predetermined end, the benefits may be distributed differently depending on which approach is used. Rich, Glass, and Selkon (1976) found that in comparing two different methods of screening school girls for bacteriuria, the most efficient method also happened to be the one that differentially found cases in middle-class girls. What was originally thought to be an obvious goal (screening school girls efficiently) turned out to be controversial. The planners had to decide whether they wanted to find cases efficiently, regardless of socioeconomic class, or whether they wanted to give girls of all social classes an equal chance of having their cases found.

Many of the strategies that have been quite effective in reducing costs may also turn out to be quite discriminatory. For example, the use of copayments, coinsurance, and deductibles is widely recognized to reduce excessive demand for services. However, if a wealthy and a poor person both must make the same copayment for a visit to a physician, it seems clear that the poorer person will experience much greater pressure to avoid the visit. Insofar as the goal is to distribute the burdens of reducing costs equitably, flat rate copayments, deductibles, and coinsurance will be unacceptable. The only alternative would be to use a graduated scale. For example, if everyone using an insurance plan had a deductible equal to a constant percentage of his or her annual income, the deductible would be more fair. It would probably be even more fair if it were a fixed percentage of one's fair income tax over the past several years (Veatch 1977). The same modifications would have to be made for copayments and coinsurance requirements if they were to distribute the burdens of controlling health care costs more equitably.[1]

Egalitarianism

The third approach for deciding how finite resources ought to be used favors using scarce resources where there is the greatest need rather than where they will do the most good or where free-market forces determine. They would first eliminate care for those who need it least, and would continue to provide care where it is needed most. This seems to be what stands behind the position of the President's Commission on the Study of Ethical Problems in Medicine and Biomedical and Behavioral Research, insofar as it is committed to equitable access to care. It is also the moral principle underlying the work of many of the philosophers working on the ethics of health care distribution, especially those working self-consciously out of the Judeo-Christian tradition (Childress 1970; Outka 1974; Ramsey 1970, 239–75; Veatch 1976).

There are two serious objections to those who advocate cutting health care costs using the criteria of greatest need to determine what care should not be eliminated. The first is the "bottomless pit" argument. If the patients with the greatest need are identified, and care is differentially channeled to them, it would appear that the entire health care budget would be diverted to the first group of patients who have great need and who have incurable illnesses. They would be bottomless pits commanding all of our health resources. Surely it cannot be right to commit all health resources on the basis of need in those cases where providing care for the most needy will do little or no good.

The first response is often to concede that care need not be delivered when it would do no good. Still, that leaves the dramatic problem of cases where resources will do some good, but in a way that is much less efficient than using the resources on better-off patients for whom much more good could be done with the same resources.

Advocates of the egalitarian basis for allocating care have several further responses. They point out that sometimes justice itself sets some limits. If all funds were diverted from immunization programs to pay for artificial hearts for patients critically ill with heart failure, some persons would eventually get infectious diseases. That would, in turn, lead to a policy of diverting funds from heart patients to now worse-off polio victims. Moreover, some of the least well-off patients might themselves consent to having some funds diverted to better-off patients when it is much more efficient to do so. The seriously ill, for whom little could be done, might voluntarily give up some care, especially if treating others would indirectly benefit them. For example, in a disaster, the worst-off victims might prefer that a better-off person be treated first if that better-off person were a physician who could, in turn, help them.

If these considerations do not place a sufficient limit on the demands generated by the egalitarian position, then perhaps a compromise between the demands of efficiency and equity will be necessary. Under that arrangement, care would be eliminated after taking into account both how much good the care does and how fairly the benefits are distributed.

A second major problem with the egalitarian agenda is determining just which patients are in the greatest need. It may not be easy to compare someone in acute pain with someone who has a chronic disease. It may be difficult to decide whether a blind person or a diabetic is worse off.

Societal Mechanisms for Choosing

As practical matters, these decisions about which persons are worst off and how equity and efficiency should be balanced may both have to be resolved by some social policy mechanism. The most plausible mechanism is probably to ask those persons who are the recipients of the benefits of a health plan, such as Medicare or Blue Cross or an HMO, what they consider to be fair and reasonable. To the extent that people cannot have all the health care that they would want or need, and that subjective choices must be made, it seems reasonable to rely on the subjective preferences of the persons funding the system and receiving the benefits.

There is one problem with such an approach. If real-life persons expressed their self-interest in funding of care, presumably they would be influenced by their knowledge of where they are in the system. Males would vote for diseases affecting males, whites would not give much attention to sickle cell disease, and so forth. People with rare diseases, especially genetic diseases for which most people would know by the time they vote that they are not at risk, would lose out. While libertarians would claim that is the misfortune of those persons, those committed to either equity or efficiency would probably want to determine the morally correct course. One way of approximating the morally correct course is to impose hypothetical blinders on those people making the choices. Ask them to design a health care plan knowing the general patterns of health and disease in the society, but pretending they do not know where they are in the system. They would pretend they did not know if they were long-lived or short-lived, rich or poor, genetically predisposed to health or illness, and so on. Advocates of this "hypothetical contract" suggest that the result would be fair (Rawls 1971; Daniels 1982). In effect, they suggest this as a device for trying to be altruistic in planning. The assumption is that if we are concerned about what is fair or ethical, all persons' interests should count equally, and the imaginary blinders are a device for trying to get all persons' interests to be given equal consideration.

The implications of this method of asking persons to set priorities are complex. It is not clear, for example, that rational persons making such choices would automatically favor either high-technology or low-technology interventions. It is not clear that they would favor basic care or tertiary care, emergency care or chronic care, or care for the elderly or the critically ill neonate. It seems likely that some mix of all of these would be included, depending on individuals' judgments about the proper mix of efficiency and equity.

Certain kinds of care would certainly be eliminated. For example, no rational person would favor a plan that delivered care that competent patients were trying to refuse. The absurdity of forced aggressive care on terminally ill, objecting cancer patients would surely be excluded, as would care that is considered ineffective by the vast majority of people. Peer review mechanisms to eliminate such apparently useless care would probably be supported with the qualification that the broader society might recognize that certain forms of care could be opposed by the majority of orthodox practitioners and still be seen as beneficial by lay people. Care that is marginally beneficial and very expensive would also be eliminated, especially for persons who are already relatively well-off.

For example, intensive psychotherapies, medically supervised health farms, and most kinds of cosmetic surgery would probably not be included in a rational society's limited resource health care plan.

One kind of marginal care is aggressive care for the critically and terminally ill, especially the elderly. Would rational persons having to decide before they knew of their needs want to fund an insurance scheme for providing ongoing supportive care for persons in permanent vegetative states? With costs of $10,000 per month, and the possibility of many years of survival, a good case could be made that rational persons would not include such coverage in their insurance package beyond the time needed to make a clear diagnosis of irreversibility and the time needed for family to adjust to their loved one's fate.

It has been argued that, since the elderly have already lived long lives in comparison with younger patients, those of the elderly with chronic, incurable illnesses should have a low priority (Veatch 1987). This argument has been used to justify a health care system that excludes certain expensive chronic care treatments for the elderly, such as hemodialysis, bypass surgery, or artificial and transplanted hearts, based on age rather than a person's future usefulness or the amount of good that would be done with the intervention.

While some expensive chronic care for the elderly might be passed up by rational, altruistic people planning their health care system in a context of limited resources, it is clear that these persons would not eliminate all care for the elderly, no matter how well-off they have been in the past. They would, for instance, continue to provide basic palliative and comfort care to persons of any age. They would also want to provide safe, simple, and sure cures for acute illness. They would probably also want to fund relatively inexpensive chronic care, regardless of age.

The net result of a system of coverage planned by rational, altruistic persons would seem to be that the system would not differentiate solely on the basis of whether the care to be provided was low-tech or high-tech, basic or complex, emergency or chronic care, care for the young or the elderly. Some of each would be included depending upon whether it benefited the needy and whether it was efficient in producing benefits. Rational participants in a health care plan would eliminate marginally beneficial, expensive care, and some care that produces benefits (even significant benefits) for persons who are not really particularly needy.

Under these circumstances, it is interesting to consider whether the diagnosis-related group (DRG) system should include separate groups with different weightings for reimbursement based on age. Consider, for example, DRGs 346 and 347. Each is for malignancy of the male reproductive system. The former is for patients age 70 or greater and the latter is for patients age 69 or younger. It is interesting that different weights (and therefore different reimbursements) are provided for the two different groups. Let us assume that it is morally appropriate for the hospital to spend the average amount for patients in each group at the same level as the reimbursement. A good case can be made that morality requires that hospital expenditures match the reimbursement level; or else other patients will be required to subsidize the care of the overtreated group (Veatch 1986).[2] This, in effect, means that the policy judgment made in setting the DRG weights ought to reflect society's judgment about how much care older and younger men with prostate cancer should receive. Assuming that the same benefit can be provided for a lower cost in younger patients and that that treatment will provide more years of life expectancy per dollar invested, a utilitarian would set the DRG weights so that more money (possibly all the money) goes into the care of younger patients. If the goal were to consider the needs of the patients at a moment of time, then more money would have to go into the DRG for the older patients (in order to give them an equal chance to benefit). If, however, the goal was to give everyone an equal chance to get to the same age, then anyone who had already reached that age would have a very low reimbursement, probably only enough to provide palliative care. Costs will be curtailed under any plan. It seems clear that for these two groups of patients, neither should get all the care that they could possibly desire. But different ethical commitments lead to different reimbursement ratios.

THE ROLE OF THE CLINICIAN

The discussion thus far suggests that not everyone will receive all the care that he or she desires or needs, and that different ethical principles will lead to different ways of curtailing health care costs. The final question is what the role of the health care clinician should be in this cost curtailment. Consider a DRG in which the reimbursement level is below the level that would be required if all the clinicians on the service provided all the care that they thought could benefit their patients. One possibility is that the DRG weight is too low and that it should be raised, so that the clinicians would be free to practice medicine as they saw fit. However, in a world of finite resources, it is almost certainly wrong for some people to have everything that would be beneficial for them. Perhaps the sacrifice should come from other spheres of life, leaving health care as an area in which everybody gets every possible benefit, no matter how expensive per unit of benefit. This does not seem likely, since health care, like other spheres of life, is decreasingly beneficial at the margin. In some health care services it is probably unwise for physicians to be permitted to deliver everything they think is beneficial (Neuhauser and Lewicki 1973).

An alternate strategy would be to make clinicians the ones who decide where to cut costs. The advantages are apparent: physicians are the ones closest to the scene, and they are particularly knowledgeable. They should be able to know where the excesses are and where benefits are small in comparison to costs.

There are problems with this approach, however. Physicians may make the trade-offs differently from others in the population. They will have to make judgments such as whether the eleventh day of hospitalization after a myocardial infarction does more or less good than, say, spending the funds on a highway program. Physicians are unique in that they are committed to the importance of health. They have given their lives to providing health care. Even excluding the possibility that physicians would make choices based on their financial interests in having patients receive care, we still expect professionals in any field to place a greater value on the amount of good their work can do.

Even within the health care sphere, we can expect that physicians would value particular services in a way that may differ from the general public. Surgeons may place a higher value on surgery than lay people do, but the problem cuts even deeper. They may value the preservation of life more (or less) than lay people. They may trade off morbidity and mortality differently so that they might, for example, spend more on life preservation and less on palliation than lay people (or the other way around). The point is that physicians would be making value judgments, not judgments that require their particular skill. Deciding the ratio of funding for elderly and younger prostate cancer patients depends on how one relates efficiency and equity and how one assesses equity. Those are not issues for which medical skill is decisive.

Moreover, if physicians are asked to be society's cost-containment agents, they will have to undergo a radical change in their traditional ethical mandate as clinicians. Since the days of the Hippocratic oath, the clinician's ethical duty has been to focus on the patient. True, the physician's ethical duty was stated as a duty to bring benefit to the patient, even if the patient did not want to be benefited; and today that has changed to a duty to benefit the patient within the scope of protecting the patient's rights, including the right to be left alone. Nevertheless, in either case the clinician's ethical mandate has always been to serve the patient, not to be society's agent in denying potentially beneficial services to the patient. If the physician takes on the new role of being society's cost-containment agent, this will require abandoning the traditional patient-centered ethic. The Hippocratic oath will have to be removed from the waiting room wall and replaced with a sign that reads,

"Warning all ye who enter here. I will generally serve your interests, but in the case of marginally beneficial, expensive care, I will abandon you in order to serve society as their cost-containment agent." I am not sure that either clinicians or the rest of us really want physicians to change their ethical commitment in this way.

If they do not, and if some constraints must be placed on the expenditures of marginally beneficial care, then someone else in the society must set the limits on cost containment. I am suggesting that the only ethically acceptable way for this to happen is for the members of society to set the limits themselves, adopting the stance of altruistic, hypothetical contractors who must ask themselves what would be fair and reasonable limits to place on a health care plan. Once society has determined which services are covered and which are not, the clinician is freed to do the best possible job of serving the patient, albeit with some limits on the resources that will be available in the effort.

NOTES

1. See Veatch, 1977, for an exposition of the ethical issues involved in graduated incentives such as this.
2. See Rawls, 1971, upon which much of this approach is based. I have developed this argument in "Ethics and the Elderly," in *Contemporary Issues in Gerontology* edited by David Schnall, forthcoming. This is a somewhat different argument from that of Daniels, who builds a case for the justice of age-based differentiation in health care coverage, but based solely on the fairness of the hypothetical contractor method and not on the substantive claim that the elderly have already had long lives while others who are equally needy at a moment in time have not.

REFERENCES

Acton, J. P. (1976). "Measuring the Monetary Value of Lifesaving Programs." *Law & Contemporary Problems* 40: 46–72.

Avorn, J. (1983). "Needs, Wants, Demands, and Interests: Their Interaction in Medical Practice and Health Policy." In *In Search of Equity: Health Needs and the Health Care System*, ed. R. Bayer, A. L. Caplan, and N. Daniels, 183–98. New York: Plenum Press.

Baram, M. S. (1980). "Cost-Benefit Analysis: An Inadequate Basis for Health, Safety, and Environmental Regulatory Decisionmaking." *Ecology Law Quarterly* 8: 473–531.

Bayer, R.; Caplan, A. L.; and Daniels, N. (eds.) (1983). *In Search of Equity: Health Needs and the Health Care System.* New York: Plenum Press.

Bayer, R.; Callahan, D.; Fletcher, J.; Hodgson, T.; Jennings, B.; Monsees, D.; Sieverts, S.; and Veatch, R. (1983). "The Care of the Terminally Ill: Morality and Economics." *New England Journal of Medicine* 309: 1490–94.

Beauchamp, T. L. (1979). "Utilitarianism and Cost/Benefit Analysis: A Reply to MacIntyre." In *Ethical Theory and Business,* ed. T. L. Beauchamp and N. E. Bowie, 276–83. Englewood Cliffs, NJ: Prentice-Hall.

Childress, J. F. (1970). "Who Shall Live When Not All Can Live?" *Soundings* 53: 339–54.

Daniels, N. (1982). "Am I My Parents' Keeper?" *Midwest Studies in Philosophy* 7: 517–40.

———— (1983). "Health Care Needs and Distributive Justice." In *In Search of Equity: Health Needs and the Health Care System,* ed. R. Bayer, A. L. Caplan, and N. Daniels, 1–42. New York: Plenum Press.

Engelhardt, H. T. (1981). "Health Care Allocations: Responses to the Unjust, the Unfortunate, and the Undesirable." In *Justice and Health Care,* ed. E. E. Shelp, 121–37. Dordrecht, Holland: D. Reidel.

———— (1986). *The Foundations of Bioethics.* New York: Oxford University Press.

Fein, R. (1971). "On Measuring Economic Benefits of Health Programmes." In *Medical History and Medical Care,* ed. G. McLachlan and T. McKeown, 181–217. London: Oxford University Press.

The Hastings Center, Institute of Society, Ethics and the Life Sciences (1980). "Values, Ethics, and CBA in Health Care." In *The Implications of Cost-Effectiveness Analysis of Medical Technology,* Office of Technology Assessment, United States Congress, 168–85. Washington, DC: Office of Technology Assessment.

Klarman, H. E. (1973). "Application of Cost-Benefit Analysis to Health Systems Technology." In *Technology and Health Care Systems in the 1980's,* ed. National Center for Health Services Research and Development. Washington, DC: U.S. Government Printing Office.

Landefeld, J. S., and Seskin, E. P. (1982). "The Economic Value of Life: Linking Theory to Practice." *American Journal of Public Health* 72: 555–66.

Levit, K. R.; Lazenby, H.; Waldo, D. H.; and Davidoff, L. (1985). "National Health Expenditures, 1984." *Health Care Financing Review* 7: 1–35.

MacIntyre, A. (1977). "Utilitarianism and Cost-Benefit Analysis: An Essay on the Relevance of Moral Philosophy to Bureaucratic Theory." In *Values in the Electric Power Industry,* ed. Kenneth Sayre, 217–37. Notre Dame, IN: University of Notre Dame Press.

Mooney, G. H. (1980). "Cost-Benefit Analysis and Medical Ethics." *Journal of Medical Ethics* 6: 177–79.

Neuhauser, D., and Lewicki, A. M. (1973). "What Do We Gain from the Sixth Stool Guaiac?" *New England Journal of Medicine* 293: 226–28.

Nozick, R. (1974). *Anarchy, State, and Utopia.* New York: Basic Books Inc.

Outka, G. (1974). "Social Justice and Equal Access to Health Care." *Journal of Religious Ethics* 2: 11–32.

President's Commission for the Study of Ethical Problems in Medicine and Biomedical and Behavioral Research (1983). *Securing Access to Health Care.* Washington, DC: U.S. Government Printing Office.

Ramsey, P. (1970). *The Patient as Person.* New Haven, CT: Yale University Press.

Rawls, J. (1971). *A Theory of Justice.* Cambridge, MA: Harvard University Press.

Rhoads, S. E. (ed.) (1980). *Valuing Life: Public Policy Dilemmas.* Boulder, CO: Westview Press.

Rice, D. P., and Cooper, B. S. (1967). "The Economic Value of Human Life." *American Journal of Public Health* 57: 1954–66.

Rich, G.; Glass, N. J.; and Selkon, J. B. (1976). "Cost-Effectiveness of Two Methods of Screening for Asymptomatic Bacteriuria." *British Journal of Preventive and Social Medicine* 30: 54–59.

Sade, R. M. (1971). "Medical Care as a Right: A Refutation." *New England Journal of Medicine* 285: 1288–92.

Schelling, T. C. (1968). "The Life You Save May Be Your Own." In *Problems of Public Expenditure Analysis,* ed. S. B. Chase, 127–62. Washington, DC: Brookings Institution.

Shepard, D. S., and Thompson, M. S. (1979). "First Principles of Cost Effectiveness Analysis in Health." *Public Health Reports* 94: 535–43.

Stason, W. B., and Weinstein, M. C. (1977). "Allocation of Resources to Manage Hypertension." *New England Journal of Medicine* 296: 732–39.

U.S. Congress. Office of Technology Assessment (1980). *The Implications of Cost-Effectiveness Analysis of Medical Technology.* Washington, DC: Office of Technology Assessment.

Veatch, R. M. (1976). "What Is a 'Just' Health Care Delivery?" In *Ethics and Health Policy,* ed. R. M. Veatch and R. Branson, 127–53. Cambridge, MA: Ballinger Publishing.

——— (1977). "Governmental Population Incentives: Ethical Issues at Stake." *Studies in Family Planning* 9: 100–8.

——— (1980). "Justice and Valuing Lives." *Valuing Life: Public Policy Dilemmas,* ed. S. E. Rhoads, 147–60. Boulder, CO: Westview Press.

——— (1986). "DRG's and the Ethical Allocation of Resources." *Hastings Center Report* 16 (3): 32–40.

——— (1987). "Two Concepts of the Role of Values in Medical Decisions." *Delaware Medical Journal* 59 (7): 433–35.

Weinstein, M. C., and Stason, W. B. (1977). "Foundations of Cost Effectiveness Analysis for Health and Medical Practices." *New England Journal of Medicine* 296: 716–21.

VIEWPOINTS OF BUSINESS, ORGANIZED MEDICINE, GOVERNMENT, AND THE MEDICAL-INDUSTRIAL COMPLEX

Chapter 6

The Needs, Desires, and Demands of Employers and Employees for Cost-Conscious Medical Services

Donald M. Hayes

Editor's Note—Most private medical insurance is purchased by employers, and the total that employers pay has accelerated rapidly over the last 15 years. The result in the auto industry is that as much as 10 percent of the cost of producing a moderate-priced American car is accounted for in expenditures for employees' families' medical care. Hayes (who was a professor of medicine at Bowman Gray School of Medicine before he became medical director at Burlington Industries) states that industry is paying as much as it can; yet, industry and private insurers are asked to bear much of the burden from cost-shifting that results from government cost-containment efforts and the disenfranchisement of the poor and near poor from public programs.

In a unique description of how a large industry views health insurance and services, Hayes points out that healthy, loyal employees are an industry's greatest asset. But it is employees' dependents who are responsible for most medical expenditures, and 10 percent of Burlington Industry's insured clients accounted for 80 percent of expenditures.

While industry health care expenditures are increasing at a rate at least as rapid as federal expenditures, business and insurers do not have the legislative and regulatory control that government can wield. These observations lead to the conclusion that business must now approach medical care expenses with the same type of managerial analysis and innovation that have been applied to other expensive overhead costs.

American employers see their employees as their number one asset. Thus, their major concern regarding health care for employees is its

FIGURE 6.1

Changes in Total Health Care Costs for Burlington Industries'
80,000 Employees and 47,000 Dependents, 1972–84

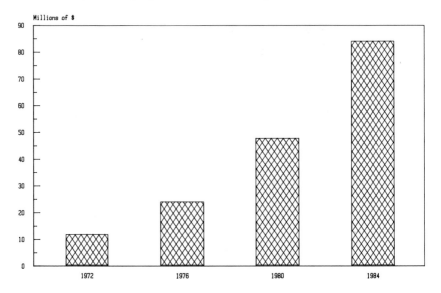

adequacy and quality. Like other lay people, employers have had no
yardstick by which to measure quality of medical care: they have been
forced to accept professional judgments about it. However, in recent
years the cost of medical care has increased at such a rate that it threatens the competitiveness of many businesses and industries. In some
cases, it even threatens their survival.

How have such changes affected individual companies? In 1983,
Chrysler paid $373 million in health insurance premiums, making Blue
Cross/Blue Shield their largest vendor. To pay the health care bill for
Chrysler employees, dependents, and retirees will require each active
worker to produce $6,000 this year. The total health care bill that Chrys-
ler pays annually amounts to over $600 for each car they sell, approxi-
mately 10 percent of the sticker price of a "K" car. That is eight times
the $75 per car health care cost at Chrysler in 1970 (Kolimaga 1984).

Burlington Industries, the largest publicly held textile manufac-
turer in the United States, has seen its health care costs go up by 468
percent in the past ten years. In 1972, when the work force was 80,000,
the medical bills were $12 million. In 1984, with a work force of 47,000,
the medical bills were $84 million (Figure 6.1). In an industry which
operates on a very narrow profit margin, such costs can spell the difference between survival and bankruptcy.

Finally, what are the dimensions of concern about health care costs for the individual employee? In 1983, more than one of every ten dollars spent in the United States went to health care, or more than $1,300 per person (Kolimaga 1984, 1). Although not all of this expense is out-of-pocket for every individual, these are imposing figures. Even those individuals who are moved to tithe to their church are not similarly inclined toward the health care system.

THE DEVELOPMENT OF INDUSTRY-SPONSORED HEALTH CARE

The railroads were the leading industry in developing extensive employee medical programs. This began in the 1880s and was later taken up by mining and lumber companies, and subsequently by others. Such developments were not, of course, entirely altruistic. The existence of an employee medical program was often helpful in avoiding costly workers' compensation claims. It was also used to build "company loyalty" and thus eliminate a foothold for union organizers. Perhaps it was this last consideration which prompted the American Federation of Labor to label all forms of compulsory medical care through employers as "paternalistic" (Selleck and Whittaker 1962).

Meanwhile, in the early 1900s, the beginnings of prepaid practice were stirring in the Northwest. Some peculiarities of the workers' compensation laws in Washington and Oregon prompted employers there to contract out medical services for their workers to for-profit "hospital associations." These companies provided medical and hospital care to workers for a fixed prepaid sum. Although many legal battles arose from this arrangement, it was the forerunner of today's HMO (Goldberg and Greenberg 1978).

A similar and related form of medical practice arose at the same time in immigrant communities in the northeastern United States. In the early 1900s some eight million Americans belonged to fraternal orders or benefit societies. These lodges often offered life insurance to their members. Many of them later found they could offer medical coverage for members and their family members for an extra dollar or two per month. This practice led to the development of what were called "lodge practices" by many physicians. The pay was usually very low but it offered a convenient safety factor for the income of a physician already in a marginal practice. By the beginning of World War I, fraternal orders were offering their members medical benefits not only in the Northeast but also in Pennsylvania, Michigan, Illinois, and California. However, lodge practice eventually died because of the poor remuneration (Rosen 1977).

During the decades before and after 1900, new developments were occurring in the area of insurance which are still having an impact in the 1980s. Politicians have long recognized that protection against the costs of illness is a strong tool in turning benevolence into power. Likewise, employers and unions often use medical care (or insurance) to recruit new workers and instill loyalty.

In America, health insurance first became a political issue on the eve of World War I. After Germany (1883), Austria (1888), Hungary (1891), Norway (1909), Serbia (1910), Britain (1922), Russia (1912), and the Netherlands (1913) had all adopted some form of compulsory sickness insurance, reformers in the United States thought the time propitious for it here (Robinson 1916, 224–50). However, to this day, there is no such program in the United States. For a variety of reasons not germane to this discussion, business, labor, and the health professions were all opposed to the development of such programs.

The early focus of sickness insurance programs was on income replacement or stabilization rather than on the costs of medical care. By the thirties, most authorities regarded the latter as more important. Some early statistics supporting this change were cited by Michael Davis. He noted that, among 211 families surveyed in 1918 in Columbus, Ohio, by the U.S. Bureau of Labor Statistics, hospital costs averaged only 7.6 percent of a total annual medical bill averaging $48.41, and about half went to physicians (Davis 1934). By 1929, according to a larger national survey, hospital charges (not including doctors and private nurses) were 13 percent of a total annual family medical bill averaging $108 (Falk, Rorim, and Ring 1933, 89).

As it became apparent that hospital costs were a great economic threat in the event of illness, a strange creation called hospital insurance appeared on the insurance market. One of the earliest of these plans, and surely the best known, was a program whereby the Baylor University Hospital offered to provide 1,500 schoolteachers with up to 21 days of hospital care a year for $6 per person. This arrangement was soon extended to other groups of people in the Dallas community. Spurred on by the American Hospital Association, similar plans developed all over the country in short order. Because of the success of Blue Cross in hospital care reimbursement, private companies which had avoided the hospital field earlier also entered this market. By 1940, the insurance companies had 3.7 million subscribers, while the 39 Blue Cross plans in operation had a total enrollment of more than 6 million (Somers and Somers 1961, 548).

Blue Shield plans, for physician reimbursement, found their development much more difficult. As late as 1942, the American Medical Association (AMA) hierarchy was unalterably opposed to Blue Cross and Blue Shield. The early Blue Shield plans in California and Michigan encountered many difficulties. By the end of 1945, Blue Cross had more than 19 million subscribers nationally, while Blue Shield had only about 1 million (Sinai, Anderson, and Dollar 1946, 73).

At the end of World War II, the unions became more active in the health care arena. The inclusion of health care benefits in contract negotiations furthered the development of private insurance programs, those directly sponsored by the unions, some prepaid plans, and the Blues. As a fringe benefit, health insurance benefited the employer as well as the worker, solved problems in the marketing of private insurance, gave the providers protection against a government program, and offered the unions an alternative to national health insurance and a means of demonstrating concern for their members.

CONTRASTING NEEDS AND WANTS OF EMPLOYEES AND EMPLOYERS

Although it is generally assumed that the needs and wants of employees and employers from the health care system are disparate and conflicting, this is not necessarily true. It is important to remember that both groups are composed of people with shared interests, and that the fundamental needs for medical care are the same whether one wears a blue collar or a white one. Thus, it is important to examine what the expectations are of the health care system from as many vantage points as possible.

A study by Hayes (1978) confirms the lack of difference between needs and wants in the health care system. After querying a large number of patients and professionals about the attributes of effective care, there were several interesting observations to note. One of these was that most people are not primarily concerned with economics when seeking care for serious illness. The general perception is that, in our society, someone will pay for the care if it is truly needed. Another item of interest was that most people take technological proficiency for granted in health professionals and thus value personal traits more highly as selection variables in choosing a physician. The old reliance on "bedside manner" apparently persists even today. The third finding of interest from this study was that "needs" as expressed by professionals and "wants" as expressed by nonprofessionals often represent the same things couched in different terms.

Whenever the American people are asked, they say they would like to see more, rather than less, money spent on health care. But they do not want just more money going to the providers for the same services. They want more and better services, more research and new technology, and more and better prevention services (Stein 1986). A detailed report by Louis Harris found a significant degree of dissatisfaction among the American people about the health care system. Almost half of them said that while there are some good things about it, there are fundamental changes needed to make it work better. Fifty-six percent of Americans believe that the prices charged by doctors and hospitals, and the costs of drugs and laboratory tests, are unreasonable. Hospital charges came under particular fire, with 70 percent of the people believing they are unreasonable (Business Week 1984).

When asked which ways of controlling costs were acceptable, 70 percent said "yes" to "encouraging uniform, preset fees based on the treatment required," 69 percent to "joining a prepaid health maintenance organization," and 60 percent to "establishing government price controls on doctors and hospitals." Only 50 percent responded affirmatively to "increasing the patient's deductible," and only 37 percent to "making the patient pay a higher percentage of the cost of treatment" (Business Week 1984).

Although impressed by the millions spent for health care, by the government, insurance companies, and employers, the average person is more immediately concerned with out-of-pocket expenses. Great changes have occurred since 1966, when the consumer paid for one-half of all health care spending, with the other half financed about equally by insurance and public programs. By 1982, public programs accounted for almost 40 percent of all spending, insurance for 32 percent, and the consumer paid only 27 percent. Despite these changing proportions, the average consumer perceives that he or she is paying more. Thus, one can conclude that total costs have gone up even more than most individuals are aware (Levit 1983).

FOR WHAT CONDITIONS DO PEOPLE SEEK CARE?

From the industry point of view, there are two ways of getting at this question. First, we can examine the records of industrial medical departments to determine utilization patterns within the workplace. Second, we can examine the insurance claims records to determine conditions for which insurance dollars were spent. Combining these two should yield a fairly clear picture of medical care needs expressed in terms of utilization of the available facilities.

Within Burlington Industries, much of the first-line care for occupationally related and non-occupationally related conditions is delivered by occupational health nurses. For the present work force of 36,000 there are 78 nurses staffing 60 medical departments. These nurses, all RNs (23 of whom are certified in occupational health nursing, and 7 of whom are nurse practitioners), operate on standing orders to care for employees within their own plant. All medical records are kept centrally in a computerized data bank, and all entries are coded by ICD-9 system. During 1985, there were 103,745 encounters recorded for nonoccupational conditions. Of these, the condition was specified by ICD-9 code in 86 percent of instances. The ten most frequent diagnoses are shown in Table 6.1 and constitute 48.8 percent of the total.

Occupationally related disorders were seen in 63,998 encounters during 1985. This figure includes many instances in which individuals were given personal protective equipment (e.g., ear plugs, safety glasses), and thus only 27 percent of these give rise to ICD-9 codable diagnoses. Of these, the ten most frequently seen are shown in Table 6.2.

In addition to the care given in occupational medical departments, the balance of medical care received by employees is accounted for by the insurance claims filed for them. Since Burlington Industries is self-insured, it is possible to monitor these figures also. The two years for which the most complete data were available were 1982 and 1983. Figure 6.2 shows the average expenditures in medical dollar benefits for male employees for these two years, subdivided into disease groupings. It is noteworthy that over one-fourth of the dollars spent were for circulatory diseases (including cardiovascular).

For female employees, the number one group of disorders covered was genitourinary, followed closely by expenses for pregnancy and child-

TABLE 6.1
Conditions Treated in Burlington Industries in 1985:
Ten Most Frequent Nonoccupational Visits

Condition	Percent (of total*)
Acute nasopharyngitis (common cold)	20
Headache	9
Acute pharyngitis	5
Dyspepsia	3
Acute sinusitis	3
Nausea and vomiting	2.6
Tension headache	1.7
Pain in limb	1.6
Chronic sinusitis	1.5
Dysmenorrhea	1.4
Total	48.8

*Total N = 103, 745.

TABLE 6.2
Conditions Treated in Burlington Industries in 1985:
Ten Most Frequent Occupationally Related Visits

ICD Name	Number	Percent (of total*)
Lumbago	290	1.65
Sprain/strain: wrist	300	1.7
Sprain/strain: lumbar	339	1.9
Sprain/strain: back	327	1.86
Open wound: finger	3,100	17.7
Splinter: finger	399	2.3
Other superficial injury: finger	461	2.6
Contusion: hand	373	2.1
Contusion: finger	815	4.6
Foreign body: eye	957	5.5

*Total N = 63,998. 46,447 would generally be "protection issued" encounters. No ICD code used.

FIGURE 6.2

Employee Medical Dollar Benefits by Disease (men): Burlington
Industries, 1982–83

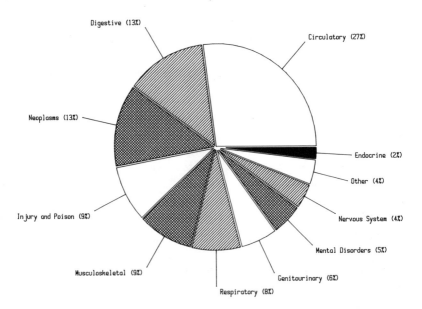

FIGURE 6.3

Employee Medical Dollar Benefits by Disease (women): Burlington
Industries, 1982–83

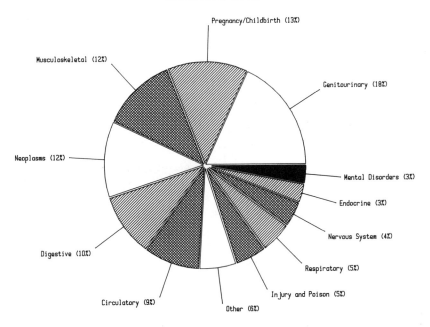

birth (see Figure 6.3). In a related observation concerning total medical
care dollars spent, the high dollar users of the system are employee
dependents, and the single highest cost category is intensive neonatal
care.

Examination of the proportion of medical care dollars spent for
male dependents shows that genitourinary and digestive disorders were
those covered most often (see Figure 6.4). This is not surprising since
the average age of this group is considerably less than that of the male
employee group.

On the other hand, the most prevalent diagnostic grouping for
female dependent coverage was circulatory disorders (see Figure 6.5).
This is related to the sizable proportion of this group who are in older
age categories. The significant contribution of congenital anomalies to
the medical care expenses of both male and female dependent groups
is related to the earlier observation that high expense areas included
intensive neonatal care.

Another observation from industry, which is qualitative rather than
quantitative, addresses the pervasive concern about coverage for the

FIGURE 6.4

Dependent Medical Dollar Benefits by Disease (men): Burlington
Industries, 1982–83

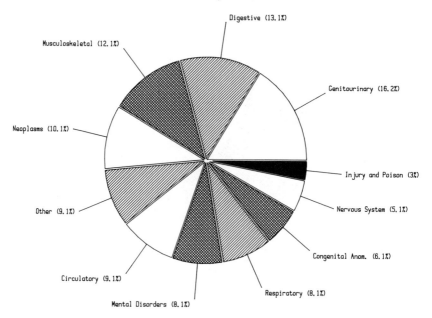

costs of medical care. In the turbulent economy of the 1980s, many
industries have been forced to close manufacturing facilities or to move
them elsewhere, leaving sizable groups of workers unemployed. Without
exception, the one question that always arises in such circumstances is
not "Where will I find another job?" but "How will we take care of
medical expenses?"

One final study from the viewpoint of the employee or the user of
medical care was addressed in a *New England Journal of Medicine* article
titled "Does Free Care Improve Adults' Health?" (Brook 1983). The
authors found that for persons with poor vision, and for low-income
persons with high blood pressure, free care brought an improvement in
those categories. For the average participant, no significant effects were
detected on eight other measures of health status and health habits. In
general, the study concluded that the more people have to pay for medical care, the less of it they use. Although there are a number of fasci-
nating aspects which might be explored, this study certainly confirms
that there are many significant variables other than cost in determining
usage and outcome of medical care. From the standpoint of the consumer, cost is not everything.

FIGURE 6.5

Dependent Medical Dollar Benefits by Disease (women): Burlington
Industries, 1982–83

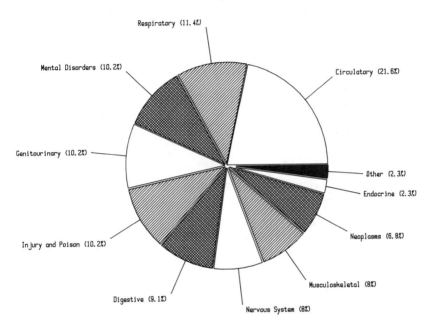

THE PRESENT STATUS OF EMPLOYER CONCERNS

Employers who, in the 1950s, legitimately pondered whether they
should include health benefits as part of their compensation scheme are
now finding that the cost of such benefits in the 1980s is a significant
portion of their overhead. The Burlington experience is shown in Figure 1. The next logical question is: What are we buying for these dollars?
A survey conducted in 1984 by the Department of Labor is summarized
in Table 6.3 (U.S. Department of Labor 1985). This survey showed that,
although most employers provided a benefit called "health insurance,"
there was great variability in its provisions. This variability was related
to such items as degree of coverage, ancillary coverage, alternatives to
hospital care, deductibles, copayments, out-of-pocket ceilings, and lifetime maxima.

After looking at what sorts of coverage they were buying, industry
began to examine the medical care system for more specific information

TABLE 6.3
Department of Labor Health Benefits Survey, 1984

Health Benefit	Percent of Employees
Health insurance	97%
Paid sick leave, sickness and accident insurance (or both)	94%
Short-term disability	47%
Retirement disability	46%
Retirement health insurance	63%
Individual coverage	100%
Contribute to health ins. premium	36
Don't contribute to premium	64
Family coverage	100%
Contribute to premium	58
Don't contribute to premium	42
Hospital care	100%
No deductible (basic)	17
Deductible required (major med)	28
Major medical and basic	54
Outpatient care	100%
Basic	12
Major medical	27
Both	60
Surgery	100%
Basic	32
Major medical	29
Both	39
Physician visits	96%
Basic	6
Major medical	86
Both	7
X-Rays and lab	100%
Basic	25
Major medical	42
Both	33
Prescription drugs	98%
Private duty nursing	96%
Mental health	99%
Dental	77%
Vision	30%

Continued

TABLE 6.3
Department of Labor Health Benefits Survey, 1984

Health Benefit	Percent of Employees
Alternatives to hospital	
Extended care facilities	62%
Home health care	46%
Hospice care	11%
Major medical deductibles	100%
Set dollar amount	94
Varied with salary	5
Annual per person	
$50	17%
$100	46%
$150 or more	12%
Coinsurance percentage	100%
80%	86
85%	5
90%	4
Other	5
Out-of-pocket maximum	75%
(stop loss)	
$2,000 or less	15%
$2,001–$4,000	27%
$4,001–$6,000	33%
$6,001–$8,000	10%
$8,001–$10,000	10%
$10,000 or more	5%
No out-of-pocket max	24%
Coinsurance decreased after certain level	1%
Lifetime maximum benefit	72%
$250,000	32
$500,000	12
$1,000,000	19
$25,000–$1,000,000	37
Medicare and Medicaid supplemental	
coverage provided by	
Blue Cross/Blue Shield	57%
Self-funded	33%
HMO or combination of plans	1%

Source: "Employee Benefits in Medium and Large Firms, 1984." DOL Bulletin 2237; Stock Number 029-001-02852-1. Washington, DC: U.S. Government Printing Office.

about the product for which they were paying. Resulting perceptions by industry were that the medical care system is:

—Sick care oriented with insufficient emphasis on prevention;

—One in which physicians are rewarded for the degree of "sickness" of their patients;

—One with no incentive for efficient delivery of their product(s);

—Equipped with no penalties for users with unhealthy life-styles;

—One in which no or inadequate purchasing criteria are used;

—A system in which the user is not only his/her own "purchasing agent" but also one over which there are few or inadequate controls; and

—One in which impulsive access to the services is encouraged by its arrangement.

Further, many companies found a disproportionate use factor at work. All populations have a subgroup of "high dollar users" of the health care system. Burlington Industries, for example, found in 1978 that 10 percent of their health insurance clients used 75 percent of the medical care purchased. The 1982 figures showed that 10 percent of the plan members used 80 percent of the care purchased, possibly indicating a trend. More specifically, 8.4 percent of the members in 1982 used 75 percent of the care. It is clear that one researchable area has to do with identifying and quantifying these "high dollar users."

A survey of a large number of companies was performed in 1983 to take a more global look at some of the factors involved in increased health care costs (Hansen Benefits Survey 1983). Based on their own experience, companies ranked the causes for health care increases in order of importance as shown in Table 6.4. "Increased utilization," although ranked an average of fourth by all companies, was considered the most important cause by a full 17 percent of them. This judgment confirms the experience of Burlington Industries, suggesting that a segment of "high dollar users" could be responsible.

What about other companies? Are their experiences similar? The Goodyear Tire and Rubber Company certainly indicates that this is so. Their health care bill was $166 million in 1983, which meant that $2 of the $57 price of the average tire goes to pay for employee health care. Robert E. Mercer, Goodyear's chairman, states: "When you look at all our expenses, health care jumps right out of the stack. It is the one that has increased most dramatically" (Cover Story 1984).

In Cleveland, nine major corporations—Stouffer, General Electric, Lubrizol, Standard Oil (Ohio), AmeriTrust, Sherwin-Williams, Parker-Hannifin, Eaton, and TRW—are pooling their hospital-claims infor-

TABLE 6.4
Relative Importance of Possible Causes of Increased Health Care Costs
for Large American Businesses (Hansen Benefits Survey 1983)

Cause	Rank
Hospital costs	1 (most important)
Inflation	2
Physician costs	3
Increased utilization	4
Medical technology	5
Administrative costs	6
Government regulation	7
Employee life-styles	8
Benefit changes	9 (least important)

mation to slash their $40 million annual health bill. By reviewing how 80,000 employees and dependents use health services, they expect to identify cost-efficient hospitals and providers (Cover Story 1984).

Around the country, the number of companies that are experiencing health care cost problems is indicated by the number that are modifying benefits plans and planning new strategies. These latter include a host of programs and approaches, ranging from HMOs to mandatory second opinions. Clearly, the proliferation of such programs is symptomatic of the degree of fiscal discomfort being experienced by the corporations, both large and small.

The findings of Burlington Industries' data analysis are such that a number of changes have been made and are projected for the future. Findings which prompted action include a 10 percent increase in hospitalization rate from 1983 to 1984. Although the average length-of-stay was less, this still resulted in a total number of hospital days per thousand insured of 720 in 1984, up from 706 in 1983.

Not only was there an increase in hospital utilization recorded during 1984, there was also a strong increase in utilization of the outpatient surgical setting. This increase of 104 percent in outpatient surgical utilization might otherwise have been interpreted as positive but, in this case, it was accompanied by an increase of 19 percent in the number of hospital confinements for surgery. Confirming this disturbing finding was the fact that the average total charge per confinement increased from $2,061 in 1983 to $2,180 in 1984—an increase of 6 percent.

"Ancillary charges," including laboratory fee. and x-rays, strain the accountability mechanisms of many systems, and Burlington's is no exception. In 1984, ancillary charges increased 10 percent over those of

1983. This represents an increase of $121 per confinement. During 1984, ancillary charges accounted for approximately 60 percent of the average hospital bill.

A different look at the "high dollar user" fraction of the population was afforded by the finding that the female spouse category, ages 25 to 64, and the dependent child category, ages 1 to 14, are responsible for 30 to 40 percent of all claims and charges. During 1984, for example, these two groups were responsible for 34.6 percent of all claims and approximately 30 percent of all claim charges. This points up the need for any communication program which is developed to be directed toward the employees' homes.

The analyses just discussed led Burlington to an intensive examination of its health care benefit package. The objective of this analysis was to determine ways of containing costs while maintaining or improving the level of employee benefits. The objective was examined in light of two relevant factors. First, they recognized that their ability to contain health care costs is limited, since many of the "drivers" influencing health care costs are outside Burlington's control. Among these are fee inflation, technological advancement, increased demand for health care, and increased supply of services. Recognizing this limitation, Burlington concluded that it would settle for a rate of growth in its health care costs that was no greater than inflation.

The second factor that the company recognized was that Burlington's corporate culture must accept improved employee health as an important goal. This value is manifested in the activities of plant nurses, management's interest in improving employee benefits, and the implementation of programs for health promotion and employee assistance.

Given these two factors—limited ability to influence costs and the value seen in improving employee health—a more appropriate objective was thought to be "to obtain maximum benefits from the dollars spent on employee health." This objective recognizes management's concern for health care costs, but places the emphasis on the area where management has the most control—how health care dollars are spent.

Logical goals following from this objective are:

1. To reduce the cost to Burlington for a given health care intervention to the minimum level consistent with assuring that employees seek adequate care;

2. To encourage health care intervention at the earliest stage in the disease process, where the maximum benefit can be obtained for the lowest treatment cost; and

3. To promote healthier life-styles for employees in order to obtain the benefits of a healthier work force and to minimize future acute care treatment costs.

These goals imply a shift in the philosophy underlying the health care benefit package from providing treatment for existing illnesses toward preventing the occurrence of those illnesses. The strategies adopted by Burlington and by many other corporations are consistent with this shift.

INDUSTRY AVENUES AND STRATEGIES

The approaches adopted by Burlington Industries are presented here, not because they represent the norm for industry (many approaches have been taken by many corporations), but as a single case example. The company's overall goals are to change the behavior of medical care consumers (employees and dependents) in the purchase of medical care and, secondarily, to influence the practice styles of physicians. The following objectives represent both short-term and long-term activities to aid in achieving these goals:

A. To reduce the demand for medical care, particularly acute hospital care

B. To reduce the risks of illness and accidental injury among employees and dependents

C. To reduce excess capacity (and growth) of the delivery system

Objective A: To Reduce Demand will be pursued by several strategies which are interrelated. Although they cannot be described in detail here, they can be enumerated as follows:

1. Obtaining utilization data in order to define patterns of care;

2. Gathering information and creating prudent buyer education programs for employees and dependents;

3. Expanding health promotion activities throughout the worker population and their families;

4. Developing programs for off-the-job accident prevention;

5. Providing employee assistance services for dealing with substance abuse and emotional problems;

6. Supporting community health planning for rationalization of services;

7. Supporting community dialogue between providers and payers (e.g., business/medical coalitions);

8. Providing alternative programs and settings for delivery of care wherever possible (e.g., HMOs, PPOs, ambulatory surgery units); and

9. Providing economic incentives to employees to promote making the best choices in their own medical care.

Objective B: To Reduce Risks will also be approached with several interrelated strategies. They are:

1. Developing a data base of health-related information on each individual in order to know the overall risks at start-up time;
2. Developing an educational program which will promote an awareness of need for individual risk management;
3. Creating a risk assessment program for measuring and following controllable risk factors;
4. Establishing risk management programs to enable individuals to manage their own risks with appropriate assistance from health professionals; and
5. Developing economic incentives to encourage individuals to take charge of their own health.

Objective C: To Reduce Excess Capacity is subject to misinterpretation and, therefore, requires clarification. This objective is based on the perception that the present medical care system is structured in inefficient ways in some locations. Because of this perception, it is reasonable to believe that it is appropriate for employers (payers) to contribute to measures for more rational and efficient distribution of medical care resources. This can be done in the following ways:

1. Identifying patterns of medical care on a community-by-community basis;
2. Encouraging the development of standards for care by consensus among providers within communities, including agreement on cost-beneficial limits for procedures;
3. Identifying "outliers" by peer review, including providers and users who habitually overutilize the system;
4. Assuring an appropriate mix of professionals, facilities, and services to meet the medical care needs in the community; and
5. Creating a public understanding of the need to rationalize the medical care system and to control the costs associated with it by educational programs.

In common with other industries, Burlington believes that they, and their employees, retirees, and dependents, have a major opportunity to reduce medical costs over the short and long term by following these strategies. They also believe that, by more efficient and visionary management of their health, medical, and disability resources, they can reduce out-of-pocket medical expenses, as well as improve their health and the quality of their lives.

FUTURE CHANGES IN HEALTH CARE

Employers are now evincing concern regarding both occupational and nonoccupational health matters, but it has become clear that the division is artificial. An emphasis on long-term prevention presents an opportunity to combine programs that will influence life- and work-styles in a manner that will improve health.

Employers will see continued changes in medical benefits programs and reimbursement procedures with substantial impact, including:

—Medical necessity tests such as precertification of care;

—More provisions for "first dollar" coverage by the consumer rather than the employer or insurer;

—Systematized standards of care, by diagnosis or diagnostic grouping, developed by peer review organizations;

—Multiple benefit options for employees, including prepaid care, high-risk/low-risk, and "cafeteria-style" programs;

—Prevention incentives with emphasis on early risk identification and aggressive risk management programs;

—Encouraging alternative settings for care by incentives for use of less-expensive alternatives; and

—Use of health care advisors or managers to assist purchasers with options and choices and to reinforce positive behaviors.

One thing has become very clear regarding the role of employers in the medical care marketplace. The majority of them are now paying as much of the cost as they believe possible, and they will take whatever measures are necessary to limit further expansion of this item of overhead expense.

REFERENCES

Brook, R. H.; Donald, C. A.; Goldberg, G. A.; et al. (1983). "Does Free Care Improve Adults' Health?" *New England Journal of Medicine* 309: 1426–34.

Business Week/Harris Poll (1984). "Americans Prescribe Radical Surgery." *Business Week*, October 15.

Cover Story (1984). "The Corporate Rx for Medical Costs." *Business Week*, October 15, 139.

Davis, Michael M., Jr. (1934). "The American Approach to Health Insurance." *Milbank Memorial Fund Quarterly* 12: 214.

Falk, I. S.; Rorim, C. R.; and Ring, Martha D. (1933). *The Cost of Medical Care.* Chicago: University of Chicago Press.

Goldberg, Lawrence G., and Greenberg, Warren (1978). "The Emergence of Physician-Sponsored Health Insurance: A Historical Perspective." In *Com-*

petition in the Health Sector: Past, Present and Future, 288–321. Washington, DC: Federal Trade Commission.

Hansen Benefits Survey (1983). *Health Care Cost Containment Survey Results.* Deerfield, IL: A. S. Hansen, Inc.

Hayes, Donald M. (1978). "Perceptions of Care by Professionals and Nonprofessionals." *Evaluation and the Health Professions* 1: 29–56.

Kolimaga, Jane (ed.) (1984). *Health Cost Management Handbook.* Raleigh, NC: North Carolina Foundation of Alternative Health Programs, Inc.

Levit, Katherine R. (1983). "Personal Health Care Expenditures by State." *Health Care Financing Review* 6: 4.

Robinson, J. M. (1916). *Social Insurance.* New York: Henry Holt.

Rosen, George (1977). "Contract or Lodge Practice and Its Influence on Medical Attitudes to Health Insurance." *American Journal of Public Health* 67: 374–78.

Selleck, Henry B., and Whittaker, Alfred H. (1962). *Occupational Health in America.* Detroit, MI: Wayne State University Press.

Sinai, Nathan; Anderson, Odin W.; and Dollar, Melvin L. (1946). *Health Insurance in the United States.* New York: Commonwealth Fund.

Somers, Herman N., and Somers, Anne R. (1961). *Doctors, Patients and Health Insurance.* Washington, DC: Brookings Institution.

Stein, Jane (1986). "What Americans Think About Health Care." *Business and Health,* January/February.

U.S. Department of Labor (1985). *Employee Benefits in Medium and Large Firms.* D.O.L. Bulletin 2237. Washington, DC: U.S. Government Printing Office.

Chapter 7

The AMA's Role in Cost Containment: Leadership or Target Practice?

M. Roy Schwarz

Editor's Note—There are six causes for increased health care costs: inflation, population increases, development of expensive medical technologies, increased numbers of nonphysician and physician medical care providers, escalating cost of liability insurance and size of malpractice suit awards, and exploitation of the third-party reimbursement system by providers. A seventh, potential cause is the development of new and costly health problems, such as acquired immunodeficiency syndrome (AIDS). Schwarz, who was Dean of the University of Colorado School of Medicine before he became Assistant Executive Vice President at the American Medical Association (AMA), believes that the AMA has attempted to address each cause, but with limited success. Physicians have concerns, moreover, that overshadow those of medical cost increases; namely, the quality of medical care, and insuring that providers are competently trained and qualified to do their work.

The AMA, as the only organization that can claim to speak for all medical practitioners, has attempted to lead its profession and society toward greater concern for the quality of care, as well as greater control over costs. In its position as the highly visible leader for medical practitioners, however, the AMA has been the target of criticisms that are not borne out by its record of involvement in cost containment.

The United States is undergoing a period of unprecedented change in its health enterprise. Driven by rapidly rising health care costs, a poor public image of physicians, concern by business about health care costs, and a massive federal budget deficit, these changes are fundamentally altering the fabric of health care in this country. No segment of the health community is free from the relentless onslaught of forces that many do not understand. Because of the dramatic nature of the increases in health care costs, a clarion call has come from those who pay for this care for new, more vigorous efforts to contain the rate of increase and the total expenditures for health care.

This chapter will (a) review the causes of the rising health care costs and the AMA's response to each of the factors, (b) discuss the successes and failures of the AMA in cost containment, (c) examine physicians' attitudes concerning cost containment and the options that a professional association has in this environment, and (d) answer the question posed by the title of this chapter.

HEALTH CARE COSTS: CAUSES FOR INCREASES AND AMA RESPONSES

There are at least six major reasons that the cost of health care in the United States has increased in such a dramatic and, from some perspectives, alarming fashion over the past decade. While complex, the causes are not mysterious and are susceptible to analysis. They include inflation in the general economy, the advent of new technologies, population growth including a dramatic increase in the number of elderly citizens, the excessive consumption and provision of health care services, increases in the number of health professionals, and, for most physicians, alarming increases in the costs of liability (malpractice) insurance.

Inflation

A major cause of the increasing health care costs has been the inflation in the general economy. Inflation has totaled 38 percent from 1980 to 1984, with increases as high as 13.5 percent (1980) and as low as 3.2 percent (1983). To respond to medical care's contribution to the inflation problem, the AMA called for a voluntary freeze on physician fees. As many as 77 percent of practicing physicians responded in 1984 with savings of $3.1 billion, an amazing degree of compliance when one considers that about one-half of all physicians are dues-paying AMA members. It suggests that members and nonmembers alike will respond when asked by the AMA and when they perceive the request to be justified.

Population

There has been a steady increase in the population of the United States over the past decade, and this is expected to continue into the next century. The result will be a 30 percent increase by the year 2025, including a doubling of the number of people over 65, a tripling of the number over 75, and a fourfold increase in the number of people over 85. Since the elderly consume significantly larger amounts of all varieties of health care service than do the nonelderly, the increased number of elderly will continue to drive health care costs, probably in an accelerating fashion in the future, unless a limit is placed on the number and kinds of services that society will provide to this age group.

The AMA has attempted to study and predict our future health care requirements, especially those of the elderly, and to evaluate how they will be met and paid for. The AMA's Ethical and Judicial Affairs Council has also studied a variety of ethical issues relating to the costs of health care delivery, including those that are especially important in the care of the elderly, and has drafted new or revised guidelines. An example is the recent statement on withdrawing life-support systems, including feeding tubes, from irreversibly comatose patients.

An aggressive attempt to develop a national health policy for the United States was completed in late 1986. This Health Policy Agenda Project should provide a blueprint for health policy development, with input provided by representatives of over 150 organizations including labor, business, the elderly, health professions, educational institutions, and government.

Technology

The United States has seen a revolution in health care technology in the past 20 years, developments so numerous and so spectacular that society has begun to expect them as a matter of course. However, some of these technologies have increased health care costs to a very considerable degree. For example, in 1973, 11,000 patients were treated with chronic renal dialysis at a cost of $229 million. In 1982, the number of patients had increased to 69,000, and the costs had escalated to $1.8 billion. Similar increases are projected for liver transplants, heart transplants, and coronary-bypass procedures in the next decade.

The AMA has responded to these new technologies by promoting increases in the National Institutes of Health budgets, in the belief that the best hope for controlling diseases and the attendant health care costs (to say nothing of the lost productivity) is to continue the nation's research and development efforts. In addition, the AMA has embarked upon an extensive evaluation of medical technology, using panels of outside experts who make judgments relative to the safety and efficacy of the technology in question. The results are published in the *Journal of the American Medical Association* and are widely cited. The AMA has also been active in national policy development on the proper applications of new technologies.

Numbers of Health Professionals

Over the past 20 years, there has been a disproportionate increase in the number of health professionals in the United States. In medicine, the entering class size of U.S. medical schools has doubled, and the number of physicians in graduate medical education, including a large number of foreign medical graduates, has increased even more. In addition, there been an increase in the number of nurses, pharmacists, and allied health practitioners, all of whom expect (and in most cases have received) sustenance from the health care dollar.

In response to the growing concern about numbers of health professionals, the AMA has emphasized maintenance of high educational standards for health professionals through the accreditation of schools of medicine, residency programs, continuing medical education programs, and allied health training programs. The AMA monitors the numbers of professionals and, in the case of physicians, it monitors their geographic distribution, practice patterns, income levels, and practice behaviors. Various councils of the AMA have studied issues related to manpower and have recommended manpower policies that do not violate the Federal Trade Commission's principle of open competition.

Liability

Physicians have been aware for over a decade of a growing problem with liability insurance and malpractice awards. Specifically, the cost of liability insurance has increased sharply, the frequency of malpractice claims and suits has increased, and there has been an alarming escalation in the size of the awards or settlements in disputes over medical outcomes. This crisis, which began in the 1970s and has worsened in the 1980s, is altering the practice patterns of certain subspecialists, forcing physicians to practice medicine defensively with an increased cost of $17 billion per year, and transforming the physician-patient relationship from one of mutual trust to one of suspicion.

In response to this crisis, the AMA has undertaken the enormous effort of collecting accurate and current data, including the number of claims, suits, settlements, and awards, and documenting the experiences of the liability insurance industry. A public education effort has been designed to educate policymakers about the crisis and potential solutions, and a federal proposal for tort reform has been developed to provide incentives to state governments to modify their laws.

In addition, the AMA has been establishing coalitions among affected groups to effect broad-based demand for reform. To help prevent expensive litigation, working through 164 state and specialty societies, the AMA has embarked upon a variety of risk management activities aimed at elucidating the nature of the suits, their causes, and the ways in which they can be avoided.

Abuse of the Reimbursement System

Over 90 percent of Americans have some form of health insurance, often in the form of generous fringe benefits negotiated between labor and industry. Until recent years, these programs did not contain significant deductions or copayments by patients, and there were financial incentives to physicians to provide as much care as was demanded. Thus, there were encouragements for both consumers and providers to overuse federal health services.

In response, the AMA has embarked on a variety of health education programs aimed at decreasing unnecessary utilization through life-style changes and self-care. In addition, the association has worked with the health insurance industry and government to develop an equitable plan of consumer payments and deductible methods known to decrease utilization of health services.

The AMA has evaluated regional variations in health care, has urged more stringent peer review efforts by physicians, and has attempted to educate the Federal Trade Commission as to why professional self-discipline is the most effective way to handle "provider abuse." An innovative project designed to detect and remediate the excessive prescribing of drugs by physicians, known as the PADS program, has led to the education of poorly informed physicians and the loss of licenses by those who purposely abuse prescribing privileges.

The association has been monitoring the cost-containment programs and policies put in place by the federal government, with a special interest in the impact of these procedures on the quality of health care. The association also established a diagnostic-related group (DRG) monitoring project that recorded physicians' impressions of the impact of DRGs. In general, there is a growing concern on the part of physicians over the deterioration in the quality of health care under DRGs, especially in the care of elderly individuals who have multiple medical disorders or who are severely ill. Other concerns expressed by physicians are the premature discharge of ill patients into ill-equipped nursing homes or home health care settings, inadequate reimbursements for care of severely ill patients, and adverse impacts on smaller hospitals. Finally, the data suggest a serious deterioration in relationships between physicians and hospital administrators who press for early patient discharge in order to realize profits through the DRG system.

The association has also monitored professional review organizations (PROs) and their impact on health care and has been an active participant in delineating the supervisory body ("super PRO") which is reviewing all state PROs for the Health Care Financing Administration (HCFA).

The association has attempted, through practice management seminars and consultation, to enhance physicians' ability to cope with new economic forces. It has also evaluated how new health care delivery systems, including for-profit chains as well as the not-for-profit HMOs, independent practice associations (IPAs), and preferred provider organizations (PPOs), affect physicians and health care costs.

Finally, the association has conducted extensive research in the socioeconomic aspects of health care, including the characteristics of practice, differential costs of care, physicians' incomes, and changes in health care delivery.

Physician Fees. When considering the rising costs of health care, one must consider the extent to which physician fees contribute to the overall increases in these costs. An analysis of the figures suggests that these fees are not a major factor in rising costs, although certain specialties with technical procedures are reimbursed at high levels compared to the reimbursement for other physician efforts. In 1985, the United States spent $424 billion (estimated) for health care. Of this amount, 20 percent or $84.8 billion were physician charges. This $84.8 billion paid for office and practice overhead as well as the personal income of physicians. Since 47 percent of every dollar billed as gross charges for physician services was used to pay practice expenses, including office overhead, physicians received $44.9 billion in pretax, personal compensation in 1985. This represents slightly more than 10 percent of the total health care costs. In addition, the purchasing power of physicians has been declining since 1970 at the rate of approximately 1 percent per year, while the costs of operating a practice have continued upward. Hence, "controlling" physician fees would have, at best, a small impact on the overall growth of health care expenditures.

HAVE THE AMA's EFFORTS BEEN SUCCESSFUL?

The answer to this question must be mixed. Certainly one would give an affirmative answer after examining the impact of the AMA's voluntary fee freeze. Data suggest that as many as 77 percent of the practicing physicians in the United States cooperated with the voluntary freeze, with a savings of $3.1 billion in health care expenditures. The efforts to educate physicians about the cost problem have had an impact, as have efforts to educate public policymakers. Furthermore, there has been little disagreement that the development of AMA initiatives such as the Health Policy Agenda Project, the proposed tort reform, legislation for liability, and vaccine compensation efforts have all been helpful.

There is also a negative side to this question, however. If success is judged from the standpoint of adoption and implementation of major initiatives to address the problem of reducing costs without compromising the quality of care or long-term behavior changes in professionals, then the AMA's efforts have not been as successful as desired. It has not successfully eliminated much of the waste from the health care system, and the AMA's efforts have not achieved the goal of having physicians speaking in a unified voice. While some gains have been made in educating policymakers, the AMA has not been successful in preventing the implementation of short-sighted initiatives that will have a profound impact on health care but will undoubtedly cost more in the long run than they will save over the short term. Much remains to be done.

PHYSICIAN ATTITUDES AND FUTURE OPTIONS

While it is hazardous to generalize about the admittedly diverse attitudes of physicians toward cost containment, there are a number of perceptions that have been repeatedly shared with the AMA that are worth noting. It is clear that all physicians wish to provide high-quality care for American people at reasonable cost. However, if physicians are required to choose between quality of care and cost containment, they will universally and without hesitation choose quality first.

Furthermore, while physicians are willing to do their part in controlling rising health care costs, they are not willing to have the health sector bear more than a fair share of the budget reductions relative to other sectors of the economy. One has to look no further than the president's 1987 budget proposal to see this inequity, in that the president exempts 50 percent of the federal budget from reduction, while the other half, including health, would suffer severe reductions.

Physicians are also not willing to have minimally or inadequately trained health professionals providing medical care in the name of economizing. Physicians are convinced that this will put the welfare of patients at risk and that such initiatives as therapeutic substitution by pharmacists, the diagnosis and treatment of disease by nurse practitioners, and expanded roles for chiropractors and other health professionals will ultimately result in the same outcome. Physicians are outraged at the unconstitutional Medicare fee freezes placed on the profession and by the liability crisis generated by the unrealistic expectations of the public and the greed of some lawyers.

Physicians are also concerned about the poor quality of health care provided by some physicians, by the unreasonable fees that are charged by some individuals, and by governmental interference in the self-discipline process of the profession. The practicing world wonders what the academic reaction would be if the Federal Trade Commission announced that the evaluation of student and resident academic performance and the evaluation of faculty performance as a part of the appointment and promotion process were in violation of anti-trust statutes and, therefore, must be discontinued. A sense of disbelief, frustration, and outrage would follow such a conclusion, and this reaction comes close to the feelings that practicing physicians have about restrictions on peer review. Finally, physicians are puzzled by the poor public image that physicians have. They question why people think that physicians are primarily responsible for rising health care costs and why they think doctors can control these costs.

Turning to future options that are available to a professional association, the most critical need is the need for a definition of what constitutes "quality health care" and how such care can be measured. The profession must also collect and analyze data on costs of health care and the performance of the various delivery systems of health care. The association must evaluate new developments in health care delivery as to effectiveness, safety, and cost efficiency. The AMA must continue to educate the profession and the public policymakers about the policies of the profession and the rationale behind them. Above all else, the association must defend the quality of patient care and the welfare of people who put their trust in the profession. In short, the AMA must promote the art and science of medicine and the betterment of public health, the purpose for which it was established in 1846.

THE AMA's ROLE IN COST CONTAINMENT: LEADERSHIP OR TARGET PRACTICE?

The AMA is the only organization in America that can claim, with some legitimacy, to speak for the entire "House of Medicine." It is the largest, most visible, most influential, and most experienced of all professional societies. It is understandable, therefore, that the AMA has become the target for "cheap shots," criticisms, envy, scorn, ridicule, and public admonitions of every conceivable variety. If the AMA is to achieve its stated purpose, however, it must—as a leader—absorb unfair criticism.

The association should encourage others to join it in pursuing matters of concern to the profession and to its members. It is imperative that this be done because this is the only way the profession can continue to have an impact on the politics of health, whether in regard to cost containment, access to health care, quality control, development of new knowledge, education, or ethics of medicine. We must insistently ask, "What is it we wish to provide in health care, at what quality level do we want the care provided, and at what cost?" Once the answers to these questions are provided, we may discover that the best care is not the cheapest care and that we do not wish to spend less on health care.

BIBLIOGRAPHY

The following AMA reports are available upon request from the American Medical Association.

American Medical Association. Council on Long-Range Planning and Development. *The Environment of Medicine.* Chicago, IL: American Medical Association, 1985.

American Medical Association. Council on Long-Range Planning and Development Report C. *Implications of Trends in Physician and Public Attitudes.* House of Delegates Annual Meeting. Chicago, IL: American Medical Association, 1985.

American Medical Association. Council on Ethical and Judicial Affairs. *Current Opinions of the Council on Ethical and Judicial Affairs of the American Medical Association.* Chicago, IL: American Medical Association, 1986.

American Medical Association. Board of Trustees Report P. *Health Policy Agenda for the American People—Current Status.* House of Delegates Annual Meeting. Chicago, IL: American Medical Association, 1986.

American Medical Association. Council on Medical Education. *Future Directions for Medical Education.* Chicago, IL: American Medical Association, 1982.

American Medical Association. Board of Trustees Report BB. *Study of Professional Liability Problems.* House of Delegates Interim Meeting. Chicago, IL: American Medical Association, 1984.

American Medical Association. Board of Trustees Report MM. *Special Task Force on Professional Liability and Insurance.* House of Delegates Interim Meeting. Chicago, IL: American Medical Association, 1985.

American Medical Association. Board of Trustees Report R. *AMA's DRG Monitoring Project and the Prospective Pricing System.* House of Delegates Annual Meeting. Chicago, IL: American Medical Association, 1985.

American Medical Association. Group on Health Service Policy. *Physician Reimbursement under DRGs. Problems and Prospects.* Chicago, IL: American Medical Association, 1984.

American Medical Association. Council on Medical Service Report H. *Peer Review Organization (PRO) Program Status.* House of Delegates Annual Meeting. Chicago, IL: American Medical Association, 1985.

American Medical Association. Board of Trustees Report QQ. *AMA Initiative on Quality of Medical Care and Professional Self-Regulation.* House of Delegates Annual Meeting. Chicago, IL: American Medical Association, 1986.

Reynolds, R. A., and Duann, D. J. *Socioeconomic Characteristics of Medical Practice, 1985.* Chicago, IL: American Medical Association, 1985.

Roback, G.; Randolph, L.; Mead, D.; and Pasko, T. *Physician Characteristics and Distribution in the US.* Chicago, IL: American Medical Association, 1984.

Chapter 8

Economic Aspects of the Medicare and Medicaid Programs

Alan L. Sorkin

Editor's Note—The major impetus for medical cost-containment legislation has come from the growth in federal and state expenditures for Medicare and Medicaid programs. Dramatic increases both in prices and utilization of Medicare hospital insurance (HI or "part A"), only part of which are explainable by general inflation and the aging of the American population, will deplete the trust fund by 1990 and result in a negative balance of over $90 billion by 1995—even if current cost-containment efforts within diagnosis-related groups (DRGs) yield the savings expected by legislators. Despite these expected losses, increases in the social security payroll taxes that support HI, and substantial copayment or coinsurance, the benefits of Medicare HI fall short of an ideal medical insurance, failing in particular to protect the elderly and their families from the financial consequences of a catastrophic illness. Medicare supplementary medical insurance (SMI or "part B"), which covers physician and outpatient services, is funded by monthly premiums ($24.50 in 1988) which have been increased each year, and by a contribution from general federal revenues to make up the difference (historically, this difference exceeds 75 percent of the total SMI outlays). It is predicted that nearly 6 percent of total general revenues may be required to fund SMI by 1988.

Only 55 to 60 percent of the people living in poverty in the United States are covered by Medicaid, for which federal and state funding has increased over tenfold since 1968. Increased costs have resulted from greater utilization (especially by Aid for Dependent Children recipients), medical price inflation, and the higher costs of institutionalization of the elderly and disabled. Medicaid reimbursement for medical services is inequitably distributed: nearly half of funds are dispensed in five large industrialized states, while the nearly half of the poor who live in southern states receive about 22 percent of funds. Cost-containment efforts have introduced a serious risk of discouraging providers from serving the poor, whose medical needs are documentably greater than more affluent persons.

The Medicare program, designed to finance acute medical care mainly for elderly Americans, also covers some categories of the disabled and those with end-stage renal disease. The program is divided into two parts: Part A, which is hospital insurance (HI), and Part B, which is supplementary medical insurance (SMI). The HI component covers short-term hospitalization, skilled nursing care, and home health services, while the SMI portion covers physicians' services, outpatient hospital care, and laboratory fees, as well as home health care. The program does not cover long-term nursing home care, dental care, or outpatient drugs.

Cost sharing is imposed on Medicare beneficiaries who use medical services. Under HI, a deductible amount approximately equal to the cost of one day in a hospital ($540 in 1988) must be paid by beneficiaries who are hospitalized. Aside from this deductible, the HI program pays in full the cost of the first 60 days of hospitalization for an episode of illness. From the sixty-first day through the ninetieth day, a 25 percent coinsurance payment of $135 per day was required as of 1988. For stays of more than 90 days, each beneficiary has a lifetime reserve of 60 additional days but must pay $200 for each day that is used (Hsiao and Kelly 1984, 209).

HI also covers up to 100 posthospital days in a skilled nursing facility (SNF). After 20 days, the beneficiary is required to pay an amount per day that is equal to 12.5 percent of the inpatient hospital deductible ($67.50 in 1988).

Under SMI, as of 1988, beneficiaries paid $15.50 per month plus an annual deductible of $75, beyond which Medicare would pay 80 percent of the "reasonable charges" for covered services. If the provider's charges were reasonable according to Medicare standards, then the patient's share was the remaining 20 percent of the total. If the charges exceeded such standards, the beneficiary was liable for the excess amount in addition to his 20 percent share (except when the physician accepted assignment).[1]

State Medicaid programs frequently serve to complement Medicare for low-income elderly persons (Burwell et al. 1987, 1). Medicaid may finance cost-sharing amounts as well as other noncovered services for eligible Medicare beneficiaries who are too poor to pay these bills.

A major weakness of Medicare's benefit structure is that it violates the primary purpose of insurance, which is to protect the beneficiary from destitution. The cost-sharing provisions of the HI and SMI mean that elderly people face unlimited liabilities if a catastrophic illness occurs. Under HI, patients are required to pay the entire hospital cost after 150 days of hospitalization. Moreover, they have already paid relatively high coinsurance rates beginning on the ninety-first day. Furthermore, SMI requires patients to pay 20 percent of reasonable charges for physician visits as well as other outpatient services. For expensive surgery, the 20 percent coinsurance rate could be a costly financial burden on an elderly patient. Consequently, even though the probability of a large financial outlay is low, there is an incentive for beneficiaries to buy supplementary insurance coverage. This weakness in Medicare's benefit structure helped to create the demand for what is presently called Medigap insurance (Hsiao and Kelly 1984, 217).

Medigap insurance pays a substantial portion of the health care costs that are not covered by Medicare. It permits those elderly persons who can afford this insurance roughly the same degree of insurance protection as that obtained by employed nonaged persons.

MEDICARE COST CONTROLS

Both overall national health expenditures and Medicare expenditures have been rising rapidly since enactment of the latter in 1965 (see Table 8.1). In 1984, Medicare's HI expenditures were almost nine times the 1970 level, and SMI expenses were more than seven times the amount spent in 1970. Over the same period, non-Medicare hospital expenditures (total expenses less expenditures under Medicare's HI) rose nearly six times, and expenses for non-Medicare physicians' services increased by five times. Part of the reason why Medicare expenditures have risen more rapidly than non-Medicare expenses is the growth and aging of the elderly population. Another reason for the differential expenditure growth results from covering the disabled and persons with end-stage renal disease under Medicare after 1972. Finally, increases in Medicare utilization rates and prices explain only a small portion of the differential growth between Medicare and non-Medicare expenditures.

COST CONTAINMENT: A LEGISLATIVE HISTORY

In order to increase controls on utilization, the Professional Standards Review Organization (PSRO) program was enacted in 1972. Provisions were also adopted to limit increases in physicians' fees allowed by Medicare. Furthermore, the legislation authorized limits on which costs incurred by hospitals could be reimbursed.

From 1972 to 1981, there was a gradual but not very stringent

TABLE 8.1

National Health Expenditures, Hospital and Physician Insurance
Expenditures, and Medicare Expenditures, 1960–84*
(billions of dollars)

Year	Total Health Expenditures	Percentage of GNP	Hospital Insurance	Insurance for Physician Services	Total Medicare	Medicare Hospital Insurance	Supplementary Medical Insurance
1960	$ 26.9	5.3	$ 5.7	$ 2.0	—	—	—
1965	41.7	6.1	13.9	8.5	—	—	—
1970	74.7	7.6	27.8	14.3	$ 7.4	$ 5.3	$ 2.1
1975	132.7	8.6	52.1	24.9	16.0	11.6	4.4
1980	249.0	9.4	100.4	46.8	36.8	25.6	10.7
1981	286.6	9.8	118.0	54.8	43.6	30.7	12.9
1982	322.3	10.5	134.7	61.8	51.1	36.7	11.4
1983	355.4	10.7	148.8	68.4	57.8	40.4	13.4
1984	387.4	10.6	157.9	75.4	64.6	44.4	14.6

Source: Katherine Levit, Helen Lazenby, Daniel Waldo, and Lawrence Davidoff, "National Health Expenditures, 1985," *Health Care Financing Review* 7, no. 1 (1985): 3, 17, 18, 20.

*For periods ending June 30.

administrative tightening of Medicare rules that reduced to some extent the rate of growth of expenditures. However, estimates of program expenditures indicated an increasing gap between those expenditures and the revenue to pay hospital bills. This contrasted with large increases in general revenue support for SMI. Greatly increased control of all hospital costs was sought by the Carter administration, but Congress would not pass the enabling legislation.

While physician fee payments were being constrained, a limit was placed on the rate of increase in SMI premium rates. Because of this limit, beneficiary premiums fell from 50 percent of the total expenditures for SMI to 25 percent. Legislation passed in 1982 has prevented, for the time being, a further decline in the proportion of total SMI expenditures accounted for by premiums.

Despite the legislative controls on physician fee increases, SMI expenditures have continued to rise rapidly because of volume growth and the ineffectiveness of the regulation. The physician fee limitation was applied without developing a federal definition of the various services subject to fee controls. As a result, some bypassing of regulations occurred due to the introduction of new services, and changes in the content of services, including "unbundling" (submitting separate charges for parts of a service that were previously billed as a unit).

One of the reasons why it is so difficult to control physician fees is that if the physician bills the patient rather than billing Medicare, the physician can charge any amount he deems appropriate. This, in effect, shifts more of the costs of Medicare-covered services to the patient. This change in billing practice has tended to slowly reduce the portion of the physician charges covered by Medicare, thus preventing the imposition of more stringent controls on physician fees by program administrators.

The Omnibus Reconciliation Act of 1981 increased the Medicare HI deductible to a level more than 12 percent higher than mandated under the automatic adjustment procedure set by previous legislation (Long, Settle, and Link 1982, 222). This change reduced federal Medicare expenditures by approximately $360 million in 1984 (Svahn 1981, 3–24).

The Tax Equity and Financial Responsibility Act (TEFRA) of 1982 was the first federal legislation explicitly designed to reduce Medicare costs. This law profoundly changed Medicare's hospital reimbursement methods (Lave 1984, 253). First, the basis of reimbursement was shifted from an implicit per diem system to an explicit per case system; second, case mix was incorporated into the payment system; and third, a limit was placed on the rate of allowable increase in costs per case (Dobson et al. 1986, 3). While reimbursement continued to be based on reasonable costs, the application of this concept was radically altered. Costs per case which were higher than 120 percent of the average (adjusted for wages and case mix for comparable hospitals), or which rose by more than the target rate over the past year, were no longer considered reasonable. TEFRA also required that a prospective payment system be developed by the Secretary of the Department of Health and Human Services (HHS).

The 1983 Social Security legislation included the substitution of a hospital prospective payment system for the former reasonable cost basis of reimbursement. This action represents the largest change in reimbursement policy since the establishment of Medicare. Significantly, the cost-control aspect of this policy focuses on hospitals, not beneficiaries. The 1983 legislation only applies to the Medicare program. Thus, despite limits on Medicare payments, hospitals have the opportunity to earn additional revenue from non-Medicare patients. This opportunity for cost-shifting enables the hospitals to offset losses in revenue resulting from treating Medicare patients. However, legislators favoring controls on all hospital costs included in the law a provision through which states could obtain waivers from the basic Medicare prospective payment plan if they instituted a prospective payment proposal that covered all hospital patients.

Because the new system applies on a per case basis, it generally results in the same payment regardless of the length-of-stay or the volume of services provided. This should reduce the incentives for hospitals to increase their patient load.

THE DRG PROSPECTIVE PAYMENT SYSTEM

The basic features of the Medicare prospective payment system are: (1) all patients are classified into one of 468 diagnosis-related groups (DRGs); (2) with few exceptions, the hospital receives a fixed payment per DRG to cover operating costs; (3) the payment per DRG received by a hospital is a function of regional wages, whether the facility is located in a rural or urban area, and the number of full-time interns and residents on its staff; and (4) capital costs and direct education are excluded, but the Secretary of HHS is to report to Congress on methods of including these costs in the prospective rates. There was a three-year phase-in period during which the payment rates shifted from being essentially based on retrospective reimbursement to being set prospectively on a national basis with adjustments based on region, staff size, and local wage rates. Thus, by 1987, reimbursement to an individual hospital to pay for the operating costs of producing services to Medicare beneficiaries became fully based on a national prospective payment system.

The current law explicitly determines how payment rates should be increased. Basically, payment rates on the average are to increase by the "market basket plus one." The market basket is a measure of the rate of increase in the prices that hospitals have to pay for their inputs, and the additional one percentage point (the intensity factor) is to provide some room for "technological change." Since the market basket price index has consistently increased more than the overall consumer price index, the new law insures that the payment rate for a Medicare illness episode will continue to increase at a faster rate than that of goods and services in general.

The probable effects of the Medicare prospective payment system are outlined below (Lave 1984, 261).

1. There are incentives to decrease the services provided to patients. In addition, some hospitals have eliminated some services completely and no longer treat certain conditions that are too expensive to provide in comparison with expected payments (Schwartz 1983, 15–21).

2. Lengths-of-stay for particular diagnoses should continue to decrease because the hospitals get no additional revenue for long stays as compared to short stays, but use of home health agencies, nursing home beds, and rehabilitation centers will likely increase. After the introduction of prospective payment, the average length of stay of Medicare patients in hospitals fell from 9.5 days in 1983 to 7.5 days in 1984.[2]

3. The number of admissions and readmissions will likely increase. Some patients who could be treated as outpatients may be treated as inpatients. In addition, there will be some incentive to space treatments or operations (if possible) rather than to do all of them during the same hospital episode, because the hospital will be reimbursed for each admission.

4. Preadmission testing should increase, as it will occasionally be possible through unbundling to charge for it under Part B and collect the full DRG rate under Part A of Medicare. The law makes it illegal to unbundle services while the patient is hospitalized, but does not include outpatient services under this prohibition.

5. Since every DRG represents a collection of different diagnoses and conditions along with their associated treatments, it is possible that some providers may attempt to admit only certain types of patients within a particular DRG. Thus, the hospital may try to select only the patients who are not relatively costly to treat within a given DRG and send the sicker patients to another facility.

6. Services that have been cross-subsidized by other activities are likely to be reduced since the DRG system does not include reimbursement for the former. Thus, programs in social services, nutritional counseling, health promotion, and prevention may be curtailed because, while they contribute to a decrease in the cost of posthospital care, they cause increases in inpatient costs.

Medicare projected a $68 billion savings over the first three years (1986–1988) of the prospective payment system, although no one knows what the cost of Medicare *would* have been without the DRG system (U.S. Senate 1983). While that hypothetical savings may only postpone the insolvency of the trust fund by one year, $68 billion is still a substantial amount of money. It should be noted that the proposal to establish uniform national DRG prices by 1987 projected no net savings to the trust fund whatsoever (Vladeck 1984, 272). For every hospital or group of hospitals that is penalized by the establishment of a single national standard, there is a corresponding hospital or group of hospitals that receives a financial gain.

Because no uniform system of price setting can ever be ideal, one can argue that the most sensible policy is to base at least some percentage of a hospital's rates on its historical cost patterns. For example, in New Jersey, a relatively complex formula has produced a pattern in which each hospital's rate for any given DRG is based roughly 50 percent on a uniform standard and roughly 50 percent on the hospital's own historical cost experience.

Losses in hospital revenues resulting from the DRG payment system could be offset if physicians increased hospital admissions to generate additional income and still conformed to acceptable standards of medical practice. If physicians generally acted to raise hospital admissions, the net effect of a DRG program would be to worsen hospital cost inflation (Wennberg, McPherson, and Caper 1984, 295). Thus, in order to successfully contain costs, hospital admission rates will need to be carefully monitored.

THE CURRENT METHOD OF PAYING PHYSICIANS

With few exceptions, Medicare uses the customary-prevailing-reasonable (CPR) charge method to determine how much it will pay for each service provided by a physician (Bovbjerg, Held, and Pauly 1982, 134–72). About 6,000 different services are identified, and payment for each is determined by comparing the amount of physician charges with both physician and area-specific ceilings for that service.

On each claim, physicians have the option of accepting or rejecting assignment of the benefit due. Accepting Medicare assignment limits the amount the physician can charge the beneficiary in exchange for a federal guarantee to pay part of the bill (usually 80 percent). Rejecting assignment allows the physician to charge the beneficiary as much as he wants, but Medicare does not guarantee collection of the billed amount.

As mentioned previously, the 1972 Social Security amendments included a provision to limit the growth in community-wide prevailing charges to a rate determined by an economic index that reflects national increases in incomes and physician practice costs. In spite of this index, Medicare's payments for physician services have grown faster than its payments for hospital services (see Table 8.2). The share of Medicare's total spending for personal health care allocated to physician services increased from 21.4 percent in 1975 to 23.1 percent in 1984. Although much smaller than hospital care's 1984 share of 70.4 percent, payments for physician services are substantial.

A major criticism of physician payment under Medicare is that it provides little incentive for physicians to utilize cost-effective treatment methods. First, as a fee-for-service system, it provides an incentive to provide more rather than fewer services. Second, CPR-determined fees for procedures do not decline as the costs of providing those services fall over time due to technological change. Third, the CPR system provides more favorable reimbursement for complex procedures performed by specialists as opposed to less costly primary care services (Juba 1987, 57).

MEDICARE FINANCING

Revenues for the funding of HI come primarily from a portion of the Social Security payroll tax. Employers and employees covered by the program each contribute 1.3 percent of earnings up to a maximum level (in 1984, the first $37,800 of earnings), with the rate scheduled to increase to 1.35 percent in 1985, and 1.45 percent in 1986. Under current law, general revenues cannot be used to make up any shortfall between outlays required to pay benefits and the balance in the trust fund (Ginsburg and Moon 1984, 167).

In contrast, SMI revenues are obtained from premiums and general revenues. The premium amount (in 1985, $15.50 per month) is increased by law every year, with a contribution from general revenues making up the difference between premium income and outlays. In fiscal year 1982, general revenues required to meet this difference totaled about $14 billion, or 77 percent of SMI funding (Ginsburg and Moon 1984, 167–68).

TABLE 8.2
Medicare's Spending for Hospital Care and Physician Services:
Amounts and Rates of Growth, 1975–84

Year	Hospital Care		Physician Services	
	Dollars (billions)	Percent of Total Medicare Spending	Dollars (billions)	Percent of Total Medicare Spending
1975	11.6	74.4	3.3	21.4
1979	21.7	73.8	6.4	21.8
1980	26.0	72.8	7.8	21.8
1981	31.0	72.0	9.7	22.3
1982	36.8	72.0	11.4	23.1
1983	40.5	70.6	13.4	23.3
1984	44.4	70.4	14.6	23.1

Percentage Growth		
Years	Hospital Care	Physician Services
1979–84	104.6	128.1
1975–84	282.8	342.4

Sources: Robert Gibson, "National Health Expenditures, 1979," *Health Care Financing Review* 2, no. 1 (Summer 1980): 29–32; Robert Gibson, Daniel Waldo, and Katherine Levit, "National Health Expenditures, 1982," *Health Care Financing Review* 5, no. 1 (Fall 1983): 13–15; Katherine Levit, Helen Lazenby, Daniel Waldo, and Lawrence Davidoff, "National Health Expenditures, 1984," *Health Care Financing Review* 7, no. 1 (Fall 1985): 28–29.

The Medicare program has begun to encounter serious funding problems. Under current policies, the HI trust fund will be entirely depleted around 1989 or 1990, while required contributions from general revenues to support physician benefits will continue to grow at a much more rapid rate than the growth in general revenues. The basic problem is that spending on medical care is growing much more rapidly than national income, with demographic trends, such as the aging of the population, explaining only a small part of the difference. Moreover, because of the 1985 federal budget deficit of more than $200 billion, the amount of additional financial resources that might be allocated to Medicare is severely limited.

Under the DRG program in which payments per admission are increased by only one percentage point more than the rate of increase of hospital input prices, the projected depletion date would be three years later (1992). The projected deficits would still grow larger each year, even with this restricted growth in outlays. By 1995 the annual deficit would be about $30 billion and the negative balance over $90 billion.

From 1985 to 1995, Medicare outlays are projected to grow at a 12.4 percent annual rate, while revenues are projected to increase at a 7.9 percent rate. This increase reflects the influences of general inflation, growth in the eligible population and its aging, and changes in the nature of hospital care. General inflation accounts for a significant portion of the increase in hospital costs, but does not itself contribute to the financing problem since it is also reflected in revenue growth.

Changes in the age composition of the population are projected to account for 2.2 percentage points of the growth in HI outlays. Of this, 1.9 percentage points reflect growth in the number of enrollees, while 0.25 percentage points are caused by the expected aging of the elderly population. Real outlays per enrollee have increased approximately 4 percent per year since 1985. This figure reflects a higher admission rate for each Medicare recipient and additional expense per hospital stay.

SMI FINANCING

Between 1975 and 1984, total SMI benefits rose 231 percent. About one-tenth of this growth was caused by expansion in the enrolled population, and the remainder by a combination of increases in prices and utilization of services.

Although it is difficult to separate increases in the price from increases in quantity, changes in the latter account for almost half of total per capita growth in SMI outlays. For example, total per capita physicians visits—which represent over 72 percent of SMI benefits—grew 342 percent from 1975 to 1984 (Levit et al. 1985, 28–29).

Concerns raised by the rapid growth expected in SMI are closely related to the size of the federal budget deficit since, by law, appropriations from general revenues to SMI must be sufficient to guarantee solvency of the trust fund. Outlays for SMI are projected to increase rapidly, by almost 16 percent per year through 1988. To finance this increase, general revenue contributions must rise even faster, averaging about 17 percent per year. Thus, the proportion of general revenues required to finance the SMI trust fund is expected to rise from 3.7 percent to 5.7 percent between 1982 and 1988. If the share of general revenues contributed to the SMI trust fund were not permitted to increase, expenditures would have to be reduced or premiums increased by almost $27 billion from 1984 to 1988, which represents about 19 percent of all SMI expenditures for that period (Levit et al. 1985, 170–71).

If both revenues and SMI outlays were to continue growing at the same annual rates now projected through 1988, SMI would require a transfer of more than 11 percent of general revenues now allocated to other purposes in 1995. Alternatively, even if SMI outlays only rose at an annual rate of 12 percent and general revenues rose by 8 percent annually, the share of such revenues necessary to fund SMI would still rise to more than 7 percent in 1995.

MEDICAID

Medicaid is a combined federal and state program that provides medical assistance to certain categories of low-income persons, including those on welfare and some of the medically indigent (persons whose incomes are too low to pay for medical care). The program is administered and roughly half the costs are absorbed by the state and local governments.

Medicaid, like Medicare, has based reimbursement of providers on market prices or costs, paying hospitals according to the Medicare cost-based standard. However, they were permitted to pay physicians at rates below Medicare reimbursement levels. Mandatory covered services (which could not be subject to patient copayment or deductible) included hospital care, physicians' services, diagnostic services, family planning advice, and nursing home care in skilled nursing facilities. Screening and treatment of children were subsequently added to the mandatory coverage category. Optional coverage items included services in intermediate care facilities, dental care, drugs, eyeglasses, and some other medical services. Cost sharing was eventually permitted for some of these optional services and for hospital and physicians' services provided to the medically indigent (Stevens and Stevens 1974, 156–60; 282–99).

Mandatory eligibility is now required for persons receiving cash assistance under federally funded income transfer programs. Therefore, persons eligible for income transfers under Aid to Families with Dependent Children (AFDC) are automatically eligible for Medicaid. States have considerable flexibility in establishing income levels or other conditions for AFDC eligibility, and are indirectly able to control the number of persons who qualify for Medicaid assistance. While AFDC is limited in a majority of states to families without a father residing in the home, 24 states and two jurisdictions also extend AFDC and Medicaid coverage to families with unemployed fathers who are not receiving unemployment compensation. Seventeen states and three jurisdictions cover all children in families with income below AFDC eligibility level, regardless of the family composition or the employment status of the parents. Persons who are mandatory recipients of Supplemental Security Income (SSI), a federal program for the aged, blind, or disabled, are also automatically eligible for Medicaid, although the income limits for SSI are established by the federal government.

Optional Medicaid beneficiaries are those for whom states may receive federal matching funds but whose coverage is not required by federal legislation. This group includes medically needy families with dependent children whose incomes are above the state AFDC limit, as well as elderly persons who do not qualify for cash assistance. Many of the latter have large medical or nursing home bills.

The 30 states offering Medicaid coverage for the medically needy establish income, asset, and family-composition tests similar to those for public assistance recipients. Medically needy income levels for a family of four as of March 1983 ranged from $9,600 in California to $2,460 in Tennessee (Muse 1983, 39). Under the so-called spend-down provision, families with incomes above these levels may also be eligible if their incomes are below this amount after deducting medical expenses incurred.

In 1984, an estimated 21.5 million people received services covered by Medicaid. This was the same number who received services in 1979. However, between 1979 and 1984 the number of people living in poverty rose from 25 million to nearly 35 million. Thus, as a result of the complex set of eligibility requirements, only 55 to 60 percent of the poverty population was covered by Medicaid in 1984 (Health Care Financing Administration 1983).

Medicaid Costs

The cost of the Medicaid program has increased rapidly. Combined federal and state-local expenditures increased from $3.5 billion in 1968 to $38.7 billion in 1984 (see Table 8.3). Three factors explain almost all the increases in expenditures: (1) the increase in the number of Medicaid recipients covered under the AFDC program; (2) sustained medical care price inflation; and (3) the high cost of skilled nursing facilities and intermediate care facilities for the aged, poor, and disabled. Expenditures for these two items more than doubled between 1973 and 1984.

The rapid growth in the number receiving welfare payments in the late 1960s and early 1970s accounted for a large portion of the increased cost of Medicaid. Since the economy was relatively prosperous at that time, most of the increase was due to the increased number of eligible people applying for benefits (Palmer 1976, 43). Estimates indicate that the percentage of eligible people participating in AFDC increased from 60 percent to more than 90 percent.

TABLE 8.3
Number of Recipients, Total Payments, and Payments per Recipient
under Medicaid: Fiscal Years 1968–84

Fiscal Year	Number of Recipients (millions)	Total Federal and State Payments (billions)	Payments per Recipient	Medical Care Price Index 1968 = 100	Payments per Recipient in 1968 $
1968	11.5	$ 3.5	$ 300	100.0	$300
1969	12.1	4.4	361	106.9	338
1970	14.5	4.1	354	113.7	311
1971	18.0	6.4	356	121.0	297
1972	18.0	7.4	411	124.9	329
1973	19.6	8.6	440	129.8	339
1974	21.1	10.0	474	141.8	334
1975	22.2	12.3	554	158.9	348
1976	22.9	14.1	615	173.9	354
1977	22.9	16.3	710	192.9	368
1978	22.2	18.0	810	207.8	390
1979	21.5	20.5	953	228.0	418
1980	21.6	25.7	1,190	252.9	471
1981	22.1	30.4	1,376	280.2	491
1982	21.8	32.9	1,509	312.7	483
1983	21.5	35.6	1,656	342.0	484
1984	21.5	38.7	1,800	363.2	496

Sources: U.S. Department of Health, Education, and Welfare, Health Care Financing Administration, *Data on the Medicaid Program: Eligibility, Services, Expenditures, Fiscal Years 1966–1977* (Washington, DC: Institute for Medical Management, 1977), p. 34; Donald Muse and Darwin Sawyer, *The Medicare and Medicaid Data Book, 1981* (Washington, DC: U.S. Department of Health and Human Services, 1982), pp. 13, 20; Robert Gibson, Katherine Levit, Helen Lazenby, and Daniel Waldo, "National Health Expenditures, 1983," *Health Care Financing Review* 6, no. 2 (Winter 1984): 20–21; U.S. Bureau of the Census, *Statistical Abstract of the United States*, 1986, 106th Edition (Washington, DC: U.S. Government Printing Office, 1985), p. 100.

The second major factor is the sustained inflation in medical care prices. From 1975 to 1983 medical care prices rose an average of 10 percent annually, with the prices of hospital services rising slightly faster. These higher prices were reflected in increasing Medicaid expenditures.

Annual Medicaid payments per recipient in constant 1968 "medical dollars" (expenditures divided by the medical care price index) averaged $496 in 1984, as compared to $338 in 1969 (see Table 8.3). From 1969 to 1977, there was little growth in real per capita expenditures. However, since 1977, payments per recipient have risen rapidly, reflecting greater utilization.

The final source of expenditure increases under Medicaid is the high cost of institutionalization for elderly, poor, and disabled people who are unable to carry out normal daily activities without nursing assistance. The aged are the only sizable group for which there has been any substantial increase in expenditures in recent years. More than two-thirds of Medicaid expenditures are for services to aged or disabled adults (Health Care Financing Administration 1983).

Medicaid Recipients

The largest group of Medicaid recipients consists of dependent children under the age of 21. However, this is the group that is least costly (per recipient) to serve (see Table 8.4). Dependent children and the adults in their families constitute 69 percent of Medicaid recipients, but are responsible for only about 26 percent of Medicaid expenditures. The largest share of Medicaid payments—37 percent—is for services to the elderly, reflecting the cost of long-term nursing home services as well as the greater need for medical services within this age group. The disabled category, which includes terminally ill persons under age 65, the mentally retarded, and poor individuals with work-related disabilities, includes less than 14 percent of recipients, but accounts for about 35 percent of Medicaid payments.

Most of the recent increases in Medicaid payments have gone to the aged and disabled. From 1980 to 1983, 46 percent of the total growth in Medicaid payments was for disabled persons, and 36 percent was for other persons over age 65. Adults in families with dependent children represent the only category of persons eligible for Medicaid in which the number of recipients has been rising. A significant source of growth in Medicaid payments for the disabled is the recent trend toward deinstitutionalization of the mentally retarded. The rate of growth in mentally retarded Medicaid recipients using intermediate care facilities (ICFs) has been greater than that for any other service. When the mentally retarded leave state institutions, they may become eligible for Medicaid benefits in ICFs or the community. The resulting increase in Medicaid expenditures comes from shifting costs away from state-funded institutions to the federal-state Medicaid program. In addition, this change frequently results in an upgrading from the largely custodial care of state institutions to the more rehabilitative care in Medicaid-funded ICFs (Granneman and Pauly 1982, 11).

Although there has been appreciable aging of the nation's population, it has not affected the growth of Medicaid costs. In fact, the number of recipients over age 65 actually declined from 1980 to 1983.

TABLE 8.4
Medicaid Recipients and Payments by Eligibility Category:
Fiscal Year 1983

Basis of Eligibility	Recipients		Payments*		Average Payment per Recipient (dollars)
	Number (thousands)	Percentage of Total	Dollars (millions)	Percentage of Total	
Age 65 or over	3,247	15.1	11,954	37.0	3,682
Blindness	76	0.4	183	0.6	2,408
Permanent and total disability	2,956	13.8	11,183	34.6	3,783
Dependent children under age 21	9,418	43.8	3,822	11.8	406
Adults in families with dependent children	5,467	25.4	4,483	13.9	820
Other	1,325	6.2	725	2.2	547
Total	21,494†	100.0†	32,351‡	100.0	1,505

Source: Unpublished tabulations provided by the Health Care Financing Administration.

*Payments are Medicaid vendor payments made to providers of service for care rendered to eligible individuals. Amounts include both state and federal share.

†Categories do not add up to total because of a small number of recipients who are in more than one category during the year.

‡Detail does not add up to total because of rounding.

Effect on Medical Services Use and Health

A number of studies have clearly demonstrated that the Medicaid program improved the medical and dental care utilization of program participants (Davis and Reynolds 1976, 404; Olendzki, Grann, and Goodrich 1972, 204; Leverett and Jong 1970, 139). In some cases, Medicaid beneficiaries used services about as frequently as middle- and upper-income people. A smaller fraction of those visits by Medicaid patients (as compared to the nonpoor), however, are to physicians in private offices, and relatively more occur in hospital outpatient departments. Considering the poor population alone, visit rates tend to be higher for those receiving Medicaid, but Medicaid recipients tend to be sicker than the poor as a whole. Davis and Reynolds suggest that the poor receiving public assistance (Medicaid-eligible) use physicians' services slightly more frequently than other persons, and at a much higher rate than the non-Medicaid-eligible poor (Davis and Reynolds 1976). Moreover, there are considerable interstate differences in Medicaid requirements, benefits, and usage.

Direct evidence of Medicaid's effect on the health of recipients is limited and conflicting. Friedman, Parker, and Lipworth found no effect of either Medicaid or private insurance on the rate of early diagnosis of breast cancer (Friedman, Parker, and Lipworth 1973, 485–90). Kehrer and Wolin found no significant effect of Medicaid eligibility on birth weight of infants born to participants in the Gary income-maintenance experiments (Kehrer and Wolin 1979, 434–62). Grossman and Jacobowitz provide evidence that Medicaid coverage of first pregnancies accounts for about 7 percent of the reduction in neonatal mortality rates for nonwhites between 1964 and 1977, but their evidence suggests that such coverage is associated with higher neonatal mortality rates for whites (Grossman and Jacobowitz 1981, 708; 710).

Thus, there are few improvements in health statistics that can be clearly attributed to Medicaid, but the program probably has had positive effects even if they are difficult to measure. One must realize that it is always difficult to separate the effects of improved medical care on health from that of general socioeconomic improvement.

For Medicaid recipients, health status has been found to be the strongest predictor of physician visit utilization and expenditures (Buczko 1986, 25). The importance of health status as a predictor suggests that expansion of the medically needy population, whose members tend to be in poor health, will increase Medicaid expenditures per enrollee for physician services.

Medicaid Expenditures

Medicaid expenditures are largely concentrated in a few northern industrial states. In 1983, New York spent 19.4 percent of all Medicaid funds, and California, with the second largest program, spent 11 percent. These two states, together with Michigan, Illinois, and Pennsylvania, accounted for 44 percent of total Medicaid expenditures (Health Care Financing Administration 1983). The state distribution of Medicaid funds does not correspond to the prevalence of poverty or sickness. The south, with approximately 45 percent of the nation's poor, receives 22 percent of all combined federal-state Medicaid funds (Health Care Financing Administration 1983).

Differences among states arise because some states cover a greater fraction of their poor population and because some have more comprehensive benefits for eligible Medicaid recipients. Average payments per Medicaid recipient in fiscal 1983 ranged from $1,030 in Mississippi to $2,632 in Nevada. The national figure was $1,505. The aged in Alabama receive services costing Medicaid an average of $1,612 per person, but in Pennsylvania the cost is $5,065 per person (Health Care Financing Administration 1983).

The fiscal 1983 medical benefits per family eligible for AFDC averaged $742 in South Carolina and $1,698 in New York, although the national average was $1,048 (Health Care Financing Administration 1983). These differences would be of less importance if they actually reflected differences in medical care prices or statewide differences in morbidity, but benefit patterns are unrelated to health care needs or the costs of health and medical care. For example, the average payment for physicians' services in fiscal 1983 was $491 in Alaska and $56 in Pennsylvania. In Oregon, 13 percent of the state's Medicaid recipients were hospitalized; in Texas and Tennessee, the figures were 25 and 27 percent, respectively. Iowa, Louisiana, and Maryland place few of their elderly in skilled nursing homes, but over half of the elderly Medicaid patients in Connecticut are in nursing homes. Average payments for skilled nursing facilities are $3,535 in Tennessee, but $11,545 in Connecticut. The national average is $8,051 (Health Care Financing Administration 1983).

Medicaid data show large differences in payments by race. The average payment on behalf of whites is about double the average payment for nonwhites (Muse and Sawyer 1982, 19; 25), and racial differences in average payment levels under Medicaid appear to be widening. Sizable differences also exist between Medicaid benefits in urban and rural areas. Anderson et al. found that average Medicaid expenditures (and other minor sources of free care) were $76 per poor child in central cities, and $5 per poor child in rural areas. Benefits for the elderly poor in central cities are twice as large as for those living in rural areas (Andersen et al. 1973, 52).

Provider Reimbursement

From the late 1970s through the 1980s, states have tried unsuccessfully to contain costs of the Medicaid program through the use of more stringent eligibility requirements, imposition of service cutbacks and limitations, tighter administrative controls, and postponement of increases in physician reimbursement.

Under the Omnibus Budget Reconciliation Act of 1981, federal Medicaid grants to states were reduced by 3 percent in 1982, 4 percent in 1983, and 4.5 percent in 1984; and Medicaid's rules for eligibility, benefits, and payment were altered. As a result, 750,000 beneficiaries became ineligible for Medicaid services with an estimated Medicaid savings of $2.9 billion from 1982 to 1985 (Iglehart 1983, 868–69). The act also modified the long-standing freedom-of-choice policy that gave individual Medicaid recipients the freedom to obtain services from any qualified provider. States may now enter into arrangements to purchase laboratory services or medical devices through competitive bids, or restrict beneficiary's choice to low-cost providers.

Spending for nursing home services is the largest and most rapidly growing component of national Medicaid outlays. Most state Medicaid programs have now adopted various forms of prospective reimbursement in which rates and rate increases are negotiated or determined by formulas prior to each new fiscal year. There are only ten states that use traditional retrospective methods for Medicaid reimbursement of nursing homes (Muse 1983, 123).

With respect to hospital reimbursement, by 1983 only 26 states (accounting for 23 percent of inpatient expenditures) still used cost-based reimbursement methods for Medicaid patients. Some states, such as New Jersey and Georgia, are using experimental systems of prospective reimbursement based on diagnostic-related groupings. Most of the other states have used facility-specific budget review, rate of increase control, and other forms of prospective rate setting (Muse 1983, 137).

Because state Medicaid authorities have not had to accept customary fees since 1981, the average Medicaid reimbursement for a visit to a physician has fallen to approximately 60 percent of the average charge for non-Medicaid patients. As a result, many physicians refuse to accept Medicaid patients or greatly limit their Medicaid patient load, and their willingness to accept such patients is related to the level of Medicaid payments (Sloan, Mitchell, and Cromwell 1978, 211–45). On the other hand, even though they are paid considerably less than the market price, many physicians still provide services to Medicaid patients. If Medicaid expenditures are cut by further reducing physicians' fees, however, the poor will no longer have ready access to physicians.

Attempting to save money by limiting payment to physicians for their services is an inefficient way to reduce program costs. Payments to physicians for their services constitute less than 10 percent of total Medicaid outlays. However, many other services are used in conjunction with physician care, and the doctor controls the use of those services to a considerable degree.

With the passage of the 1972 amendments to the Social Security Act, there began a gradual but consistent trend toward paying less than actual cost to hospitals with above-average costs; these reimbursement limits may have encouraged the transfer of costs for caring for public patients to states and to private insurance companies.

If the amount Medicaid will pay to hospitals is further reduced through a prospective payment system, several responses can be expected. First, access by Medicaid patients is likely to be reduced, with some hospitals, when legally permissible, refusing to accept public patients. Second, a reduction in quality or intensity of care may occur. If hospitals are required to provide service when revenue is less than cost, they must make up the deficit. If they consume working capital, they will eventually be forced to shut down. Charging other patients higher prices for care is inequitable and may not be feasible in an increasingly competitive environment.

Nearly 60 percent of all Medicaid patients treated in private physician practices receive services from doctors whose patient volume is composed of at least 30 percent Medicaid patients (Council of Economic Advisors 1986, 155). Despite irresponsible accusations that these physicians are operating "Medicaid mills," visit length in large Medicaid practices is similar to that of non-Medicaid physicians, and prescribed ancillary services do not appear to be excessive. Medicaid doctors generally earn less than other private physicians, although they are more likely to be older, non-Board certified, and graduates of foreign medical schools.

Medicaid Reform

Proposals for Medicaid reform can be classified into three broad categories: alteration of eligibility criteria and coverage of the poor; reduction in Medicaid benefits; and a changed federal role.

The optimal federal role is vigorously debated. For example, a shift in federal policy might involve eliminating matching federal grants and substituting block grants to the states. Those who advocate block grants maintain that they give the states greater flexibility in deciding how to use Medicaid funds, but they might also encourage Medicaid recipients to migrate from states with meager benefits to states with high benefit levels.

Another policy alternative is to tie the federal contribution to a program of basic Medicaid benefits considered essential in all states, and states desiring to supplement basic benefit levels would be required to do so with their own funds (Council of Economic Advisors 1986, 156). A third option is to steadily reduce the federal contribution to Medicaid by a fixed percentage, as was done in the Omnibus Budget Reconciliation Act of 1981.

Another attempt to limit Medicaid hospital expenditures is to contract with selected hospitals on a competitive bid basis, as California is currently doing. Arizona is requiring nearly all recipients to choose between prepaid organizations that are reimbursed on a capitation basis; all care must be provided or authorized by the health care organization, which is also at financial risk for the provision of health services.

The Medicaid program has also begun to enroll participants in health maintenance organizations (HMOs). Enrollment of Medicaid recipients in HMOs rose from 349,000 in June, 1984, to 561,000 in December, 1985 (Waldo, Levit, and Lazenby 1986, 9). There are some indications that Medicaid enrollees are dissatisfied with HMOs. Disenrollment rates for this group are high, perhaps due to frustration in dealing with a health care institution that is oriented toward limiting utilization of health services.

SUMMARY

The Medicare program finances a large share of the health care costs of older people, the disabled, and those with end-stage renal disease. Medicare costs have risen extremely rapidly since the inception of the program in 1965.

The Medicare program makes extensive use of coinsurance and deductibles. While these are intended to deter unnecessary utilization, a majority of the elderly purchase supplementary insurance which negates the cost-sharing provisions of Medicare.

Medicare has gradually increased its cost-containment policies. Since 1981, there has been an increase in cost sharing and the imposition of a prospective payment system for hospitals based on DRGs. The DRG system will likely result in shorter stays for most hospitalized elderly patients with some decrease in provided services. Moreover, services such as health promotion, which traditionally have been cross-subsidized, are likely to be cut back or eliminated.

The Medicare program faces major financing problems in the near future. Without major increases in revenues or decreases in expenditures, the hospital insurance (HI) trust fund will be completely depleted by 1990. Moreover, the proportion of general revenues needed to finance supplementary medical insurance (SMI) will have to increase rapidly to avoid fast-rising premiums. While a number of policy options exist, given the current political climate in the United States, it is likely that the elderly will be called upon to finance an increasing share of Medicare costs.

Medicaid is a combined federal-state program which provides medical assistance to about two-thirds of all low-income persons. Because of state differences in eligibility criteria and access to providers, Medicaid benefits are concentrated in a small number of northern industrial states. California, which used to have a generous Medicaid program, has become increasingly restrictive.

The rapid increase in Medicaid costs, which reflects both medical care price inflation and higher utilization, has caused both state and federal government to impose budget cutbacks and a variety of cost-containment measures. In many states, hospitals and nursing homes are no longer reimbursed on a retrospective cost basis, but on the basis of prospective costs. Reimbursement rates for physicians are being scaled back in relative terms and many states are restricting the beneficiary's freedom of choice of provider in order to encourage patients to utilize certain low-cost providers. This may reduce the willingness of some physicians to accept Medicaid patients.

Several proposals to reform Medicaid were discussed. Block grants are advocated by those who desire more flexibility for state programs, but differences in state benefit levels could encourage interstate migration. State contracts with selected hospitals on a competitive bid basis may help to slow the growth in Medicaid expenditures.

NOTES

1. Public Law 92-603, section 223, excludes from the definition of reasonable cost "any part of incurred cost found to be unnecessary in the efficient delivery of needed health services." The open-endedness of this provision has led some to suggest it as a possible means of sharply reducing payments to hospitals without the need for further legislation.
2. See "Medicare Quick Release Criticized," *Baltimore Evening Sun*, 26 February, 1985, A–9.

REFERENCES

Andersen, Ronald; Kravits, Joanna; Anderson, Odin; and Daley, Joan (1973). *Expenditures for Personal Health Services: National Trends & Variations.* U.S. Department of Health, Education, and Welfare Publication No. (HRA) 74-3105. Washington, DC: U.S. Government Printing Office.

Bovbjerg, R.; Held, P. J.; and Pauly, M. V. (1982). "Procompetitive Health Insurance Proposals and Their Implications for Medicare's End-Stage Renal Disease Program." *Seminars in Nephrology* 2: 134–72.

Buczko, William (1986). "Physician Utilization and Expenditures in a Medicaid Population." *Health Care Financing Review* 8 (Winter): 17–25.

Burwell, Brian; Clauser, Steve; Hall, Margaret Jean; and Simon, James (1987). "Medicaid Recipients in Intermediate Care Facilities for the Mentally Retarded." *Health Care Financing Review* 8 (Spring): 1–12.

Council of Economic Advisors (1986). *Economic Report of the President, 1985.* Washington, DC: U.S. Government Printing Office.

Davis, Karen, and Reynolds, Roger (1976). "The Impact of Medicare and Medicaid on Access to Medical Care." In *The Role of Health Insurance in the Health Services Sector,* ed. Richard Rossett, 391–425. New York: Neale Watson Academic Publications.

Dobson, Allen; Langenbrunner, John; Pelovitz, Steven; and Willis, Judith (1986). "The Future of Medicare Policy Reform: Priorities for Research and Demonstrations." *Health Care Financing Review* 7 (Annual Supplement): 1–7.

Friedman, Bernard; Parker, Paul; and Lipworth, Leslie (1973). "The Influence of Medicaid and Private Health Insurance on the Early Diagnosis of Breast Cancer." *Medical Care* 11 (November–December): 485–90.

Ginsburg, Paul, and Moon, Marilyn (1984). "An Introduction to the Medicare Financing Problem." *Milbank Memorial Fund Quarterly* 62: 167–82.

Granneman, Thomas, and Pauly, Mark (1982). *Controlling Medicaid Costs.* Washington, DC: American Enterprise Institute for Public Policy Research.

Grossman, Michael, and Jacobowitz, Stephen (1981). "Variations in Infant Mortality Rates among Counties of the United States: The Roles of Public Policies and Programs." *Demography* 18 (November): 695–713.

Health Care Financing Administration (1983). "Medicaid Recipients by Maintenance Assistance Status and by HHS Region and State: Fiscal Year 1983." Unpublished tabulation.

Hsiao, William, and Kelly, Nancy (1984). "Medicare Benefits: A Reassessment." *Milbank Memorial Fund Quarterly* 62: 207–29.

Iglehart, John (1983). "Medicaid in Transition." *New England Journal of Medicine* 309 (October 6): 868–69.

Juba, David (1987). "Medicare Physician Fee Schedules: Issues and Evidence from South Carolina." *Health Care Financing Review* 8 (Spring): 57–67.

Kehrer, Barbara, and Wolin, Charles (1979). "Impact of Income Maintenance on Low Birth Weight: Evidence from the Gary Experiment." *Journal of Human Resources* 14 (Fall): 434–62.

Leverett, Dennis, and Jong, Anthony (1970). "Variations in Use of Dental Care Facilities by Low-Income White and Black Urban Populations." *Journal of the American Dental Association* 80 (January): 137–40.

Lave, Judith (1984). "Hospital Reimbursement under Medicare." *Milbank Memorial Fund Quarterly* 62: 251–68.

Levit, Katharine; Lazenby, Helen; Waldo, Daniel; and Davidoff, Lawrence (1985). "National Health Expenditures, 1984." *Health Care Financing Review* 7 (Fall): 1–35.

Long, Stephen; Settle, Russell; and Link, Charles (1982). "Who Bears the Burden of Medicare Cost Sharing?" *Inquiry* 19 (Fall): 222–34.

Muse, Donald (1983). "Analysis of State Medicaid Program Characteristics." Washington, DC: La Jolla Management Corporation. Mimeographed.

Muse, Donald, and Sawyer, Darwin (1982). *The Medicare and Medicaid Data Book, 1981.* Washington, DC: U.S. Department of Health and Human Services.

Olendzki, Margaret; Grann, Richard; and Goodrich, Charles (1972). "The Impact of Medicaid on Private Care for the Urban Poor." *Medical Care* 10 (May–June): 201–6.

Palmer, John (1976). "Government Growth in Perspective." *Challenge* 19 (May–June): 43–48.

Schwartz, W. (1983). "The Competitive Strategy: Will It Affect the Quality of Care?" In *Market Reform in Health Care,* ed. J. A. Meyer, 15–21. Washington, DC: American Enterprise Institute.

Sloan, Frank; Mitchell, Janet; and Cromwell, Jerry (1978). "Physician Participation in State Medicaid Programs." *Journal of Human Resources* 13 (Supplement): 211–45.

Stevens, Robert, and Stevens, Rosemary (1974). *Welfare Medicine in America: A Case Study of Medicaid.* New York: The Free Press.

Svahn, J. (1981). "Omnibus Reconciliation Act of 1981: Legislative History and Summary of OASDI and Medicare Provisions." *Social Security Bulletin* 44 (October): 3–24.

U.S. Senate Special Committee on Aging (1983). *Prospects for Medicare's Hospital Insurance Trust Fund.* Washington, DC: U.S. Government Printing Office.

Vladeck, Bruce (1984). "Comment on Hospital Reimbursement under Medicare." *Milbank Memorial Fund Quarterly* 62: 269–78.

Waldo, David; Levit, Katherine; and Lazenby, Helen (1986). "National Health Expenditures, 1985." *Health Care Financing Review* 8 (Fall): 1–21.

Wennberg, John; McPherson, Klim; and Caper, Philip (1984). "Will Payment on Diagnostic-Related Groups Control Hospital Costs?" *New England Journal of Medicine* 311 (August 2): 295–300.

Chapter 9

The Evolution of For-Profit Medical Institutions and Cost Containment

Thomas F. Frist, Sr., and Samuel H. Howard

Editor's Note—The traditional not-for-profit hospitals and clinics have evolved from religious and philanthropic institutions, and generally did not have the business orientation and techniques required for modern medical care delivery. Investor-owned (for-profit) hospitals have thus been pioneers in the use of business practices and systems models that are now standard for the entire medical care industry—for-profit and not-for-profit institutions alike. Frist and Howard assert that not-for-profit hospitals would not be able to survive in this era of medical cost containment if they did not adopt the strategies of investor-owned institutions: management practices directed by business discipline; multihospital systems that facilitate operating efficiencies; the development of health care executives who have had graduate training in the special knowledge and skills of hospital management; and integrating of medical insurance with medical care delivery to allow experimentation with new models of managed medical care delivery networks.

In this unique description of how the investor-owned hospital business views itself, the authors point out that the techniques of modern hospital management are in their infancy. Not only do not-for-profit hospitals owe much to these pioneering efforts, the authors believe that further development and refinement of techniques used by for-profit hospitals should yield greater efficiencies in the future as medical providers learn how best to respond to a demand-driven market.

Investor-owned hospitals have made valuable contributions to the health care industry's attempts to achieve new system and efficiency goals under prospective payment and other cost-containment strategies. First, investor-owned hospitals brought a new business discipline to health care, providing management expertise needed to achieve the industry's new cost-containment goals. Second, investor-owned hospitals pioneered the use of the multihospital system model to achieve important financing and operating benefits. Third, investor-owned hospitals created a new breed of health care executive with the tools and analytic abilities needed to transform a loosely coordinated cluster of social welfare providers into more efficiently run businesses.

Fourth, we believe important cost and operating efficiencies achieved by investor-owned hospitals demonstrated to government that the industry no longer needed protection under cost-based reimbursement, which was producing unacceptable escalations in health care costs. This demonstration may have encouraged the introduction of prospective payment and the creation of a competitive, market-driven industry. Fifth, by combining the insuring and delivery sides of the business, investor-owned hospitals created opportunities for experimenting with new forms of health care delivery, including alternative delivery systems and managed delivery networks.

Ultimately, investor-owned hospitals demonstrated that health care, a social service industry traditionally financed by philanthropy and government, could be run as a business, and that business discipline would improve access to services and needed capital while ensuring high levels of patient care quality.

DELIVERING HEALTH CARE: THE EVOLUTION FROM SOCIAL WELFARE PROVIDERS TO BUSINESSES

The management practices and organizational forms which dominated nonprofit hospitals since the turn of the century simply could not meet the financial demands imposed by prospective payment and other cost-containment initiatives introduced during the early 1980s. Previous corporate structures were not suited to the expansion and diversification required if hospitals were to survive in a newly evolving competitive, market-driven environment. Nor could they provide access to the kinds of capital needed to finance expansion and diversification on such large scales, since investors could not justify their investments given the financial risks associated with prospective payment.

Nonprofit hospitals had long been suspected of suffering from "managerial slack." In fact, several studies in the mid- to late 1970s were documenting the fact that the investor-owned hospitals were more efficient than their nonprofit counterparts. Knowles (1979), for example, found that although investor-owned hospitals had lower expenses and fewer patients than voluntary hospitals, they offered only slightly fewer services. Clarkson (1972) suggested that nonprofit managers were avoiding unpleasant but efficiency-relevant tasks, and that they had access to information that was easy to obtain but more crudely calibrated to performance than the information used by investor-owned hospital managers.

Business Discipline

One basic premise for the investor-owned hospitals that were emerging in the late 1960s was that business methods and management practices from other industries could be used to make hospitals efficient and profitable operations at a time when efficiency was not a major concern, and before profits were a measured part of the hospital's balance sheet.

Investor-owned hospitals began by adopting new accounting and forecasting methods. They introduced cost-efficiency, productivity, and utilization systems to quantify and measure these items. They imported new financial systems to better manage their assets. Cost containment, as a strategy for achieving a better return on assets, was already a primary goal for investor-owned hospitals before the prospective pricing concept was introduced.

Labor productivity is extremely important to the profitable operation of a hospital, and crucial under prospective payment, since labor accounts for the largest portion of hospital costs. By introducing new operating measures, improved resource allocation and utilization systems, and eventually, the concept of product line management, investor-owned hospitals began achieving early reductions in ratios of full-time employees (FTEs) to patients, averaging approximately 2.0 to 2.5 FTEs per patient, compared to an average of over 3.0 FTEs in nonprofit hospitals. Efficiency achievements were also realized in labor costs as a percentage of total operating costs, where these costs typically were 60 to 70 percent of the total for nonprofit hospitals, and 50 to 55 percent for investor-owned hospitals. These and other labor-related savings were achieved primarily through the use of industrial engineering techniques that correlate labor force to number of patients (Anderson 1976).

These new management practices were already producing important cost savings. While in 1978, for example, per diem charges at investor-owned hospitals were somewhat higher, the average total bill charged for patient stay per procedure was lower, because procedures tended to be performed more efficiently, and patients released more quickly (American Hospital Association 1979). Additionally, studies noted that, despite lower occupancy rates, investor-owned hospitals were generating lower costs because of uniform shorter average lengths-of-stay and fewer cost-generating resources (i.e., capital assets and personnel) (Vignola 1978, 24). Without access to these systems and procedures, and without the cost-containment incentives under which investor-owned hospitals were already operating, nonprofit hospitals were, on average, showing significantly greater value in assets per bed, had more personnel per patient, and tended to be more capital intensive than their investor-owned counterparts.

Multihospital System Management

Investor-owned hospitals also pioneered the use of multihospital system management models, and demonstrated that system benefits, including standardized management applications, common accounting systems, distributed data processing capabilities, joint purchasing arrangements, and other mechanisms that achieved economies of scale and reduced redundancies, would be the hospitals' best line of defense in the new market-driven environment.

By the early 1970s, investor-owned hospitals were experimenting with national purchasing contracts; standardized employment procedures and staffing controls; budgetary control and financial planning systems; common accounting and patient management systems; regional specialization; sophisticated market research and planning techniques; and advanced management tools from other industries. They also were recruiting managers more attuned to bottom line performance and quality services through the use of incentives.

By the late 1970s, investor-owned hospitals were creating integrated information systems to produce accurate and relevant cost-accounting data that would be extremely useful when prospective payment was introduced. A large percentage of a hospital's expenditures are related to information processing, and much of this tends to represent redundant handling. The efficiencies gained from the use of integrated information systems at the department and system levels has proven to be successful in reducing lengths-of-stay and identifying procedures which can be performed less expensively on an outpatient basis.

Another operating efficiency for which investor-owned hospitals saw an early need was in the area of cash management. The Hospital Corporation of America (HCA), for example, realized that it must minimize collection time while maximizing disbursement time, and developed a cash management system through banks which, because of their multifacility capabilities and size, were able to achieve these cash management goals (which became increasingly important as short-term interest rates began rising). HCA used these banks as central collection and disbursement points, and reduced collection time from 2½ days to one day, saving over $4.3 million a year.

So effective are system benefits that nonprofit hospitals quickly followed suit. In the late 1970s, larger nonprofit hospitals began restructuring, and forming multihospital systems. Today, they are creating larger alliances not just to compete with investor-owned systems but also to realize system benefits needed to survive economically under new cost-containment strategies.

New Breed of Health Care Executives

The new multihospital system model and the business discipline brought to health care by investor-owned hospitals required a new breed of health care executive with superior analytic abilities and management skills. During the 1970s, hospitals were quickly becoming complex business operations as the first signs of expansion, diversification, and consolidation emerged. It became apparent that hospitals needed more than "administrators" if they were to survive in a radically reconfigured industry.

By the mid-1970s, only about one-third of all hospital administrators had undergone formal training for their positions. While 70 graduate programs were training future managers, these programs concentrated on the traditional approach to hospital management (i.e., administering rather than changing and controlling the system). The administration model had served well until this time, since hospitals were the organized settings for medical services, and functioned as 24-hour physician support systems. In this medical workshop, the manager's role was to direct the administrative side of organized medical practice. Administrators recruited staff, provided information-gathering services, helped secure funding from government and philanthropic sources, shared the costs of technology, and kept the physical plant running smoothly. Administrators typically followed the lead of physicians in developing service lines, and in this capacity acted primarily in a support role. System control and operating efficiencies were not overriding concerns for administrators (Bentley 1985).

By the mid-1970s, investor-owned hospitals were introducing system control and operating efficiency measures, business practices which permitted effective asset management and proved crucial for surviving under prospective payment. Given the increasing technical sophistication of health services, escalating costs, and increasing demands for accountability and coordination, hospital administrators needed at least moderate sophistication in a number of technical areas, including basic medical vocabularies and procedures, management methods, quantitative indices of hospital functioning, and government regulation. They also needed a working knowledge of social, demographic, and economic trends, and familiarity with projected health needs. It was clear that the characteristics required for successful hospital administration were changing, and that managers with new skills and resources were needed. By 1975, HCA and other investor-owned hospital companies had identified these characteristics and developed standardized selection criteria and assessment mechanisms based on areas of interest, knowledge, personality, and behavioral skills.

With the introduction of cost-containment mechanisms by several states in the late 1970s, prospective payment nationally in 1983, and various cost-containment strategies by business and industry in the following years, administrators were also charged with expanding the hospital's revenue base by taking on functions previously performed by others. They found themselves competing with physicians, other hospitals, and insurance companies, and with the new alternative delivery systems that were being created and tested in almost every hospital's market.

System control and efficiency goals meant that hospital administrators must become chief executive officers in the corporate sense. They needed marketing, financial, and system-building skills, expertise provided more by an MBA than by most traditional graduate hospital administration programs at the time. Investor-owned hospital companies had been recruiting executives from other industries and were building a cadre of executives with analytic abilities and strategic-thinking skills who could, through the new planning and management methods, bring financial, interpersonal, marketing, and organizational expertise to bear on hospital operations.

Nonprofit hospital systems have followed suit, and are moving rapidly from the administrative to the corporate management model. Within all areas of health care there is a growing emphasis on the administrator as health care executive, and on meeting the training and experiential needs of this new breed of manager. It is estimated that, by 1990, 90 percent of all hospital administrators will have master's degrees, while 8 percent will have an MD or a PhD. In an industry driven by cost containment and change, these new executives will be able to direct and adapt their systems as new organizational forms and models emerge in response to growing competition and further evolutionary changes in the marketplace.

Innovative Alternative and Managed Delivery Networks

Investor-owned hospitals have also facilitated the formation of innovative alternative delivery systems and managed delivery networks. This was a crucial development, since it permitted an unprecedented level of experimentation with new forms of health care delivery in which different relationships and organizational models can be market tested. Much of this testing involves new health insurance products based on variations of health maintenance organizations (HMOs), preferred provider organizations (PPOs), and indemnity plans, and uses insurance vehicles to funnel patients into and through a particular system. Investor-owned hospitals encouraged this experimentation through their innovations and willingness to take risks, with the new models being tested primarily by insurance companies that had begun aligning with HMOs and other managed care plans. Investor-owned hospitals also furthered the development of these models by taking the lead in integrating the insurance and delivery functions into a single system. Most nonprofit providers and alliances are now following suit, given the growing demand for these managed delivery models.

The goal of these new managed delivery networks is to control cost and service utilization. Rather than focusing on price discounts, they encompass convenience, quality, common entry points, comprehensive services, range of service and insurance options, simplified administrative procedures, and management systems to control utilization and costs. Hence, management efficiency and patient control rather than deep price discounts are overriding goals. These are the kinds of managed networks that major purchasers (business, government, and insurance companies) are demanding and, in many cases, mandating. From a practical standpoint, they constitute the most effective model for achieving operating efficiencies, prudent use of system resources, and cost-containment goals.

These innovative delivery networks reflect the new form that competition is taking in health care. The issue is no longer who controls the hospital, but who can enter a market with the capability to capture and retain patients through insurance functions (HMOs, PPOs, and other hybrid plans). The most effective and cost-efficient strategy is to link the delivery and financing sides of the business into an integrated managed network with strong insurance products. Managed delivery networks, and their evolving alliances with other networks and providers, address this new form of competition, and enable networks to capture and retain customers within single systems while controlling service delivery, utilization, and costs.

Improving Access to Care and Capital

Investor-owned hospitals have improved access to health care services by their initial focus on acquiring and opening smaller hospitals in rural and suburban markets. Through their organizational and managerial innovations, investor-owned hospitals also opened new investment opportunities not just for themselves, but also for the health care industry as a whole. This became a crucial development for nonprofit hospitals, which were facing a capital-financing crisis of enormous proportions.

Investor-owned hospitals are not distributed randomly throughout the country, but are overrepresented in smaller markets where health care services are needed but often difficult to obtain. HCA's first 15 hospitals, for example, were acquired in such secondary markets as Salem, Virginia; Carthage, Tennessee; Selma, Alabama; and Lubbock, Texas; and not in major urban areas. Additionally, the first hospitals constructed by HCA were in similar second-tier communities.

The extent to which physicians congregate in larger and more profitable urban markets, thus creating shortages in smaller, less profitable rural markets, is well known. But by opening new hospitals in these markets and acquiring and maintaining existing hospitals, investor-owned companies ensured access to quality health services when access was seriously jeopardized.

Investor-owned hospitals were also formed to take advantage of new investment opportunities. Until the late 1960s, hospitals were basically a "tin-cup" industry, relying upon philanthropy and the government for support. But during the 1970s, investor-owned hospitals demonstrated to America's investment communities that health care could be run as an efficient and profitable business, and that investments wisely made in this industry would bring a reasonable return. By demonstrating that hospitals operated with the discipline of a business, that they could compete in the general marketplace for capital, and that they were a safe, profitable, and legitimate investment option, investor-owned hospitals opened new, more efficient and appropriate forms of capital to the entire institutional health care sector.

In 1975, after years of experience with investor-owned hospitals, the business and financial communities felt secure in opening the tax-exempt bond market to nonprofit hospital systems. This provided a new avenue of financing, one that by 1985 represented $28.6 billion. It enabled nonprofit organizations to restructure, enter new lines of business, and evolve from social institutions to business organizations providing a social service. It also laid the groundwork for new and innovative opportunities for capital formation, beyond the traditional avenues open to the hospital industry. These opportunities will become increasingly important as health care providers face new financing needs under new market conditions and, eventually, new tax laws that will force many nonprofit organizations to further restructure and pursue different financing strategies.

This development was important for two reasons. First, if the system was to be truly competitive and market driven, then providers needed access to capital to finance the development of alternative delivery systems, outpatient settings, and other alternatives. Obviously, this market-driven environment could be developed faster and more efficiently through access to venture capital and other markets that are traditionally closed to nonprofit hospitals.

Second, capital financing needs of hospitals were growing at a rapid rate, faster than traditional markets could support. In fact, by the late 1970s, capital financing was becoming one of the most serious issues facing the hospital industry. Studies were suggesting that considerably more than $100 billion would be required by community hospitals to meet their plant and equipment needs during the 1980s. The projection most often cited was between $130 and $193 billion. By comparison, community hospitals were investing approximately $50 billion in their plants and equipment during the 1970s.

THE BUSINESS MODEL AND COST CONTAINMENT

Current cost-containment initiatives in health care are being sought through radically new financing mechanisms. These mechanisms constitute a revolution in health care financing. While previous economic transformations never sought to change historic organization and delivery patterns by challenging the behavior of physicians and hospitals, the new reimbursement strategies introduced by various states in the late 1970s, and by the federal government in 1983, started from a radically different premise. As Fuchs (1986) notes, those who were paying the piper, primarily business and government, decided to start calling the tune. Both private and public sectors embraced large-scale alterations in the reimbursement of hospitals and physicians that would ultimately force health care providers to become efficient and businesslike or leave the industry.

These alterations carried far greater implications than either the introduction of private health insurance after World War II or the creation of Medicare and Medicaid in 1965. While these two innovations greatly increased demand for health care, prospective payment slowed spending by curbing demand. By opening the health care industry to competition, providers would no longer be isolated from the general economy and its market-driven dynamics.

Cost and Operating Efficiencies

At the heart of the new financing mechanism is the use of competition in combination with reduced regulation to transform health care into a market-driven industry. This is changing both the way hospitals organize and deliver their services and the way they manage their operations. Two primary operating goals are cost control and utilization control in order to achieve increased productivity, new operating efficiencies, and stabilized costs. Operating efficiency and system control are now major concerns.

Significant changes in health care financing are occurring in every sector of the economy. Prospective payment has altered hospital reimbursement for Medicare patients. Several states now regulate hospital rates for all types of patients, while others have created special cost-containment programs for Medicaid patients. HMO enrollments are growing and will increase, especially since the government's decision to open certified HMOs to Medicare participants. Providers and insurers are experimenting with new types of coverage, including PPOs and PPO-type plans, which channel users to selected providers in exchange for discounted rates. Most conventional insurers now include large deductibles and coinsurance provisions designed to encourage more prudent use of the system.

These and other changes, including the opening of the industry to competition, are moving health care delivery from the inpatient to the outpatient setting. The hospital is no longer the only organized setting for medical practice. Alternative delivery providers, including primary care centers, ambulatory surgery centers, diagnostic centers, and others, are opening in every hospital's market. In response, hospitals are specializing in diagnosis and the treatment of special health problems, and becoming centers for new and expanded health care organizations. Cost and productivity pressures are forcing hospitals to meet new financial goals. Cross-subsidizing is being eliminated as competing buyers of health care refuse to pay more than their true costs. Efficiency and system control are now top priorities.

Has prospective pricing as a model for achieving cost containment actually worked? While it is too early to generalize about the effects of recent reimbursement changes, preliminary trends suggest that prospective pricing is achieving some of its cost-containment goals. Inpatient hospital utilization rates are dropping as health care delivery shifts to the less expensive and more competitive outpatient setting. For example, in the first year of prospective pricing, hospital admissions on a seasonally adjusted basis declined by almost 600,000, from 9.47 million in early 1983 to almost 8.9 million by the end of 1984, a 7.3 percent decrease. Admission rates by late 1984 were declining by an average of 2 percent per quarter across all acute care hospitals, representing the sharpest drop in admissions ever recorded.

Adjusted hospital patient days began falling as well, registering a 9.4 percent annual decline by 1984, a trend prompted by reductions in average length-of-stay as well as by reductions in admissions. Finally, average occupancy rates began decreasing, dropping from 73.3 percent at the end of 1983 to 67.7 percent for the end of 1984. Experts feel that this decline will moderate, averaging 3 to 4 percent over the next two years as opposed to 5 to 7 percent during 1985.

The cost of hospital care is also declining. Nationally, hospital expenditures now represent a lower percentage of total national health care expenditures than they have in the past. In 1981, 46.6 percent of total expenditures were for hospital care, versus 42 percent by early 1985, and a predicted 30 to 35 percent for 1990. Hospitals are demonstrating that with advantageous organizational forms, sound management, and access to new capital markets, they can become leaner, more efficient, and less expensive providers, without sacrificing quality. Despite earlier fears, there is no convincing evidence that shorter lengths-of-stay are jeopardizing patient health.

Many of the benefits pioneered by investor-owned hospitals have enabled all providers to achieve these new cost and operating efficiencies and even to prosper under the new financing mechanisms. Using the multihospital system model, business discipline, the new breed of health care executive, and their access to new capital markets, many hospitals adjusted quickly to the diagnosis-related groups (DRGs) because of the management information and cost-accounting systems they had implemented. With these systems, hospitals could develop a synergistic approach, and innovative and well-conceived long- and short-term strategies to control costs and align finances and operations with the fixed payment rates.

One important change has been the shift to flexible budgeting, a technique not previously widely accepted within the industry, but one that becomes an important tool given volume-sensitive reimbursement methods. Under the flexible budgeting system, volume and productivity standards drive budgeting revenues, expenses, and manhours. Because volume is a principal determinant of needed resources, labor and material resources are added or decreased as volume changes.

These and other innovations brought to health care from other industries by investor-owned hospitals, and now used almost universally by nonprofit providers, constitute a business model that in a cost-conscious environment helps the hospital maintain market share, increase unit productivity, cut costs, and obtain capital—four critical objectives given the new reimbursement mechanisms and cost-containment strategies.

The business practices used by investor-owned hospitals and, with increasing frequency, nonprofit systems, do not constitute a profit-maximization model. Rather, they apply important accounting systems and management tools so that hospitals can manage their assets more efficiently, keep expenditures under control, and maximize their revenues. This is a key difference. By maximizing revenues, hospitals can achieve reasonable profits without sacrificing quality or jeopardizing access. Additionally, achieving size through system formation is not a "larger is better" strategy, but rather a strategy designed to achieve financial and managerial benefits that accrue to systems, and to permit the diversification needed to survive in a competitive marketplace.

During the 1970s, both investor-owned and nonprofit systems demonstrated their ability to more effectively access capital markets, and obtain capital on more favorable terms, than could free-standing units. In part, this success was due to their ability to hire managers and specialized staff with exceptional skills, initiative, and abilities, and then to spread this corporate overhead over a larger patient population. Moreover, the expanded size of these systems made it possible for them to influence and adapt more rapidly to environmental changes originating either from purchaser preferences or from regulatory agencies. All of this contributed to their ability to improve operating margins which, ultimately, are a major determinant of success in any business.

Achieving New Economies

While many investor-owned and nonprofit hospitals initially prospered under prospective payment, 1985 marked a turning point. It became apparent that new economies and efficiencies were needed if providers were to continue maximizing revenues and operating profitably. Providers, especially investor-owned hospitals, began experiencing steady declines in admissions and occupancy rates as the market continued to shift from the inpatient to the outpatient setting. Additionally, hospitals began engaging in intense price competition. Some hospitals began discounting their prices by as much as 10 to 20 percent. While the majority of price breaks are going to HMOs, some health care analysts feel that hospital pricing discount percentages could reach 50 or 60 percent by the late 1980s (Shaw 1985). While a better operating environment could emerge for hospitals, the late 1980s will have been the most difficult years experienced since the late 1970s.

The challenges of prospective payment and subsequent restructuring of the industry provide opportunities for investor-owned hospital companies to lead the way in streamlining their operations and making them even more efficient providers. HCA, like other major investor-owned companies, is reconfiguring its assets, segmenting markets, developing new products and new revenue sources, finding ways to achieve even greater system benefits and, most importantly, is becoming an information-driven business.

Information will be a key factor in the success of hospitals under prospective pricing and new generations of cost-containment strategies. Integrated information systems that can monitor and control patient entry into and movement through a provider network will be crucial for managing utilization and cost. These systems are also necessary if hospitals are to develop true cost-accounting data, a crucial need under prospective pricing. HCA, for example, has developed one of the industry's most comprehensive integrated information systems to obtain productivity, cost monitoring, and efficiency data. Using information generated by this system, HCA can develop appropriate asset configurations for each consumer segment by geographical area, asset mix, physician practice patterns, and consumer needs. Each of HCA's primary markets can be segmented, and key consumer groups identified so that low-cost product lines can capture substantial market share.

Access to this kind of data through integrated information systems is crucial given the dramatic change in the buying patterns of major purchasers. While fixed price and capitated programs are becoming increasingly important, major purchasers are not just seeking price discounts. They are selecting, and in some cases mandating, providers who can offer a full range of flexible and attractive service packages with simplified administrative procedures for controlling utilization and costs. Providers must be able to offer (or affiliate with) integrated managed delivery networks on a regional basis, including a full range of services and multiple financing (insurance) options if they want to meet purchaser demand and capture patients. While investor-owned hospitals are clearly ahead of the nonprofits in this area, nonprofit systems, primarily through new alliances and joint ventures with each other, with investor-owned systems, and with insurance companies, are closing the gap.

HEALTH CARE IN THE FUTURE: MANAGED DELIVERY NETWORKS

The new efficiencies demanded by current and projected cost-containment strategies present opportunities as well as challenges for all hospitals regardless of ownership form. As Ellwood (1986), Abramowitz (1986), Averill and Kalison (1986), and others have noted, managed delivery networks (or managed security organizations, as Ellwood calls them) are becoming *the* model for delivering health care. This model permits even greater levels of efficiency in order to control costs and utilization.

Averill and Kalison (1986) suggest that providers who succeed in this new demand-driven market will be fully integrated regional health care organizations which combine hospitals, nursing homes, primary care centers, home health programs, and other services, and that these organizations will themselves be part of national chains of what they call health care corporations, entities organized by existing nonprofit multihospital systems and investor-owned hospital companies. They and Abramowitz (1986) predict that even some commercial insurance companies will become health care operations by acquiring existing hospitals.

Ellwood (1986) sees the same scenario when he predicts the advent of what he calls managed security organizations, health conglomerates that manage a variety of health and economic risks. These comprehensive national organizations will combine insurance, hospital, and physician services, and will control the multitude of health "suppliers" (hospitals and other providers) that operate at the regional and local levels. While Ellwood predicts that most managed security organizations will be investor owned, he suggests that at least one could be a nonprofit firm, one an insurance company entity, and possibly one formed by physicians.

This new integrated managed delivery model addresses a new determinant in health care, where the major issue is no longer who owns the hospital, but who can enter a market with both a delivery capability and strong insurance options capable of capturing and controlling patients. The managed delivery model, made possible by system benefits, consolidation, and access to sophisticated business and management practices, is becoming the model not just for hospitals, but for all health care providers, including physicians.

However, there will be a shakeout in managed care plans within the coming decade, and during this shakeout, PPOs offering only price discounts may disappear. Some HMOs will also disappear as the same consolidation taking place among hospitals reaches HMOs and PPOs, and as new hybrid managed care models are developed and tested. Some 400 HMOs share less than one-tenth of the market, a significant amount of competition for a small parcel of the private sector. Consolidation, if not total expiration, will ultimately shrink that number over the next decade. HMOs and other managed care plans that survive will be those which are a part of strong managed health care organizations, with their superior financial and managerial advantages.

Additionally, the same cost-containment pressures driving change in the hospital industry are affecting physicians as well. Physicians are now using the same organizational structures and management methods pioneered by investor-owned hospitals to protect income, gain access to capital needed to finance technology, bargain more effectively with insurance companies and purchasers seeking discounted and predetermined rates, protect market share, and basically survive under the new financing structure.

Confronting many of the same financial and competitive pressures affecting hospitals, and faced with a projected surplus, physicians are forming and/or joining group practices at a steadily increasing rate.

They are aligning economically with HMOs and other insurance plans, and with insurance companies. These group practice systems are increasing both in number and in size.

We are also seeing alliances between group practices modeled on the alliances being formed between hospital chains and systems. Preferred Providers of America, for example, is an alliance of 13 multi-specialty group practice organizations located throughout the state of California. This may be a forerunner of the kinds of super systems that will be formed across the nation in the coming years as physicians' practice organizations unite to gain new economies and efficiencies that meet cost-containment goals.

It is safe to say that, in today's health care industry, the business practices and system models pioneered by investor-owned hospitals have been widely adopted by nonprofit systems and are serving as *the* model for health care providers. It is important to remember, however, that these practices and models are really in their infancy. The industry has just embarked on the prospective payment experiment, and we can anticipate further cost-containment strategies modeled on prospective payment that force even greater efficiencies. As a result, investor-owned hospital companies are developing new generations of business practices and delivery models, especially in the area of electronic data processing, to meet these challenges. As in the past, the entire industry will benefit.

SOCIAL WELFARE VERSUS THE BUSINESS MODEL

America is moving beyond the issue of the nonprofit versus for-profit forms for health care delivery. Prospective payment and other landmark cost-containment strategies are forcing all health care providers to become more businesslike in their behavior. In this process, providers are evolving from social institutions into businesses providing a social service. The formation of systems and the use of business practices from other industries were natural consequences of this evolutionary process, and the only viable option if providers were to achieve the efficiencies mandated by prospective payment and other cost-containment strategies.

Politically, America is moving toward the privatization of many services once provided and/or financed by the government. Additionally, the tax status of nonprofit health care providers is being challenged. While it may never be totally taken away, rigorous new tests are being proposed at both the federal and state levels that will, when enacted, make it more difficult for hospitals to retain their tax exemptions. Given this trend, it is in the interest of all hospitals to form systems and use business practices that strengthen their financial position and ensure their survival. The investor-owned hospital industry has demonstrated that hospitals can function efficiently and profitably despite tax status. Cost-containment pressures will not abate. They will continue and intensify. Hospitals must protect themselves economically at this time if they want to survive in the future. Investor-owned hospitals have pointed the way and are continuing to pioneer new financial and managerial innovations that achieve even greater efficiencies and cost savings. The most important lesson we can learn from the investor-owned hospital experience is that sound financial and business practices applied in a market-driven environment can be more effective than strict regulation of the industry in achieving efficiency and cost-containment goals.

REFERENCES

Abramowitz, Kenneth (1986). *The Future of Health Delivery in America: Strategic Analysis/Financial Forecast*. New York: Sanford C. Bernstein & Co., Inc.
American Hospital Association (1979). "Hospital Statistics" (Table 1): 4–7.
Anderson, Jack R. (1976). *The Road to Recovery*. Nashville, TN: Rich Publishing.
Averill, Richard A., and Kalison, Michael J. (1986). "Present and Future: Predictions for the Healthcare Industry." *Healthcare Financial Management* 40 (3): 50–54.
Bentley, James D. (1985). "Changing Relationships in Health Care: Implications for Managers." Speech delivered at the Seminar on the Future of Medicine. Center for the Study of Health Care Issues, University of Virginia, September 24.
Clarkson, Kenneth (1972). "Some Implications of Property Rights in Hospital Management." *Journal of Law and Economics* 15.
Ellwood, Paul M. (1986). "Ellwood Says 'Supermed' Concept Gaining Ground, Expects up to 10 within a Decade." *Federation of American Health Systems Review* 19, no. 2 (March/April): 69–70, 72.
Fuchs, Victor R. (1986). "Paying the Piper, Calling the Tune: Implications of Changes in Reimbursement." *Frontiers of Health Services Management* 2, no. 3 (February): 4–27.
Knowles, Richard (1979). "Investor-Owned Chains: Hospitals Compete More." *Modern Healthcare* (August): 24.
Shaw, Seth H. (1985). "Health Care Valuation Perspective: An Industry in Inflection, Part 1." Shearson Lehman Brothers, September.
Vignola, Peter (1978). *An Economic Analysis of For-Profit Hospitals*. Cambridge, MA: Harvard Law School Monograph, June 18.

Chapter 10

The Medical-Industrial Complex: Another View of the Influence of Business on Medical Care

Stanley Wohl

Editor's Note—Growth of the medical-industrial complex (MIC) was stimulated by a federal government–facilitated flow of investment capital into hospital ownership. Diversification from the owning and operating of acute care facilities into a wide variety of services occurred quickly and has been characteristic of the major firms in the MIC: chronic care beds, home health care, pharmacy supplies, freestanding emergency rooms and clinics, and hospital supplies are examples of the diverse health care–related services spun out by the MIC. A logical target for further diversification by the MIC, one that would serve to guarantee a supply of customers (patients) for medical services, is the medical insurance industry. The companies belonging to the MIC have thus attempted to establish health maintenance organizations (HMOs) and preferred provider organizations (PPOs) with notably less success than they experienced with their initial diversification efforts.

According to Wohl, there are dangers if large medical industry corporations, such as the ones described—Hospital Corporation of America, National Medical Enterprises, American Medical International, Humana Beverly Enterprises, ARA Holding, and Maxicare Health Plans, which are highly successful businesses—actively broker physician services and potentially play a greater role than the federal government in shaping the future of medical care. If they merge with the large medical insurers, as he predicts they will, it is they—the MIC—who will ultimately determine the future costs and content of medical care. In addition, their business practices have been so universally adopted by the non–investor-owned hospitals that they are becoming nearly indistinguishable from investor-owned institutions.

For better or worse, health care in America is now a major industry. In fact, it is the nation's largest industry, employing 5 percent of the population, directly or indirectly, in a $470 billion "operation." The term "medical-industrial complex," or MIC, refers to the 500 or so listed corporations that have been instrumental over the last two decades in converting health care in this country from a public service, cottage-type industry into a highly profitable, investor-oriented, "big business" enterprise. Nor is it a passing fad, this conversion: no health professional is presently immune from the fallout, or likely to be so in the future. The new atmosphere of entrepreneurial medicine pervades the hallowed halls of the Harvard Medical School as much as it does a private Hollywood hospital for the glamorously ill.

In a strict sense, the American health care system has always had an MIC sector, but until the 1960s, its activities were largely confined to the manufacture and distribution of health care products and pharmaceuticals. When Arnold Relman originally coined the term "medical-industrial complex" in 1980, he was essentially referring to the growing number of corporations that had entered the health care arena as providers of health services in contrast to the previously restricted role of the health care suppliers (Relman 1980). Listed corporations were moving into the business of owning and managing hospitals, nursing homes, and clinics and, for many medical professionals, these new companies alone defined the essence of the MIC (Relman 1983). This discussion of the MIC will focus on facility ownership, although it represents only a fraction of the MIC's activities.

In his important book, *The Social Transformation of American Medicine*, the sociologist Paul Starr meticulously chronicled the metamorphosis of this country's health care system into a major industry (Starr 1982). Subsequently, the companies involved in that metamorphosis were described and categorized according to their size and activities (Wohl 1984; 1986). To briefly summarize the story, by 1986, major corporations were able to acquire 20 percent of the acute care hospitals and 67 percent of chronic care facilities for four main reasons:

1. The 1965 Medicare reimbursement regulations were tailor-made for investor-owned companies, because the federal government wished to encourage the flow of private capital into hospital ownership, management, construction, and renovation.

2. Related to the above intentions, certain terms of the Medicare cost-plus guaranteed return on equity formula for hospital reimbursement permitted investor-owned companies that operated hospitals to treat the costs of borrowing money for expansion and acquisitions as part of the cost of managing facilities.

In other words, the growth of the investor-owned hospital corporations was in large part subsidized by Medicare.

3. Because the Medicare regulations were so generously written, and because the Medicare program brought 26 million newly insured subscribers into the marketplace, Wall Street investors allowed the new entrepreneurial facility owners to run much higher debt-to-equity ratios than were previously acceptable.

4. Besides benefiting from a lot of general good luck and from a generous Medicare program, the investor-owned hospital industry owes much of its success to the extraordinary accomplishments of Thomas Frist, Sr., founder of Hospital Corporation of America. Frist got his pathfinding company going in a big way, pulled it through tough times when the tough times came, and devised many of the policies and strategies that were to serve as templates for the industry.

Frist and his fellow entrepreneurs did not invent the concept of multifacility organizations. Kaiser-Permanente and the benevolent orders of the Catholic Church were managing chains of hospitals long before HCA or Humana. Neither did the MIC founders invent the profit motive in health facility ownership and management. Investors—physicians, for the most part—owned hospitals and nursing homes a full half-century prior to the establishment of National Medical Enterprises. The truly novel business ideas that the new MIC concocted for the system were: (a) the combining of the profit motive in health facility management with the chaining mechanism, and (b) going public with the enterprise of health facility ownership.

The "stock marketization" of health care—the utilization of Wall Street investment banking techniques to raise health care capital—was truly unique (Siegrist 1983). Because the joining of Wall Street and health care has in fact occurred, and because the companies involved in the relationship have been so successful, the entire health care system now functions according to new units of measure. Mergers, acquisitions, divestitures, and quarterly results have become the new health care yardsticks, much as they have always been for all other industries.

The subtleties of the health care–Wall Street marriage are easily missed and often overlooked in what are now the well-known circuitous arguments made in support of, or in criticism of, the MIC. For example, the MIC is frequently considered to be a homogeneous entity operating with singleness of purpose. The performance of the investor-owned companies taken as a whole is often compared to that of the traditional voluntary facilities—as though all hospitals listed on the stock exchange have everything else in common in addition to their Wall Street con-

TABLE 10.1
The Largest Health Facility Management Companies, 1985

Company	Number of Facilities	Number of Beds (thousands)	1985 Revenues (billion $)	Employees (thousands)
Beverly Enterprises	908	101	1.4	87
HCA*	480	74	4.9	90
NME	400	70	2.7	69
ARA Services†	276	32	3.4	115
AMI	142	26	2.4	41
Humana	100	18	2.1	44
Republic Health‡	85	8	0.4	4
Charter	51	5	0.6	8

*HCA owns 3 percent of the outstanding common shares of Beverly Enterprises.

†Only 10 percent of ARA Services' revenues and 14 percent of profits are derived from health facility (nursing homes) management.

‡Republic Health was acquired by Pesch in a leveraged buyout.

nection. In reality, though, Hospital Corporation of America is as different from American Medical International as St. Elsewhere is from Massachusetts General Hospital. The individual companies that comprise the MIC should therefore be considered as distinct, separate entities. A brief look at a few of the best-known companies in the field will help to make this point. The sundry activities of these companies, in all their variety, offer considerable insight into the true meaning of the MIC. In addition, Table 10.1 provides a capsule summary of the status of eight of the leading companies of the MIC in 1985.

HOSPITAL CORPORATION OF AMERICA

Hospital Corporation of America (HCA) is the largest investor-owned hospital management company ranked by revenues and the eleventh largest of the Fortune Service 500 companies. The company now owns or manages 480 hospitals with a cumulative total of just over 74,000 beds. One hundred and eighty-seven of the hospitals managed by HCA are not-for-profit facilities.

The general trend in the industry toward diversification is evident from looking at HCA's various activities. The company owns 3 percent of Beverly Enterprises, the largest long-term care corporation, and 25 percent of Scientific Leasing, a company that does what its name implies. It purchased Johnson and Johnson's home health care division and the Hill-Richards Companies, an insurance claims processing firm, and announced plans to purchase New Century Life Insurance.

In early 1985, HCA entered the field of health maintenance organizations (HMOs) by acquiring an 80 percent interest in Lovelace Health Plan, a 50,000-member HMO in New Mexico. Furthermore, under the name "HCA Care," HCA has plans to apply for HMO licenses in 15 other states. The company has also applied for general insurance licenses in 34 states in order to sell a wide selection of health insurance policies, including a Medicare supplemental plan. All told, HCA spent $100 million in 1985 in its effort to develop the insurance vehicle needed to penetrate the HMO market.

But not all of HCA's initiatives in its bold program to create a vast diversified health care empire have met with success. On March 30, 1985, HCA announced plans to merge with American Hospital Supply, the largest distributor of hospital supplies in the country and the fourteenth largest diversified service company, with revenues of $3.44 billion. However, the friendly merger attempt was defeated by Baxter Travenol which, in an unfriendly but ultimately successful bid, acquired American Hospital Supply for itself.

Just as Medicare sets the tone for the entire health care system, HCA has served as the bellweather for the investor-owned segment of the system. On October 1, 1985, HCA company officials announced that they expected to report only a 10 percent gain in third-quarter earnings over the previous year, and that they could foresee flattened earnings in the fourth quarter. With the realization that a health care industry shakeout was happening in earnest, the values of almost all the health care stocks dropped 10 to 15 percent over the next few trading days (Wayne 1985).

On March 4, 1986, HCA announced a joint venture agreement with The Equitable Life Assurance Society of the United States. That agreement resulted in the establishment of a new company, Equicor HCA Corporation, a combination of Equitable Group and Health Insurance Company, which provides health, life, dental, and disability insurance, and Hospital Corporation's HCA Health Plans, a health insurance unit. At its inception, the joint venture company already had 8 million subscribers and $2 billion in annual revenues.

This latest HCA undertaking represents the convergence of two recent trends within the MIC. The investor-owned facility managers have experienced significant difficulties in developing insurance products; as a consequence, their attempts to penetrate the highly competitive HMO market, dominated by Kaiser, have proven to be more costly than anticipated. As a result, a growing number of joint ventures have recently been announced involving facility owners on the one hand and major insurance companies on the other. For their part, the major insurers see in these amalgamations an opportunity to enter the health care market and to use health insurance as a loss leader for their much more profitable life insurance offerings. Examples of such unions include HCA-Equitable, Voluntary Hospitals of America–Aetna, Metropolitan Life–local community HMOs, American Healthcare Systems–Transamerica, U.S. Health Care Systems–Lincoln National, and the acquisition of Whittaker Corp, an HMO operator, by Travelers (Wohl 1986).

NATIONAL MEDICAL ENTERPRISES

Ranked by revenues, National Medical Enterprises (NME) is second only to HCA as a hospital management company, constituting the twenty-fourth largest diversified service company in the nation. For the decade 1974–83, NME ranked fourth among the Fortune Service 500 in total return to investors (51.86 percent).

Even before it become fashionable to do so, NME was the first among the listed chains to recognize the importance of diversification in health care. The company is the most diversified operation in the group, with 50 percent of its revenues derived from nonhospital operations. The company continues, of course, as a major owner of acute hospital beds. In addition, its Hillhaven Division ranks third, behind Beverly Enterprises and ARA Holding, as an operator of chronic care facilities. Furthermore, NME derives 13 percent of its profits from psychiatric hospitals, and 7 percent from health care products marketed through its Medical Products Division.

Prior to the 1985 health care shakeout, NME's goal was clearly to create an entire health care agglomeration that met every possible need of its prospective clients and patients; as one of the most diversified health care companies in America, the firm was well positioned to achieve that goal. However, the company lagged behind HCA and Humana in marketing the insurance vehicle necessary to draw more patients into the system. On June 24, 1986, as a result of mounting financial difficulties, NME announced a major restructuring program. Several acute care hospitals will be sold, and the company intends to concentrate its focus on specialty hospitals and nursing homes.

AMERICAN MEDICAL INTERNATIONAL

American Medical International (AMI) was the target of a $1.9 billion unfriendly takeover bid by closely held Pesch and Company. The latter company acquired Republic Health through a leveraged buyout.

AMI was a natural target for an acquisition. Despite its involvement in diversified activities such as surgi-centers and information systems, nearly all of its earnings are derived from acute care hospitals. In the shakeout atmosphere, many view this factor as a distinct weakness in the company profile, and recent earnings reports bear witness to the concern.

AMI grew rapidly in January 1984, after its $890 million acquisition of Lifemark, a Texas-based hospital management concern. The acquisition coincided with the onset of the health care shakeout, making the new purchase somewhat difficult for AMI to digest. It is interesting that when Lifemark decided to sell out, company officials held talks with HCA as well as with several non–health-related companies. The entire episode drove home the fact that in today's health care world, any company, whether a health concern or not, can enter the fray simply by purchasing 50.1 percent of the stock of any other.

Though perhaps overzealous, the acquisition of Lifemark served to slow down whatever attempts AMI may have had in mind to develop insurance products as a means of attracting new clients. The company lags behind both HCA and Humana in the important fields of HMO and PPO—that is, "preferred provider"—development. The company has begun marketing a variety of insurance plans under the AMICARE logo, but to date only 2,000 subscribers have enrolled. AMI is also test-marketing AMICARD—"America's Health Care Card"—a program offering streamlined admission to AMI facilities, basic emergency information on a centralized data base, and a line of credit at AMI facilities. On March 13, 1986, AMI reached an agreement to acquire Gateway Health Group, the operator of a 91,000-member HMO in the Denver region. In conjunction with Salick Health Care, AMI announced ambitious plans to develop a chain of outpatient cancer care networks.

HUMANA

Humana is in many ways a unique organization and, among the investor-owned hospital companies, has been the most interesting one to follow. Between 1974 and 1984, Humana provided a total return to investors of 58.48 percent—the second highest among the Fortune Service 500 companies. Those figures represent a spectacular performance whatever the field of endeavor, but they are especially impressive in health care. Humana knows how to make news and how to keep its name in the public eye. In 1984, it recruited the DeVries artificial heart team from the University of Utah to its Louisville hospital, and thereby bought itself months of free prime time, front page media exposure. Whether by coincidence or not, the artificial heart fireworks coincided with the launching of a superb advertising campaign for Humana Care Plus, the company's entry in the HMO sweepstakes. And then, in February of 1986, Humana ended its membership in the American Hospital Association, claiming that it had not received adequate services for the $330,000 in dues it had paid in 1985.

One-quarter of Humana's hospitals are less than seven years old, and two-thirds of them were built within the last 12 years! Humana's success is usually attributed to three factors: (a) tight centralized control (the company principals own 25 percent of the shares), (b) superb advertising and public relations, and (c) a proclivity for melodramatic medical publicity. The product the company offers is not that much different from those offered by the other chains, or any other hospital in the country, for that matter. Yet Humana's financial performance is second to none, for-profit or not-for-profit. Simply put, Humana knows how to turn a profit from hospital beds.

Besides promoting its artificial heart program, Humana promotes its new "Humana Care Plus" HMO plan to subscribers. As is true for the other investor-owned chains, this diversification into the insurance field has proved to be a far more difficult and expensive undertaking than was first anticipated. In December 1985, Humana announced pretax losses of $8.2 million for its MedFirst clinics and Care Plus insurance operations for the first quarter (ending November 30, 1985). In March of 1986, the company announced a further loss of $14 million for its health insurance business. On October 2, 1986, Humana announced a pretax charge of $232 million in its fourth quarter, the direct result of rising claims in its medical insurance division. The charge will result in an overall $100 million loss for the quarter.

With one eye on America's aging population, Humana recently acquired financially troubled International Medical Centers, the largest HMO licensed to care for Medicare patients. If there is a weakness in Humana's structure, it is the company's lack of significant involvement with chronic care facilities. In view of the country's growing elderly population, such a commitment is a virtual necessity for a company bent on offering a full range of health services to its patients. Shakeout economics also make chronic care facilities the key to efficient utilization of one's resources in order to maximize efficiency. It should not be surprising, then, to see Humana buy into or acquire a chronic care management company in the near future, as HCA and NME have already done.

BEVERLY ENTERPRISES

Beverly Enterprises, although seldom in the news, is probably the most important facility owner among the companies of the MIC. Besides being the single largest owner of facility beds (101,739), Beverly has cornered 5 percent of the nursing home market, thus making it far and away the leader in the field of chronic care. Besides nursing homes, the company operates 119 home health care agencies, 14 retirement living centers, and 76 medical equipment outlets. Beverly also acquired Pharmacy Corporation of America, a supplier of pharmacy services to nursing homes.

Chronic care lacks the flash and drama of acute care. This fact, coupled with the conservative nature of the company, has led Beverly to operating in a low-key but highly successful manner. Less news is better in the nursing home business. Yearly growth has been significant and steady, and Beverly's long-term goal is to provide a full array of services for the elderly. The rapidly growing population of the elderly should insure that, over the next decade, Beverly will probably emerge as one of the largest listed health care providers.

Historically, Beverly Enterprises has had a close relationship with HCA, with HCA owning as much as 20 percent of Beverly stock. Following HCA's unsuccessful merger attempt with American Hospital Supply, HCA reduced its stake in Beverly to 3 percent. Had the HCA–American Hospital Supply merger not been undermined by Baxter Travenol, the stage would have been set for the creation of a single entity that would have been the largest owner of acute beds, the largest owner of chronic beds, and the major supplier of hospital products. That, in a nutshell, is what the MIC is all about.

Beverly's current dilemma is the one of "patient mix." True, almost all its beds are full most of the time, but a large number of the patients are on Medicaid, which tends to reimburse poorly in all states. The patient mix, or at least the company's revenues per patient, can only improve, however, as private insurers begin writing health policies that cover services rendered in chronic care facilities, and as Medicare comes under increasing political pressure to expand the program's nursing home coverage. For the present time, Beverly itself has decided not to enter the insurance field and to remain strictly a provider. But it is a certainty that, with the great and growing shortage of such facilities, insurers and providers will need the chronic care beds managed by Beverly.

In recognition of Beverly's strategic position in the health care system, Beverly principals unsuccessfully attempted to effect a leveraged buyout of the company in the fall of 1986.

ARA HOLDING (FORMERLY ARA SERVICES)

ARA Services did not start as a health care concern but has nonetheless become the country's second-largest operator of nursing homes. The company also owns the country's largest emergency medical group—

Spectrum Emergency Care—a company that enters into staffing contracts with hospital emergency rooms. ARA was the first investor-owned company to actually buy out a medical group. With its holdings in health and family services (which account for 12 percent of its revenues), ARA is probably the most diversified service company in the United States. Going far beyond the health field, the corporation provides almost every kind of service and product imaginable, including food, transportation, correctional systems, child care centers, product distribution (including newspapers and magazines), and uniforms. It is estimated that one ARA service reaches every single American every day, either directly or indirectly.

ARA's health division is making a big effort to expand its services to the elderly. In 1983, 27 personal care units were started up in Texas; another 46 units were begun in 1984. Thirty-six of ARA's nursing homes were recently renovated in order to attract more private paying residents. The company is unique in its involvement with expanding markets at both ends of the age spectrum: it runs child care centers at the one end and nursing homes at the other.

MAXICARE HEALTH PLANS

An important current trend in health care is the rapid growth of HMOs. None has grown faster than Maxicare, now the nation's largest investor-owned operator of HMOs. By virtue of Maxicare's recent acquisitions of Healthcare USA and of HealthAmerica, Maxicare now has more than 2 million subscribers in 32 states.

While HMOs are growing rapidly in size, their profits have not kept pace with their subscriber increases. Maxicare, for example, reported a 79 percent decrease in 1986 earnings on a 75 percent increase in revenues. While the issue of physician as employee remains a hot topic in medical circles, it is not yet clear whether large HMOs will survive long enough to serve as the employers (Anderson 1987). People tend to forget that it took Kaiser-Permanente, the largest and most successful HMO in the country, 50 years to attract 5 million subscribers. Most of Maxicare's growth came by way of acquisitions, not by virtue of independently attracting more subscribers.

The new breed of HMOs, as exemplified by Maxicare, do not, for the most part, own their own hospitals. They are finding the administrative aspects of managing HMOs to be every bit as difficult as the marketing task of attracting subscribers. The HMO sector has become highly competitive, and no single large HMO has shown signs that it can mimic Kaiser's success in running prepaid health programs over several decades.

THE FUTURE OF THE MIC AND
TRADITIONAL HOSPITALS

The MIC, much like the health care system it dominates, is constantly changing. The entire industry has found itself in the midst of a Medicare-stimulated shakeout and, as a result, the MIC stands out less clearly from the traditional nonprofit sector, as each sector adopts some of the practices of the other in order to survive. It is no longer accurate, then, to portray the health care system as being divided into two camps: the investor-owned group and the traditional voluntary group. While it was possible to make clear-cut distinctions between the two as recently as 1983, that is no longer the case. The camps of today possess more similarities than differences and, in fact, often overlap.

Aggressiveness in marketing, mergers, acquisitions, affiliations, and divestitures are as common today in the traditional sector as they are in the investor-owned sector. Except for some tax differentials—which are gradually being removed—and the listing of the chains on the stock exchange, one would be hard-pressed today to distinguish on the administrative level between a chain of hospitals operated by, say, American Medical International and a chain operated by the Sisters of Charity of St. Vincent De Paul. Indeed, whatever differences continue to exist will probably be diminished even further as the nonprofit organizations lose their tax perks (Harlan 1986), the investor-owned organizations lose their easy access to capital, and the Wall Street investors lose their taste for the health care stocks in the shrinking market.

It is likely that the differences between the traditional hospitals and the new hospitals will erode still further as the for-profits and the not-for-profits develop closer working relationships with each other. The nonprofit Kaiser-Permanente health plan has an agreement with investor-owned Humana to lease Humana wards in some hospitals in order to accommodate Kaiser's exploding beneficiary list. In some areas of the country, Kaiser has also contracted with investor-owned Beverly Enterprises to lease some of that company's nursing home beds to care for Kaiser patients. In a similar vein, Voluntary Hospitals of America, and its associated American Health Capital, have entered into a joint venture agreement with Aetna Insurance to market a variety of health care plans. Voluntary Hospitals of America is itself a for-profit company, owned by shareholders, which consists of member nonprofit hospitals. Hundreds of similar examples exist that seem to indicate that there may no longer be any marketing or operational incentives for a health provider to remain strictly nonprofit or strictly for-profit. Nevertheless, one does not have to attend a great number of corporation or professional meetings to learn that each camp considers the other camp's grass to be greener. The recent flurry of accommodations reached between members of the two systems seems to suggest that some combination of the for-profit and non-profit formats works to the advantage of both sides. The serious development on Wall Street—namely, that investors have started deserting the listed health care chains—would seem to indicate that those investor-owned organizations that fail to link up in some way with the nonprofit organizations may not survive the shakeout. Institutional investors are notoriously fickle and, once they detect the slightest stall in growth on the part of a company, they tend to desert the ship; and, as a rule, they do not soon return. The pure for-profit, investor-owned company—uninvolved with traditional providers in any significant way—may very well turn out to be doomed to extinction. In fact, as the various provider organizations, for-profit and not-for-profit, come to resemble each other more and more, the profit motive itself may cease to be the burning issue it is today.

The health care system has entered the brand name era. Whether wrapped in the for-profit or the nonprofit mantle, various organizations are competing to attract patients to a logo in much the same way that computer companies and soap companies attract their clients. In the case of health care, once the patient is on board, the goal is to sell, to make available to that patient all the relevant services he or she could conceivably need, virtually from cradle to grave. Brand name health care is the result of a growing awareness on the part of all health care facilities that they can no longer afford to leave to chance, or to the largesse of community physicians, the responsibility for filling their beds. Blue Cross calls it patient management; other organizations use other attractive euphemisms. But what it all boils down to is a method of brokering physician services. The trend converts physicians to pawns in a larger game, variously termed the "plan," the "package," or the "provider organization." Whether it is a Humana Care Plus HMO, a Kaiser HMO, or a community PPO, control of the patient list ends up in the hands of someone other than the physician.

PHYSICIANS AND THE NEW MEDICAL POLITICS

Physicians will likely find that the most troublesome future consequence of the industrialization process is the continuing consolidation of facility ownership. More and more hospitals will come to be owned by fewer corporations and organizations, and big business has a habit of dealing harshly with those who are not team players. Already, many of the health care companies have legions of attorneys on retainer whose sole job is to protect the name on the company logo. The power of the company legal staff, coupled with the power of the advertising dollar, has the potential to destroy what has always been the greatest strength of the American health care system: its independence and diversity.

Physicians have legitimate differences of opinion regarding the perils and strengths of the MIC, yet the medical profession has failed to prepare its younger members for these realities. The AMA either does not see or does not want to recognize the perils of employee status for physicians (American Medical Association 1987). To this day, the vast majority of medical schools steadfastly refuse to educate their students in matters that pertain to the new medical politics. The bottom line is that the MIC represents the single greatest threat to the independence of the medical profession in the last 50 years. Cost containment, Medicare cuts, health care shakeouts, and HMOs will come and go with the political seasons (Health Care Financing Administration 1987), but these companies and organizations, in one form or another, are here to stay. The bigger they grow, the greater is the likelihood that more and more physicians will become "company doctors."

The companies for which future physicians will work are unlikely to be the current facility owners of the MIC, or even the rapidly growing HMO companies such as Maxicare. The future will belong to those with the deepest pockets. The major life insurance and diversified financial companies—Equitable, Aetna, Transamerica, Lincoln National, Travelers, CIGNA, Occidental—which are currently moving into the HMO marketplace, have enormous financial resources and are likely to emerge as the ultimate survivors of the health care shakeout. As increasing discretionary utilization power in health care is shifted from providers to insurers, the MIC of 1990 will likely be called the "medical insurance complex." Regardless of the nature of the surviving health care companies and organizations, continuing consolidation within the industry is a virtual certainty. There is no turning back the clock.

REFERENCES

American Medical Association (1987). "Employee MDs: Growing Trend." *Emergency Medicine and Ambulatory Care News* 9 (January): 6.

Anderson, W. H. (1987). "HMOs' Incentives: A Prescription for Failure." *Wall Street Journal*, January 2, 10.

Harlan, S. C. (1986). "1986 Tax Reform." *Health Care Briefing* (Arthur Young & Co.) 12: 1–4.

Health Care Financing Administration Proposal. *Federal Register.* January 13, 1987. Washington, DC.

Relman, A. S. (1980). "The New Medical-Industrial Complex." *New England Journal of Medicine* 303: 936–40.

——— (1983). "Investor-Owned Hospitals and Health Care Costs." *New England Journal of Medicine* 309: 370–72.

Siegrist, R. B. (1983). "Wall Street and the For-Profit Hospital Management Companies." In *The New Health Care For Profit*, ed. B. H. Gray, 35–50. Washington, DC: National Academy Press.

Starr, P. (1982). *The Social Transformation of American Medicine*. New York: Basic Books.

Wayne, L. (1985). "The Hospital Corp.'s Stumble." *New York Times*, October 8, 29.

Wohl, S. (1984). *The Medical Industrial Complex*. New York: Harmony Books.

——— (1986). *The Health Sector Database*. San Francisco, CA: Infomed Books.

IV

COST-CONTAINMENT EFFORTS: MIXED RESULTS OF CONTROLS ON TECHNOLOGY USE, EDUCATION, RATIONING, AND INFORMATION SYSTEMS

Chapter 11

Influencing Physicians' Decisions to Use Medical Technology

Stephen J. McPhee, Jonathan A. Showstack, and Steven A. Schroeder

Editor's Note—Medical technology has accounted for about 15 to 25 percent of the increase in the cost of hospital care over the last decade. Initial analyses concentrated on fixing blame on increased use of either "little ticket" or "big ticket" technology, but neither seems to consistently explain the rise in costs.

Evidence for unnecessary use of technology, which should be more the focus of our attention than increased use, per se, rests on observations that: some uses of technology vary substantially among countries, regions, and physicians without notable differences in clinical outcomes; HMOs tend to have lower hospitalization rates and average length-of-stay for hospitalizations; and, in natural experiments, access to technology was restricted at academic medical centers without notable differences in clinical outcomes. While these observations suggest that there may be waste in how technology is used, conclusive data are lacking, and underuse of technology, perhaps an equally or more serious issue, is unstudied.

Attempts to modify physician use of technology have generally met with failure or short-term success. McPhee et al. assert that this may not be a result of limitations of the strategies employed (education, audit with feedback, administrative maneuvers, and financial incentives) as much as lack of attention to the five major decisions that lead to use or overuse of technology: the decisions to (1) admit to hospital, (2) transfer to an intensive care unit, (3) perform sur-

This chapter is based, in part, on Schroeder, S. A. (1987). "Strategies for Reducing Medical Costs by Changing Physicians' Behavior." *International Journal of Technology Assessment in Health Care* 3; 39–50.

gery, (4) place in a long-term care facility, and (5) sustain life in a terminal illness. These five decisions must occupy more attention in future cost-containment research efforts.

More than ever before, there is the perception that there are limited resources available for health care. This perception, along with the rising costs of care, has led policymakers, researchers, and economists to assess the major factors contributing to medical care expenditures, such as general inflation, population growth and aging, and increased use of medical technology.

RISING HEALTH CARE COSTS: IS MEDICAL TECHNOLOGY THE CULPRIT?

The increased use of medical technologies has resulted from changes in how medical care is delivered (e.g., establishment of intensive care units), the development of new clinical techniques (e.g., coronary artery angioplasty), and the development of new hardware and devices (e.g., multichannel blood chemistry analyzers). Freeland and Schendler have estimated that between 1971 and 1981, 21 percent of the rise in hospital costs was due to an increased intensity of technological services per admission (Freeland and Schendler 1983). More recently, the Office of Technology Assessment estimated that between 1977 and 1982, 15 percent of the increase in costs per admission and 24 percent of the rise in hospital costs per capita were due to increased use of such services (U.S. Congress 1984).

Much of the debate about the cost of medical technology has centered on the relative contributions to the rise in health care costs of "little ticket" (high-volume, low per service cost) items such as clinical laboratory tests and simple x-ray studies, compared to "big ticket" (low-volume, high per service cost) items such as computed tomography (CT) and magnetic resonance imaging (MRI) scans. Those who argue that there is overuse of little ticket services cite the very high rate of use of clinical laboratory tests in both hospital and office settings (Scitovsky 1979; Parkerson 1978). Over the past two decades, laboratory tests comprised one of the fastest growing components of medical care, increasing at about 15 percent per year (Fineberg 1979). The great variability among physicians in use of tests implies that some of the increase is unnecessary (Freeborn et al. 1972; Schroeder et al. 1973). While some investigators have concluded that the growing volume of low-cost services accounts for a higher proportion of the burgeoning costs of care than do the large, expensive technologies (Moloney and Rogers 1979), others have suggested that rising costs are due more to the overuse of big ticket items (Steinberg et al. 1986). It is important that big ticket medical technology not be equated with devices and hardware, but that it also include new surgery (e.g., coronary artery bypass grafting), procedures (e.g., lithotripsy), or other complex services (e.g., renal dialysis).

OVERUSE OF MEDICAL RESOURCES: HOW MUCH "FAT" IS THERE?

Central to the efforts to contain expenditures for medical care is the question of whether or not medical resources are overused. If substantial overuse exists, then it may be possible to reduce the quantity and costs without lowering the quality of care.

There are three types of evidence that relate to the issue of technology overuse: variations in practice patterns; differences between practices in the fee-for-service sector and health maintenance organizations (HMOs); and case studies from specific institutions.

Variations in Practice Patterns

There are large international differences in the use of technological services. Physicians in the United States admit patients to the hospital more frequently than do their counterparts in other developed nations, and they perform surgery and other complex procedures more often (Schroeder 1984a). For example, in 1978 the U.S. Office of Technology Assessment found rates of coronary artery bypass graft surgery varying from 19 operations per million population in France to approximately 483 per million in the United States; Australia came closest to the United States, with 150 per million population (Banta and Kemp 1980). By 1982, the U.S. rate increased to 755 operations per million population (Rimm 1985). Similarly, there is considerable national variation in the rates of dialysis treatment of end-stage renal disease among elderly patients (Challah et al. 1984); of five English-speaking countries in 1980, the United Kingdom had the lowest rate (less than 1 case per 100,000) and the United States had the highest (39 cases per 100,000). With the possible exception of treatment of end-stage renal disease with dialysis, however, there is no real evidence that these markedly different performance rates have resulted in measurable differences in national health status or mortality.

Even within the United States, there is great variability in rates of performance of surgical procedures among physicians in different geographic areas. Such regional differences were first documented by Lewis (1969) and, more recently, by Wennberg and Gittelsohn (1982) and Wennberg (1984).

Similarly trained physicians within single institutions or areas also differ greatly in their use of medical services. In an early study, for example, 33 faculty internists at a university medical center HMO were found to have up to 17-fold differences in costs of laboratory tests ordered for similar patients (Schroeder et al. 1973). Another study found that laboratory test use at the Portland Kaiser-Permanente HMO varied substantially among physicians, with internists ordering the most tests (Freeborn et al. 1972). There is no evidence, however, that greater use of such services improves either quality or efficiency of care (McPhee et al. 1982; Myers and Schroeder 1981; Eisenberg and Williams 1981; Eisenberg 1985a; Grossman 1983).

Finally, practice patterns have been found to vary markedly over time despite the absence of marked changes in disease prevalence. Recent examples include the declining rates of tonsillectomies, an increasing proportion of deliveries by cesarean section, and the decreasing length-of-stay for hospitalized patients.

Contrasts between Care in Fee-for-Service and HMO Settings

Within the United States, patients enrolled in HMOs have 15 to 40 percent fewer admissions to hospital and accrue 25 to 45 percent fewer hospital days than do patients with traditional health insurance (Luft 1978). The decrease in admissions is distributed relatively evenly among surgical and medical diagnoses, as well as between urgent and elective conditions. Although data are limited, patient care appears not to suffer in HMOs because of lower hospitalization rates (Luft 1981). Similar differences between the fee-for-service sector and HMOs have been found in performance rates for a variety of surgical procedures (Luft 1978).

Case Studies from Specific Institutions

Using retrospective case review, many investigators have detected patterns of overuse of specific clinical services. These services include laboratory tests such as white blood cell differential counts (Shapiro, Hatch, and Greenfield 1984), serum lactic dehydrogenase (Eisenberg et al. 1977), thyroid function tests (Rhyne and Gehlbach 1979), blood cross match (Devitt and Ironside 1975), preoperative screening tests (Kaplan et al. 1985), x-ray studies such as upper gastrointestinal series (Marton et al. 1980), barium enema studies (MacEwan et al. 1978), chest x-rays (Hubbell et al. 1985), surgical procedures (such as tonsillectomies) (Roos et al. 1977), prescription drugs (Maronde et al. 1971), and nursing service orders (Vautrain and Griner 1978). In a recent study at our institution, faculty auditors reviewed medical records and estimated that some 21 percent of the more than 8,000 services ordered for 173 patients on the general medical wards were judged to be unnecessary. The most overused services included determinations of the partial thromboplastin time (deemed unnecessary 63 percent of the time), stat (emergency) orders (43 percent unnecessary), nuclear medicine studies (26 percent), and platelet counts (25 percent) (Myers et al. 1985).

Dixon and Laszlo, at the Veterans Administration Hospital in Durham, North Carolina, analyzed use of clinical laboratory tests for 25 patients on a general medical ward. They evaluated the value of each test according to four criteria of test utility: (1) did it generate an order for medication or other care? (2) were the test results considered in planning for subsequent care? (3) if test results were abnormal, was the test repeated? and (4) if test results were normal, did it exclude certain diagnoses? They found that only 5 percent of the tests met one or more of these criteria (Dixon and Laszlo 1974). Reports from other teaching and community hospitals have confirmed that as few as 3 to 5 percent of diagnostic tests are actually used in patient management (Griner and Liptzin 1971; Williams, Alexander, and Miller 1967).

Unplanned "natural experiments" have also allowed study of overuse of clinical technology. Griner, for example, compared the use of resources for adult patients with acute pulmonary edema the year before and the year after the opening of a medical intensive care unit at Strong Memorial Hospital in Rochester, New York. Although mortality remained constant at 8 percent during the two periods, the length of hospital stay increased by 2.3 days, the average hospital bill increased by 46 percent, and the use of clinical laboratory tests increased dramatically (including a fivefold increase in arterial blood gas determinations) (Griner 1972). In another example, at the Massachusetts General Hospital, an acute nursing shortage led to a marked reduction in medical intensive care unit beds, particularly for patients with potential new myocardial infarctions. The reduction in availability of beds led to tighter diagnostic criteria and a higher proportion of positive diagnoses among the patients admitted to the unit, but there were no significant differences in mortality rates (Singer et al. 1983).

These institutional case reports have four major limitations. First, they derive almost exclusively from academic medical centers and, within those centers, from internal medicine services. Whether similar results would be found in nonacademic centers and on noninternal medicine services is unclear. Second, these reports come predominantly from inpatient, as opposed to outpatient, settings. Third, they focus more upon little ticket items than upon big ticket services. Fourth, virtually all are studies of the fee-for-service sector. Finally, these case reports are asymmetric, reporting examples of service overuse much more often than examples of service underuse. One report from our institution reminds us of the potential for underutilizing necessary services: a group of clinical pathologists analyzed the care of 258 patients with anemia. They concluded that 29 percent of the cases had inadequate follow-up, and estimated that 25 percent had documented underuse of laboratory tests, while only 10 percent had overuse (Wheeler et al. 1977).

MAJOR DETERMINANTS OF PHYSICIAN USE OF MEDICAL TECHNOLOGY

What Are the Decisions Along the Way?

Figure 11.1 is a simplified schematic representation of the usual referral chain for a patient developing a serious illness (such as chronic renal failure) requiring diagnostic evaluation and subsequent ongoing management. The boxes are shaded according to the theoretical cost of the referral, with highest cost services and outcomes shaded darkest. Initially, the patient may present to a primary care physician, such as a family practitioner or internist. After a series of tests, the physician arrives at a diagnosis. The patient may then be treated medically, referred to a specialist (e.g., nephrologist), admitted to the hospital if necessary, or referred to an institution (renal dialysis unit or nursing home). The specialist may decide, independently, to admit the patient to the hospital. Once in the hospital, the patient may be transferred to an intensive care unit, or sent to surgery.

Using this basic model, the decision-making process for management of a variety of conditions can be better understood. Two other examples are illustrated in Figures 11.2 and 11.3. Care for a patient with symptomatic nephrolithiasis is shown in Figure 11.2: here the choice is between expectant (symptomatic) therapy and referral to a urologist for stone extraction, or, in some cases, to a center offering lithotripsy. Extraction may be performed through open surgery, endoscopically or percutaneously. Figure 11.3 illustrates care for a patient with symptomatic coronary artery disease: here the major decision is between medical therapy (generally the use of medications prescribed by the primary care physician or consulting internist or cardiologist) and referral for coronary arteriography. Based on the arteriography, coronary artery angioplasty or bypass grafting may be performed.

Obviously, in each of these examples, the early decisions (e.g., the patient's decision to seek care, or the physician's decision to refer) carry in their wake a series of further likelihoods and consequent costs. For example, the primary care physician's decision to refer the patient with

FIGURE 11.1

Simplified Example of the Referral Path
of a Patient with Symptoms

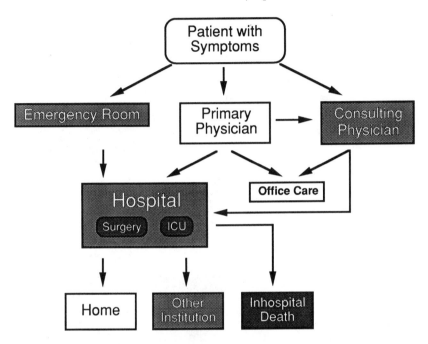

angina to a cardiologist carries a fairly high probability that the patient will have coronary angiography done, and once the anatomy is known, coronary artery bypass graft surgery or angioplasty. Yet many cost-containment efforts have been directed at physician decisions fairly far along the chain, such as the use of laboratory tests once the patient has been hospitalized. Perhaps because hospital administrators and other nonphysicians have been so involved in cost-containment efforts, and because it has not been apparent that the initial decisions could be readily debated, the most costly decisions (e.g., the decision to hospitalize the patient or to perform surgery) have been largely ignored in efforts to contain health care expenditures. Thus, given the number of treatment alternatives available, a major question now looming is whether expectant (symptomatic) therapy will continue to have a major role, for example, in the management of nephrolithiasis. A new technology is often adopted and used widely even before its benefits (and risks) have been proved (consider, for example, intracoronary streptokinase infusion) (Muller et al. 1981).

FIGURE 11.2

Simplified Example of the Referral Path
of a Patient with a Urinary Tract Stone

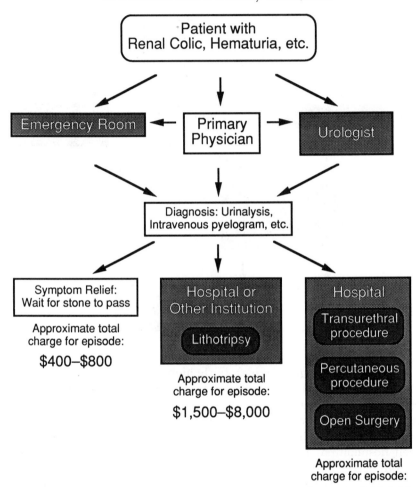

How and Why Are Decisions Made?

The factors that influence physicians to order medical services
include: (1) the belief that patient care will be improved; (2) the fear of
missing potentially important information; (3) concern for the individual patient outweighing concern for conserving society's resources;
(4) uncertainty in medical decision making; (5) patient demand; (6) peer

FIGURE 11.3

Simplified Example of the Referral Path
of a Patient with Angina

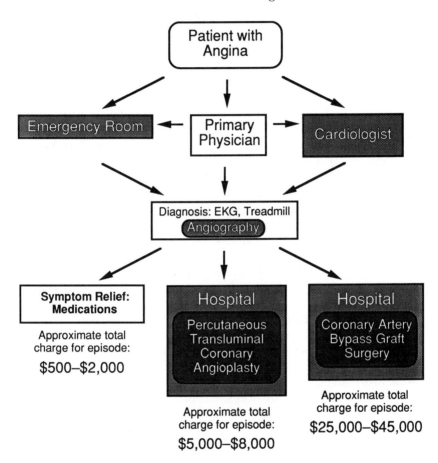

pressure; (7) medicolegal considerations; and (8) financial incentives (Eisenberg 1979; Schroeder 1980).

The first, and probably most important, of these influences is the belief that employing diagnostic or therapeutic technology will improve patient outcomes. The physician is faced with a wide, and ever-expanding, array of diagnostic tests and therapeutic procedures from which to choose in caring for patients, who are increasingly elderly and frail. Particularly in the inpatient setting, this combination creates powerful incentives to order more tests and procedures for diagnosis and monitoring.

Almost as powerful an influence is the physician's fear of missing important information. Interestingly, many physicians are more concerned about omitting a possibly useful diagnostic test or therapeutic procedure than potentially harming patients by performing an unnecessary (and risky) test or procedure; and in clinical practice, physicians often seem to order tests and procedures without clear-cut regard to their potential risks.

Medical decision making is inherently limited by uncertainty. Several recent studies have shown that many, and perhaps most, physicians have difficulty thinking in probabilistic terms; they often exhibit particular difficulty with interpreting sensitivity and specificity of diagnostic tests, and with the predictive value of positive or negative results (McPhee et al. 1982; Casscells, Schoenberger, and Graboys 1978; Tversky and Kahneman 1974). Uncertainty about the significance and appropriate clinical use of laboratory tests, hence, may contribute to their overuse.

Fear of malpractice litigation may be responsible for physicians' use of some technologies (Wertman et al. 1980). The rapid increase in use of fetal scalp monitoring has been cited as one example of such "defensive medicine." Unfortunately, no good data exist to document the importance of defensive medicine in daily clinical practice (Tancredi and Barondess 1978). However, many physicians, especially in such specialties as emergency medicine, plastic surgery, anesthesiology, and obstetrics, perceive malpractice as a persuasive reason to order services having a very low probability of contributing to patient welfare (Hershey 1972; Denson and Manning 1982).

Peer pressure to order more, rather than fewer, services exists in some settings. Physicians may be reluctant, for example, not to order tests or procedures suggested by consultants (McPhee et al. 1984b).

Financial incentives to order use of technologies may be either obvious or subtle. Internists in private practice may double or triple their net incomes by conducting more office laboratory or diagnostic procedures. Reimbursement rates for such procedures are often much higher than for physician time in direct patient care, thus further encouraging the use of such tests (Schroeder and Showstack 1978; Almy 1981). More financial pressure to order tests for inpatients existed in the era of retrospective reimbursement; hospital laboratories were relative "profit centers" in which to recover costs of other hospital services. Only recently, with the introduction of prospective reimbursement systems, have counter-incentives to the use of technologies begun to emerge, at least within the hospital setting.

The large international differences in the use of various technologies undoubtedly have complex causes, reflecting different levels of investment in physician specialists and equipment (Schroeder 1984a;

Schroeder, Myers, and McPhee et al. 1984) as well as different expectations by patients and physicians (Sox, Margulies, and Sox 1981; Challah et al. 1984). Similarly, regional differences in surgical rates may reflect differences in practice styles, differences in concentrations of specialists, and differences in patient expectations. As Eisenberg describes, there are also sociologic influences on clinical decision making, including patient characteristics, physician characteristics, the doctor-patient relationship, and the professional role of the physician (Eisenberg 1979).

Upon reflection, it is clear that most of these factors tend to encourage physicians to use new technologies as they become available rather than maintaining more traditional or conservative approaches. There may, however, be good medical reasons to restrain the adoption, or limit the use, of new technologies. Each new technology carries its own risks of untoward complications and potential for long-term unexpected outcomes. As more physicians begin to perform new techniques, there is a larger proportion of physicians who do relatively few procedures, and often lower volumes imply greater risks (Luft et al. 1979; Maerki et al. 1986). So, for example, while published estimates of in-hospital mortality for coronary artery bypass graft surgery in academic centers averages 3 to 5 percent, careful review of data from unselected hospitals shows that mortalities may be considerably higher in low-volume hospitals (fewer than 100 procedures per year) (Showstack, Rosenfeld, and Garnick 1987). Perhaps cognizant of this volume-outcome relationship, the American College of Surgeons, in its guidelines for minimal standards in cardiac surgery, states that the performance of at least 150 open-heart operations per year by an independent team is desirable (American College of Surgeons 1984).

There may also be good financial reasons to limit adoption or use of new technologies. For example, specialists performing gastrointestinal endoscopy may charge less than surgeons or general internists performing the same procedure (Showstack and Schroeder 1981), and having fewer specialists who are allowed to perform procedures also enables HMOs to limit the use of such procedures (Luft 1981).

MODIFYING PHYSICIAN USE OF TECHNOLOGY

Physicians remain the dominant clinical decision-makers. Until recently, physicians have been allowed to order tests, procedures, and therapies without regard to cost, almost as if in an expensive restaurant from a menu without prices. In trying now to affect these decisions, the health policymaker must really answer two questions. First, what are the best places to intervene along the continuum of care? And second, what are the most potent interventions?

The discussion above highlights some of the places where intervention might be effective, but the cost consequences of such interventions are difficult to predict. On the one hand, it is difficult to estimate the costs entrained by referral of a patient with angina to a cardiologist; on the other, it is difficult to assign cost values to withholding the potential benefits of angiography and surgery and allowing the patient to live out the natural history of the disease. It is even more difficult to examine the trade-offs that must be occurring now that the health care budget has become limited. Consider the dilemma imposed by realizing that the $45,000 average cost for one coronary bypass hospital stay is approximately the cost of ensuring adequate prenatal care for enough low-income women to result in the birth of one less low-birth-weight infant (who might have required a prolonged and expensive stay in a neonatal intensive care unit) or of hiring three full-time home health aides for homebound and disabled elderly.

The evidence regarding specific methods of modifying physician use of technology is reviewed in detail below. Theoretically, the most potent interventions would either offer the physician financial incentives to change behavior, or would encourage their behavioral change through organizational and structural changes. Examples of both approaches are found in managed care systems such as HMOs. The first approach is illustrated by the proposal to control health care costs by enlisting primary care physicians as gatekeepers to medical care. In such systems, primary care physicians would approve all nonemergency care provided to their patients (Eisenberg 1985b). The second approach is illustrated by the constraints imposed by HMOs (e.g., limited number of subspecialists, queues, and use of nonphysician substitutes such as nurse practitioners). More recently, in the fee-for-service sector, preferred provider organizations have provided a mechanism for restraining physicians who prove to be "high utilizers" (e.g., through exclusion from closed panels, contract nonrenewal, and so on).

What Works?

Table 11.1 shows the four broad strategies for changing physicians' use of medical technologic services: education, audit-with-feedback, barriers (and other administrative maneuvers), and rewards (financial incentives) (McPhee et al. 1982; Myers and Schroeder 1981; Eisenberg and Williams 1981).

Education. Educational strategies are predicated upon the assumption that educating physicians about service or test characteristics, indications, contraindications, yields, and costs will result in decreased, and

TABLE 11.1
Strategies for Reducing Costs by Changing Physician Behavior

Strategy	Level of Impact	Type of Intervention	Success of Intervention
Education	National/ regional	"Voluntary effort"	Unsuccessful
	Institutional	Lectures, materials, etc.	Generally unsuccessful
Audit with feedback	National/ regional	PSROs, geographic profiles, etc.	Scanty experience, mixed results
	Institutional	Medical record reviews, comparison of practice patterns	Mixed results
Barriers/ administrative maneuvers	National/ regional	Certificate-of-need, FDA approval, insurance coverage decisions	Successful, if applied rigorously
	Institutional	Restrictions, rationing, administrative barriers	Implementation difficulties limit applicability
Financial incentives	National/ regional	HMOs, DRGs, prospective payment schemes	Very successful
	Institutional	Bonuses, penalties	Little experience

more appropriate, patterns of use. Education was most notably used at the national level during the late 1970s when the American Hospital Association and organized medicine promoted a much publicized "Voluntary Effort" aimed at reducing costs in all U.S. hospitals. During this effort, educational materials were distributed as handouts, presented at rounds at hospitals, and disseminated as videotapes across the country.

At the institutional level, educational strategies have usually been aimed at physicians (most often house officers in internal medicine) and evaluated in experimental fashion. These studies have evaluated the effects upon test ordering and service use of education about the costs of various laboratory and other hospital services, about test characteristics and principles of decision analysis, and about indications for appropriate use of specific services (McPhee et al. 1982; Myers and Schroeder 1981; Eisenberg and Williams 1981). The efficacy of such educational approaches is unclear. At the national level, it seems fair to say that educating physicians failed to contain costs. During the Voluntary Effort of the late 1970s, the costs of medical care continued to rise faster than costs elsewhere in the economy. At the institutional level, educational efforts have sometimes been successful in decreasing use of services; however, these successes have often been modest or short-lived (Rhyne and Gehlbach 1979; Eisenberg 1977). In addition, some of the studies have been uncontrolled (Lyle et al. 1979; Griner 1979), while others have reported failure (Grossman 1983; Schroeder et al. 1984; Williams and Eisenberg 1986).

Audit-with-Feedback. Audit-with-feedback strategies at the regional level have most often involved distributing information about variations in practice patterns (e.g., tonsillectomy rates) to physicians within a defined geographical area (state or province) (Wennberg 1984; Roos 1984). Within institutions, a variety of feedback strategies have been employed. Some have been simply informational, highlighting differences in individual service use profiles (for example, comparing individual physicians' current service use patterns to their own past performance or to that of their peers). Others have focused upon management decisions of physicians for actual cases (Schroeder et al. 1973; Martin et al. 1980; Schroeder et al. 1984; Everett et al. 1983).

Experience with such feedback strategies has been limited. At the regional level, Brook demonstrated that audit and feedback of the patterns of antibiotic use for Medicaid patients to a group of New Mexico physicians led to less use of injections and specific antibiotics; the program failed to reduce costs, however (Brook and Williams 1976). Elsewhere, declines in surgery rates have been attributed to distribution of profiles of physicians' rates of operations (Wennberg and Gittelsohn 1982; Wennberg 1984; Dyck et al. 1977). There have been several reports of successful audit-with-feedback approaches at the institutional level. Martin and colleagues, in a study of the effect of medical record review at the Brigham and Women's Hospital in Boston, found that audited physicians decreased their use of laboratory tests by 47 percent compared to a concurrent control group (Martin et al. 1980). However, similar studies elsewhere have shown this approach to be only marginally effective (Everett et al. 1983) or ineffective (Williams and Eisenberg 1986; Schroeder et al. 1984). Another study showed that feedback of laboratory test utilization patterns to faculty internists in an outpatient general medical practice led to a short-term 29 percent reduction in costs. It was not determined if this effect was sustained (Schroeder et al. 1973).

Barriers. Barriers and other administrative maneuvers of several kinds have been used as cost-containment measures. Nationally, certificate of need and other mechanisms have been used to constrain the number of hospital intensive care units and the purchase of very expensive equipment such as CT scanners. The Food and Drug Administration influences directly the availability of new drugs. Through their decisions to pay for such services, government and third-party insurers have affected the use of medical technologies such as hemodialysis, heart transplantation, and magnetic resonance imaging. Abroad, political decisions about selection of patients for technologies such as renal dialysis and transplantation, decisions about payment and eligibility coverage for certain benefits, and decisions about the supplies of medical specialists and equipment have served explicitly or implicitly to ration services (Challah et al. 1984; Schwartz and Aaron 1984).

At the institutional level, administrative barriers of several kinds have been used as cost-containment measures. Barriers have taken the form of explicit limits (e.g., maximum numbers of laboratory tests per unit time) (Dixon and Laszlo 1974), restrictions on choice (e.g., drug formularies), obstacles to obtaining certain services (e.g., specific forms or prior approval required for specific drugs or tests) (Gray and Marion 1973), or the elimination of packaged services (e.g., the unbundling of multichannel laboratory tests).

Evidence for the effectiveness of administrative barriers at the national level has been mixed. Certificate-of-need legislation was not effective in limiting the diffusion of CT scanners. The Food and Drug Administration, however, has had considerable influence upon introduction of new drugs, and third-party payers have had a strong influence upon use of new diagnostic and therapeutic technologies. When Medicare undertook to fund the costs of care for patients with end-stage renal disease, for example, there was an unexpected increase in the number of such patients. On the other hand, the constraints upon dialysis facilities in the United Kingdom have meant that far fewer patients with end-stage renal disease receive adequate treatment (Challah et al. 1984).

Administrative barriers may be more difficult to introduce at the institutional level, but they have sometimes been efficacious. Dixon and Laszlo, by restricting the number of laboratory tests per patient, were able to effect a two-thirds reduction in test volume (Dixon and Laszlo 1974). By requiring prior approval from a hematologist, Gray and Marion decreased use of several coagulation studies (Gray and Marion 1973). Recently, at the University of California, San Francisco, the unbundling of a multichannel blood chemistry panel (the SMA-12) led to a 45 percent decrease in the use of tests on the panel, and a 35 percent decline in laboratory tests per inpatient day (Cohen 1986). Anecdotal evidence suggests that many hospitals have considered such administrative barriers, but rejected them as too difficult to implement.

Rewards. Finally, financial incentives to contain costs have been tried at the national level for both hospitals and physicians. Recent prospective payment schemes have created incentives to decrease the length of hospital stay and the costs per case. Health maintenance organizations often provide financial incentives to physicians to lower their use of medical resources, especially hospital care. Perhaps because of ethical constraints, financial incentives have seldom been used at the institutional level. Where they have been tested, incentives have usually been in the form of rewards such as textbooks, or subscriptions to journals, in exchange for lowering use of resources (Martin et al. 1980).

Financial incentives to institutions appear to be very powerful in their secondary effect upon physician behavior. Regionally, HMOs are able to limit both hospital days and hospital admissions. Nationally, the recent change to prospective hospital payment for Medicare patients has been associated with a dramatic 29 percent decline in length of hospital stay, from 10.4 days in 1981 to 7.4 days in 1984. At the institutional level, there have been few comparable trials, and the few available have generally not reported significant effects upon resource use (Martin et al. 1980).

At What Level?

Interventions to constrain physician use of medical technologies may be undertaken at several different levels: (1) at the national level (e.g., changes in the Medicare program to develop a prospective system of hospital payment, or decisions by insurance carriers to cover costs for organ transplantation or magnetic resonance imaging); (2) at the state or local government level (e.g., decisions to restrict services provided to Medicaid patients); (3) at the hospital level (e.g., decisions to acquire new and expensive technologies, such as lithotripsy); (4) at the physician level (e.g., incentives to refer or not to refer patients for coronary angioplasty); and (5) at the patient level (e.g., decisions to seek elective surgical therapy such as total hip replacement or cataract removal).

At What Price?

Are the cost savings of a program worth the effort or cost of implementing that program? While several studies have suggested that interventions aimed at containing costs may have some benefit, they also have their price. In our recent study of a hospital cost-control program, we analyzed the implementation costs of its six mutually reinforcing components. Implementation costs varied: they were high for medical record audits and periodic cost summaries, moderate for educational lectures, and low for provision of price booklets, patient bills, and reading materials (McPhee et al. 1984a). The cost savings resulting from the program, however, were relatively modest compared to the estimated dollar costs of conducting the interventions.

WHAT REMAINS TO BE DONE?

Several major questions remain unanswered. First, if cost-containment strategies aimed at physicians are successful, how will they affect quality of care? In general, cost-containment efforts stem from the perception that considerable amounts of unnecessary, and expensive, care are provided. Eliminating such unnecessary care, the theory says, would reduce costs without compromising patient welfare. The aim of cost-containment strategies, to "cut the fat, but preserve the muscle," is illustrated in a simplified fashion in Figure 11.4 (Enthoven 1978; Schroe-

FIGURE 11.4

The Relationship between Increasing Medical Care and Outcomes

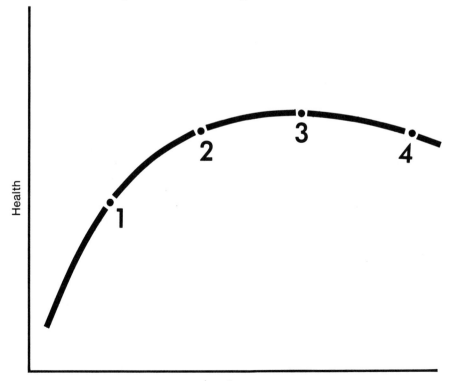

der 1985). Improved outcomes presumably result from an initial increase in medical resources provided (moving from point 1 to point 2); however, as more services are provided, the point of diminishing returns is reached (point 3); provision of still more care may then result in adverse patient outcomes (such as clinical iatrogenesis, point 4). Any reduction in costs due to restrictions of services between points 1 and 3, however, may come at the price of eliminating necessary care.

It has become clear that this theory may be too simplistic. The distribution of medical care is unequal, so that while one segment of the population is at or beyond the point of diminishing return, another is still reaping benefits from resources spent for additional care. In rural areas, in inner cities, and for the underinsured and uninsured, attempts to reduce medical costs by restricting physician use of technology may result in poorer clinical outcomes. It is important to remember that the U.S. population is more heterogeneous in demographic characteristics and health status than the populations of other Western countries, as evidenced by the twofold differences in U.S. infant mortality rates between blacks and whites and the appreciably longer life expectancy for whites than blacks.

Certainly more research is needed regarding the enhancement of quality of life by various technologies (we need both more functional status measures and better measures of quality of care in general). Research should be expanded to include the reasons for untoward events that result from the use of technological procedures (e.g., the relatively high rates of death and permanent disability in patients undergoing coronary artery bypass graft surgery). Such quality of care research will undoubtedly need to be tailored to fit the needs of the payment system (e.g., in prospective payment systems, such as HMOs, potential under-utilization must be monitored) and the various "high risk" patient groups (e.g., timely referral of the elderly for cataract removal).

Another unanswered question is whether the "little vs. big ticket" debate is too narrowly focused. At one time there was hope that costs could be substantially reduced merely by eliminating unnecessary little ticket technologies, such as laboratory tests (Moloney and Rogers 1979). Recent studies at our institution suggest that this may not be a productive cost-containment strategy. For 2,011 patients with one of ten common inpatient diagnoses, we compared the use of clinical services in 1972, 1977, and 1982. Contrary to conventional wisdom, for most of the diagnoses studied, use of clinical laboratory tests and standard radiology procedures generally remained the same or declined. Practice patterns did change in several important ways that resulted in major increases in medical costs. For example, in 1982, a much larger proportion of patients with acute myocardial infarction received Holter monitoring, coronary arteriography, coronary angioplasty, intra-coronary streptokinase, and coronary artery bypass graft surgery (Showstack, Hughes-Stone, and Schroeder 1985).

This latter study provided evidence that use of little ticket services may not be changing much over time and may not constitute a significant proportion of the hospital bill. While use of big ticket items may be increasing for some diagnoses, even these services may not account for a large proportion of the hospital bill. Indeed, as causes of rising costs, both little ticket and big ticket technologies may pale in comparison to five critical decisions: (1) to admit a patient to the hospital, (2) to transfer to the intensive care unit, (3) to perform surgery, (4) to place in a long-term care facility, or (5) to sustain life in terminal illness. Each of these decisions triggers a predictable cascade of medical expenditures. Interventions having an impact upon these five major clinical decisions are therefore more likely to be successful in containing costs than are policies aimed at the use of specific technologies. To date, few educational or administrative strategies for cost containment have focused upon any of these crucial clinical decisions. Feedback strategies have concentrated either on decisions with relatively few cost implications such as laboratory test use, or on the decisions to perform surgery. Only financial strategies (at the national level) have addressed most of these decisions.

A major limitation of virtually all of the experiences reviewed earlier is that they were conducted at a time of retrospective reimbursement. In our new era of fixed-cost contracts and prospective case-based payment systems, which may provide powerful incentives to reduce the use of services, these strategies might yield different results. The new prospective payment schemes are, in fact, potentially powerful ways both to contain costs and to ration technology use. At the same time, these new schemes create a new responsibility, to guarantee that appropriate and cost-effective treatment is provided.

As new, less invasive technologies (such as lithotripsy) are developed, they can be applied to nonhospitalized patients. This may result in increasing costs of care, both as complications from such procedures are incurred and as indications for such procedures are broadened to include patients who are minimally symptomatic or asymptomatic.

Still unknown is the impact upon hospitals of advances in diagnosis and treatment and of the pressures to contain costs. It may be that these factors result in an increase in the average severity of illness (and therefore, paradoxically, an increase in costs) for hospitalized patients, as less severely ill patients are treated in an outpatient setting.

Other important questions must be answered. How should new medical technologies enter the scene, and what happens when they do (e.g., are they, in the aggregate, additive or substitutive)? Can the effects of new technological advances upon the content of medical practice be predicted? How should physicians already in practice be trained to use new technologies appropriately, and how can they learn to deal with the increasingly rapid pace of technological change? Should incentives be provided to encourage physicians to use the least costly and least risky approaches to a given problem? How can technical quality be ensured as increasing numbers of physicians adopt new technologies, and as the numbers of procedures performed by individual physicians decline? How can we modify the patient expectations of the medical care system that developed at a time when the health care budget was not constrained? And finally, have the easy targets for cost containment already been hit, leaving much more difficult questions, such as whether care should be rationed by, for example, withdrawing care for the terminally ill?

REFERENCES

Almy, T. P. (1981). "The Role of the Primary Physician in the Health-Care 'Industry'." *New England Journal of Medicine* 304: 1413–19.

American College of Surgeons Bulletin (1984). *Guidelines for Minimal Standards in Cardiac Surgery.* Chicago: The College.

Banta, H. D., and Kemp, K. B. (eds.) (1980). "The Implications of Cost-Effectiveness Analysis of Medical Technology," Background Paper #4. In *The Management of Health Care Technology in Ten Countries,* 119–40. Washington, DC: U.S. Congress, Office of Technology Assessment.

Brook, R. H., and Williams, K. N. (1976). "Effect of Medical Care Review on the Use of Injections: A Study of the New Mexico Experimental Medical Care Review Organization." *Annals of Internal Medicine* 85: 509–15.

Casscells, W.; Schoenberger, A; and Graboys, T. B. (1978). "Interpretation by Physicians of Clinical Laboratory Results." *New England Journal of Medicine* 299: 999–1001.

Challah, S.; Wing, A. J.; Bauer, R.; Morris, R. W.; and Schroeder, S. A. (1984). "Negative Selection of Patients for Dialysis and Transplantation in the United Kingdom." *British Medical Journal* 228: 1119–22.

Cohen, S. N. (1986). Personal communication.

Denson, T. A., and Manning, P. R. (1982). "Current Problems in Medical Practice as Viewed by California Physicians." *Western Journal of Medicine* 136: 369–72.

Devitt, J. E., and Ironside, M. R. (1975). "Can Patient Care Audit Change Doctor Performance?" *Journal of Medical Education* 50: 1122–23.

Dixon, R. H., and Laszlo, J. (1974). "Utilization of Clinical Chemistry Services by Medical House Staff: An Analysis." *Archives of Internal Medicine* 134: 1064–67.

Dyck, F. J.; Murphy, F. A.; Murphy, J. K.; et al. (1977). "Effect of Surveillance on the Number of Hysterectomies in the Province of Saskatchewan." *New England Journal of Medicine* 296: 1326–28.

Eisenberg, J. M. (1977). "An Educational Program to Modify Laboratory Use by House Staff." *Journal of Medical Education* 52: 578–81.

———— (1979). "Sociologic Influences on Decision-Making by Clinicians." *Annals of Internal Medicine* 90: 957–64.

———— (1985a). "Physician Utilization: The State of Research About Physicians' Practice Patterns." *Medical Care* 23: 461–83.

———— (1985b). "The Internist as Gatekeeper: Preparing the General Internist for a New Role." *Annals of Internal Medicine* 102: 537–43.

Eisenberg, J. M., and Williams, S. V. (1981). "Cost Containment and Changing Physicians' Practice Behavior: Can the Fox Learn to Guard the Chicken Coop?" *Journal of the American Medical Association* 246: 2195–2201.

Eisenberg, J. M.; Williams, S. V.; Garner, L.; et al. (1977). "Computer-Based Audit to Detect and Correct Overutilization of Laboratory Tests." *Medical Care* 15: 915–21.

Enthoven, A. C. (1978). "Shattuck Lecture: Cutting Cost without Cutting the Quality of Care." *New England Journal of Medicine* 298: 1229–38.

Everett, G. D.; deBlois, S.; Chang, P. F.; et al. (1983). "Effect of Cost Education, Cost Audits, and Faculty Chart Review on the Use of Laboratory Services." *Archives of Internal Medicine* 143: 942–44.

Fineberg, H. C. (1979). "Clinical Chemistries: The High Cost of Low-Cost Diagnostic Tests." In *Medical Technology: The Culprit Behind Health Care Costs?* ed. S. H. Altman and R. Blendon, 145–65. U.S. Department of Health, Education, and Welfare Publication No. (PHS) 79-3216. Washington, DC: U.S. Government Printing Office.

Freeborn, D. K.; Baer, D.; Greenlick, M. R.; et al. (1972). "Determinants of Medical Care Utilization: Physicians' Use of Laboratory Services." *American Journal of Public Health* 62: 846–53.

Freeland, M. S., and Schendler, C. E. (1983). "National Health Expenditure Growth in the 1980's: An Aging Population, New Technologies, and Increasing Competition." *Health Care Financing Review* 4 (3): 1–58.

Gray, G., and Marion, R. (1973). "Utilization of a Hematology Laboratory in a Teaching Hospital." *American Journal of Clinical Pathology* 59: 877–82.

Griner, P. F. (1972). "Treatment of Acute Pulmonary Edema: Conventional or Intensive Care." *Annals of Internal Medicine* 77: 501–6.

Griner, P. F., and Liptzin, B. (1971). "Use of the Laboratory in a Teaching Hospital: Implications for Patient Care, Education and Hospital Costs." *Annals of Internal Medicine* 75: 157–63.

Griner, P. F., and Medical House Staff, Strong Memorial Hospital (1979). "Use of Laboratory Tests in a Teaching Hospital: Long Term Trends—Reductions in Use and Relative Cost." *Annals of Internal Medicine* 90: 243–48.

Grossman, R. M. (1983). "A Review of Physician Cost-Containment Strategies for Laboratory Testing." *Medical Care* 21: 783–802.

Hershey, N. (1972). "The Defensive Practice of Medicine: Myth or Reality?" *Milbank Memorial Fund Quarterly* 50: 69–98.

Hubbell, F. A.; Greenfield, S.; Tyler, J. L.; et al. (1985). "The Impact of Routine Admission Chest X-Ray Films on Patient Care." *New England Journal of Medicine* 312: 209–13.

Kaplan, E. B.; Sheiner, L. B.; Boeckmann, A. J.; et al. (1985). "The Usefulness of Preoperative Laboratory Screening." *Journal of the American Medical Association* 253: 3576–81.

Lewis, C. E. (1969). "Variations in the Incidence of Surgery." *New England Journal of Medicine* 281: 880–84.

Luft, H. S. (1978). "How Do Health-Maintenance Organizations Achieve Their 'Savings'? Rhetoric and Evidence." *New England Journal of Medicine* 298: 1336–43.

————— (1981). *Health Maintenance Organizations: Dimensions of Performance.* New York: Wiley–Interscience.

Luft, H. S.; Bunker, J.; Enthoven, A.; et al. (1979). "Should Operations Be Regionalized? An Empirical Study of the Relation between Surgical Volume and Mortality." *New England Journal of Medicine* 301: 1364–69.

Lyle, C. B.; Bianchi, R. F.; Harris, J. H.; et al. (1979). "Teaching Cost Containment to House Officers." *Journal of Medical Education* 54: 856–62.

MacEwan, D. W.; Kavanagh, S.; Chow, P.; et al. (1978). "Manitoba Barium Enema Efficacy Study." *Radiology* 126: 39–44.

Maerki, S. C.; Luft, H. S.; Hunt, S. S.; et al. (1986). "Selecting Categories of Patients for Regionalization: Implications of the Relationship between Volume and Outcome." *Medical Care* 24: 148–58.

Maronde, R. F.; Lee, P. V.; McCarron, M. M.; et al. (1971). "A Study of Prescribing Patterns." *Medical Care* 9: 383–95.

Martin, A. R.; Wolf, M. A.; Thibodeau, L. A.; et al. (1980). "A Trial of Two Strategies to Modify the Test-Ordering Behavior of Medical Residents." *New England Journal of Medicine* 303: 1330–36.

Marton, K. I.; Sox, H. C.; Wasson, J. H.; et al. (1980). "The Clinical Value of the Upper Gastrointestinal Tract Roentgenogram Series." *Archives of Internal Medicine* 140: 191–95.

McPhee, S. J.; Chapman, S. A.; Myers, L. P.; et al. (1984a). "Lessons for Teaching Cost-Containment." *Journal of Medical Education* 59: 722–29.

McPhee, S. J.; Myers, L. P.; Lo, B.; et al. (1984b). "Cost-Containment Confronts Physicians." *Annals of Internal Medicine* 100: 604–6.

McPhee, S. J.; Myers, L. P.; Schroeder, S. A.; et al. (1982). "The Costs and Risks of Medical Care: An Annotated Bibliography for Clinicians and Educators." *Western Journal of Medicine* 137: 145–61.

Moloney, T. W., and Rogers, D. E. (1979). "Medical Technology: A Different View of the Contentious Debate over Costs." *New England Journal of Medicine* 301: 1413–19.

Muller, J. E.; Stone, P. H.; Markis, J. E.; et al. (1981). "Let's Not Let the Genie Escape from the Bottle—Again." *New England Journal of Medicine* 304: 1294–96.

Myers, L. P.; Chapman, S. A.; McPhee, S. J.; et al. (1985). "Which Hospital Services are Most Overused? Results from a Medical Audit." *Western Journal of Medicine* 143: 397–98.

Myers, L. P., and Schroeder, S. A. (1981). "Physician Use of Services for the Hospitalized Patient: A Review, with Implications for Cost Containment." *Milbank Memorial Fund Quarterly* 59: 481–507.

Parkerson, G. R., Jr. (1978). "Cost Analysis of Laboratory Tests in Ambulatory Primary Care." *Journal of Family Practice* 7: 1001–7.

Rhyne, R. L., and Gehlbach, S. H. (1979). "Effects of an Educational Strategy on Physician Utilization of Thyroid Function Panels." *Journal of Family Practice* 8: 1003–7.

Rimm, A. A. (1985). "Trends in Cardiac Surgery in the United States" (Letter to the editor). *New England Journal of Medicine* 312: 119–20.

Roos, N. P. (1984). "Hysterectomy: Variation in Rates across Small Areas and across Physicians' Practices." *American Journal of Public Health* 74: 327–33.

Roos, N. P.; Henteloff, P. D.; and Roos, L. L. (1977). "A New Audit Procedure Applied to an Old Question: Is the Frequency of T&A Justified?" *Medical Care* 15: 1–18.

Schroeder, S. A. (1980). "Variations in Physician Practice Patterns: A Review of Medical Cost Implications." In *The Physician and Cost Control,* ed. E. Carels,

D. Neuhauser, and W. Stason, 23–50. Cambridge, MA: Oelgeschlager, Gunn & Hain.

———— (1984a). "Western European Responses to Physician Oversupply: Lessons for the United States." *Journal of the American Medical Association* 252: 373–84.

———— (1984b). "How Do Western European Hospitals Compare with the United States: A Case Report from Leuven, West Berlin, Leiden, London and San Francisco." *Journal of the American Medical Association* 252: 240–46.

———— (1985). "Doctors and the Medical Cost Crisis: Culprits, Victims, or Solution." *The Pharos of Alpha Omega Alpha* 48: 12–18.

Schroeder, S. A.; Kenders, K.; Cooper, J. K.; et al. (1973). "Use of Laboratory Tests and Pharmaceuticals: Variation among Physicians and Effect of Cost Audit on Subsequent Use." *Journal of the American Medical Association* 225: 969–73.

Schroeder, S. A.; Myers, L. P.; McPhee, S. J.; et al. (1984). "The Failure of Physician Education as a Cost Containment Strategy." *Journal of the American Medical Association* 252: 225–30.

Schroeder, S. A., and Showstack, J. A. (1978). "Financial Incentives to Perform Medical Procedures and Laboratory Tests: Illustrative Models of Office Practice." *Medical Care* 16: 289–98.

Schwartz, W. B., and Aaron, H. J. (1984). "Rationing Hospital Care: Lessons from Britain." *New England Journal of Medicine* 310: 52–56.

Scitovsky, A. A. (1979). "Changes in the Use of Ancillary Services for 'Common' Illness." In *Medical Technology: The Culprit Behind Health Care Costs?* ed. S. H. Altman and R. Blendon, 39–56. U.S. Dept. of Health, Education, and Welfare Publication No. (PHS) 79-3216. Washington, DC: U.S. Government Printing Office.

Shapiro, M. F.; Hatch, R. C.; and Greenfield, S. (1984). "Cost Containment and Labor-Intensive Tests: The Case of the Leukocyte Differential Count." *Journal of the American Medical Association* 252: 231–34.

Showstack, J. A.; Hughes-Stone, M.; and Schroeder, S. A. (1985). "The Role of Changing Clinical Practices in the Rising Costs of Hospital Care." *New England Journal of Medicine* 313: 1201–7.

Showstack, J. A.; Rosenfeld, K. E.; and Garnick, D. W. (1987). "Association of Volume with Outcome of Coronary Artery Bypass Graft Surgery: Scheduled vs. Nonscheduled Operations." *Journal of the American Medical Association* 257: 785–89.

Showstack, J. A., and Schroeder, S. A. (1981)."Case Study #8: The Cost-Effectiveness of Upper Gastrointestinal Endoscopy; Background Paper #2: Case Studies of Medical Technology." In *The Implications of Cost-Effectiveness Analysis of Medical Technology.* Washington, DC: U.S. Congress, Office of Technology Assessment,

Singer, D. E.; Carr, P. C.; Mulley, A. G.; et al. (1983). "Rationing Intensive Care: Physician Responses to a Resource Shortage." *New England Journal of Medicine* 309: 1155–60.

Sox, H.; Margulies, I.; and Sox, C. H. (1981). "Psychologically Mediated Effects of Diagnostic Tests." *Annals of Internal Medicine* 95: 680–85.

Steinberg, E. P.; Dans, P. E.; Keruly, J. C.; et al. (1986). "A Case Study of Physicians' Use of Liver-Spleen Scans: Are We Doing What We Think We Are?" *Archives of Internal Medicine* 146: 253–58.

Tancredi, L. R., and Barondess, J. A. (1978). "The Problem of Defensive Medicine." *Science* 200: 879–82.

Tversky, A., and Kahneman, D. (1974). "Judgement under Uncertainty: Heuristics and Biases." *Science* 185: 1124–31.

U.S. Congress (Office of Technology Assessment) (1984). *Medical Technology and Costs of Medical Care.* Washington, DC: Office of Technology Assessment, July.

Vautrain, R. C., and Griner, P. F. (1978). "Physicians' Orders: Use of Nursing Resources, and Subsequent Clinical Events." *Journal of Medical Education* 53: 125–28.

Wennberg, J. E. (1984). "Dealing with Medical Practice Variations: A Proposal for Action." *Health Affairs* 3: 6–32.

Wennberg, J. E., and Gittelsohn, A. (1982). "Variations in Medical Care among Small Areas." *Scientific American* 246: 120–33.

Wertman, B. G.; Sostrin, S. V.; Pavlova, Z.; et al. (1980). "Why Do Physicians Order Laboratory Tests? A Study of Laboratory Test Requests and Use Patterns." *Journal of the American Medical Association* 243: 2080–82.

Wheeler, L. A.; Brecher, G.; and Steiner, L. B. (1977). "Clinical Laboratory Use in the Evaluation of Anemia." *Journal of the American Medical Association* 238: 2709–14.

Williams, J. W.; Alexander, M.; and Miller, G. E. (1967). "Continuing Education and Patient Care Research: Physician Response to Screening Test Results." *Journal of the American Medical Association* 201:118–22.

Williams, S. V., and Eisenberg, J. M. (1986). "A Controlled Trial to Decrease the Unnecessary Use of Diagnostic Tests." *Journal of General Internal Medicine* 1: 8–13.

Chapter 12

*Altering Medical Resource Utilization:
The Economic Ironies of Charges and
Costs in Teaching Hospitals*

Carl B. Lyle, Jr., William D. Mattern, Edith E.
Bragdon, and Jack D. McCue

Editor's Note—When physicians limit the amount of medical
services provided to inpatients as they attempt to reduce the expense of medical
care, *charges* are reduced to third-party insurers, who will pay for about 80
percent of all hospital-related expenses. But a small portion of those charges
(usually about one-third) represents the hospital's *costs* that can be directly allocated to performing that test, and most of those costs are for labor, not for
supplies. Hypothetically, if we influence physicians to order one fewer $30 test,
the insurance company saves $30; but the hospital might lose $20 of "profit"
that would be used to subsidize other services such as social workers, education,
or patient comfort-related amenities. The materials saved by not doing the test
would be only $2, and they represent a true cost savings to the hospital. The
hospital has contracted to supply $8 of labor to draw the blood, do the test, and
record the result, so unless that labor can be deployed elsewhere, the hospital
has sustained an $8 loss in money that it must pay out whether the test is ordered
or not. In addition, it must make up for the lost $20 profit that has been used
to subsidize other services. Over time, changes work out—the labor is rede-
ployed, and laboratory space is used differently. Over the short run, however,
everyone but the insurer probably loses.

Lyle et al. argue that, as we make cost-containment recommendations, they
must be made with administrative cooperation. Otherwise, the lost charges are
just added on to the charge of some other service so that budgetary needs can
still be met. In addition, Lyle was one of the first researchers to demonstrate
that when the fat has been trimmed, only muscle and bone remain. Costs will
then rise at about the same rate as before the cost-cutting efforts were made.

The authors also point out that before major reductions in the cost of medical care can be made, we will have to seriously consider denying intensive care to many seriously ill, elderly patients. Our society and many of those who press for major cost reduction are reluctant to recognize the societal and ethical implications of reducing care to these patients, however well we may show that the benefit of such care is limited.

Physicians initiate charges that may account for up to 90 percent of all health care expenditures (Eisenberg 1985). They order medicines, decide when to hospitalize patients, order procedures or do surgery, and decide when or whether patients are to go home or to a skilled nursing facility or to receive home health services. In fact, physicians largely determine how most of the money for health care is spent—over a billion dollars a day.

It should seem obvious, therefore, that the key to controlling costs is in physician decision making. If we convince physicians to order 10 percent fewer tests—the unnecessary ones, we hope—then the medical care industry will consume fewer resources, and the amount of money expended on medical care will fall. Unfortunately, it does not work that simply. For the short term, medical costs are controlled by the hospital budget setters. Reducing hospital income by ordering 10 percent fewer tests may cause some minor labor shifts in the laboratory and a small decrease in the cost of supplies ordered, but the total cost of running the laboratory is changed imperceptibly. The budget setters must now raise some charges inside or outside the laboratory to make up the loss in income, because their expenses for the short term remain more or less the same, despite their physicians' conscientious attempts to reduce unnecessary testing.

Studies conducted at North Carolina Memorial Hospital illustrate that physicians may have much less effect on the costs of medical care than is usually assumed. One financial problem area in the 155-bed medical service was the high utilization of laboratory procedures in intensive care units, where 350 percent more procedures per patient were ordered daily than on the seven nonintensive care units. The average patient in the Medical Intensive Care Unit was being charged over $500 per day for laboratory procedures alone.

Arterial blood gases (ABGs) were found to be the largest component of total laboratory charges, and a substantial portion were being ordered by the intensive care nurses rather than by the residents. It had become common for ABGs to be drawn toward the end of a nursing shift so the "passing of the baton" could be complete with current laboratory data; the subsequent nursing shift often repeated the ABGs for confirmation of the results and clinical trends.

When an arterial blood gas requisition was instituted that simply requested, but did not require, the nurse to check off the reason and the proposed action that would be based on the results, the number of ABGs dropped by 46 percent in the first month. Fewer than 10 percent of the requisitions were fully completed, yet the immediate reduction in requests was dramatic! The hospital charge for a blood gas is $21, so that on the surface there would seem to be a savings on ABGs from that one six-bed intensive care unit of $50,400 per year—money that Medicare, Medicaid, Blue Cross/Blue Shield, commercial insurance companies, and patients would not have to pay for medical care. If such simple behavior modification were instituted for other hospital activities, one could hypothesize that the savings to society could be enormous. For the short term, however, the results were not as expected.

In the blood gas laboratory, where ABGs are carried out, the only real saving on a blood gas not ordered as a result of the intervention was $1.02 worth of reagents; so for the 200 fewer blood gases ordered that month (only a six to seven per day reduction), $204 in supplies were actually saved. For the 24-hour day, the laboratory lights were on, the water was running, the heat or air conditioning was on, the technicians were present, and the machines were undergoing the decay of amortization; and little else changed—except that the hospital was now entitled to bill and collect $4,200 less that month than the month before. The major expense in health care—labor—was certainly unaffected by a reduction in ABG ordering of about two per eight-hour shift! Those well-meaning attempts at cost containment resulted in a potentially serious loss of income for the hospital for which, in the short term at least, it could not possibly compensate.

It is estimated that about 30 percent of medical expenditures are unnecessary: successful attempts to modify physician behavior have commonly resulted in the reduction of utilization of resources by almost one-third. The net effect, however, is that while total *charges* are indeed reduced, *costs,* at least for the short term, remain the same; and some unit costs in other areas may increase to compensate for the lost income.

Before *cost* reduction can occur, clinicians must coordinate their efforts to reduce utilization with the administrators who are responsible for their hospital's ancillary services. Only phased reduction in utilization that allows adjustments within the ancillary service units, such as reduction of personnel and altering of service schedules, can maximize the cost benefits to be achieved. ABG usage patterns, for example, had evolved over a long period of time; if the misusage is to be corrected without major economic mischief, the hospital financial planners, as well as the physicians who order services, must be involved.

A HISTORY OF OUR ATTEMPTS TO REDUCE THE COSTS OF MEDICAL CARE

Between 1970 and 1973, a few faculty members of the Department of Medicine of the University of North Carolina at Chapel Hill (both full-time and clinical) undertook a study of how actual private practice habits of clinical faculty members at an urban community teaching hospital affected their patients and their patients' third-party payers. A goal of this study was to determine whether the normal behavior of this existing group practice, in which the physicians were similarly trained and handled almost identical populations, would be compatible with some form of prepayment plan. The results showed such a wide variation in clinical behavior and practice styles among physicians that a successful transition by the group from a fee-for-service practice to a prepayment capitation system seemed highly unlikely. Even when patients were paired for age, sex, and diagnosis, there was nearly a 30 percent difference in the average total charges for office encounters among the physicians. The patients whose physicians used resources most liberally had annual charges per year that were 70 percent greater than patients of the group's more conservative utilizers. Overall patient charges, per capita, varied as much as 100 percent per year between different individual physicians' practices.

This was the first documentation of the wide variations in the utilization of medical resources by physicians, which have since been recorded by Wennberg (1984) and others. Admittedly, it was a small study, but it is one that had the advantage of examining the practices of physicians who worked together, taking care of similar groups of patients in the same community and hospital setting. Despite these similarities and the apparent lack of any quality of care differences (studies on physician variations have been unable to measure quality of care), remarkable differences were noted. What was the origin of these differences?

It was the consensus of the physicians involved in the private practice study that their practice styles or habits were developed in the early phase of their house staff careers. The next step, therefore, was to explore ways to influence the resource utilization patterns of house officers in an internal medical training program at the same 900-bed community teaching hospital used by the private practice group, to determine when and how practice habits are formed. In all, 100 house officers were introduced to a "charges awareness program."

Two approaches were taken to work with house officers on their practice styles and their awareness of charges. First, the approach to *inpatient teaching* was as follows.

1. Morning report became the chief occasion for heightening the house officers' awareness of their impact on the economics of health care. Each morning the residents received a printout of the length-of-stay and accumulated cost for each patient. The three junior residents in charge of the three general medicine services met each weekday morning for an hour with four full-time faculty members, a clinical pathologist, a clinical pharmacologist, and a social worker. Each case admitted the previous day was discussed in detail from a clinical perspective, and this was augmented with discussions of alternative ways the case might have been managed to use available resources more effectively. In addition, the cases of patients who had stays of greater than nine days were reviewed and discussed in detail at each session.

2. A two-hour teaching and work round session followed morning report each day. It was attended by third-year medical students, and first-year and second-year residents. Each attending physician on these services was aware of the fact that cost was a "vital sign" of each patient's medical care.

3. At the time of discharge each patient's itemized hospital bill was reviewed with the resident and intern in charge of the case. This allowed house officers to see where the orders that they had written had demonstrated significant redundancy in laboratory and x-ray utilization, and where failure to review drug orders at appropriate intervals had resulted in waste.

The results were positive, but ultimately discouraging. During the time of this study, the average length-of-stay for patients on the medical teaching service was reduced by 21 percent, and the charges per admission rose at a rate of 4.3 percent per annum, while the charges per admission on all other medical services rose at 14.5 percent per annum. However, once this reduction in resource utilization was achieved, charges then rose annually at the same rate as those for nonteaching service patients. In other words, once the "fat" was trimmed, there was no more fat to cut! If the labor-intensive efforts continued, the participants could only hope to maintain the differential in charges. Further substantial reductions were not likely to be possible without reductions in the quality of care.

In the *outpatient setting* the following changes were made:

1. A total reorganization of the clinic enhanced monitoring of first-year residents' activities.

2. An encounter analysis system was introduced. Encounter forms, describing what took place during the encounter, which tests and procedures were ordered, and the disposition on the encounter, were recorded, and the information was analyzed on a small hand-held computer.
3. Conferences on individual and team outpatient activities and the charges generated were held at the end of each clinic day. Potential problem areas of individual house officers' styles of resource utilization could thus be identified and discussed on the same day they occurred. Specific issues that were generic to all the house officers also became topics at the afternoon clinic report.

Over a three-year period, 4,710 inpatient discharges and 28,800 outpatient encounters were analyzed and discussed with the house officers. Although outpatient activities accounted for sixfold more encounters, they represented only 10 percent of the total charges for the care delivered by the residents. Nevertheless, the outpatient setting, where house officers were making their own decisions, was important to the study because it offered a much better opportunity for the researchers to observe and interact with the house officers on a one-on-one basis. At the inpatient setting, on the other hand, consultants, supervising residents, and attending physicians frequently dictated interns' actions.

During the 36-month analysis, the use of nursing personnel to coordinate health care, the establishment of a system for rapid retrieval of patient information, the use of paraprofessionals to obtain patient histories and to staff a blood pressure maintenance clinic, and the design of a system to monitor productivity and costs of care by individual house officers produced the following results:

1. There was an increase of 29 percent in physician productivity as measured by the number of patient encounters, while during the same period there was a 19 percent reduction in the actual hours that the house officers spent in clinic.
2. There was a reduction of 35 percent in ambulatory care costs generated by physicians.

In contrast to the inpatient cost-containment efforts, the ambulatory care program led to increased physician productivity and efficiency, and costs were reduced as well. These changes occurred through physician initiatives and did not require administrative intervention and cooperation. Unlike the inpatient cost-containment program, which asked physicians to limit or justify the services provided to patients, the outpatient teaching program concentrated on the quality of medical decision making and the resultant care through individualized teaching. The greater reduction in charges occurred with the inpatient program, but the ambulatory program probably had a greater long-term effect on the cost, efficiency, and quality of medical care provided by those residents in their future practice.

The next step was to investigate whether the success of these programs could be replicated in a university setting—one in which many more faculty members and house officers were involved, and where there was more resistance to change. In part, this step was needed to test whether it was the programs that were successful, or whether it was the researchers' interest and commitment to cost containment that influenced residents to change the behaviors.

In 1983, a 19-bed general medical unit at North Carolina Memorial Hospital was designated as a study unit, and a 21-bed general medical unit on the same hospital floor served as the control. Several organizational changes were instituted on the study unit:

1. The nursing staff was changed from team nursing to primary nursing.

2. The unit became the only location in the medical services where an attending physician could admit a private patient and remain the physician of record, rather than relinquishing the patient's care to the teaching attending physician assigned to the service that month. Approximately one-half of the patients were cared for in this manner, but students and residents were responsible for evaluating and caring for all patients.

3. First-year residents did not rotate to this unit. Only second-year residents and four third-year medical students were scheduled on a monthly basis.

4. Several times weekly the house staff, students, and attending physicians were given feedback on the hospital charges that accrued on each of their patients. Price lists were made readily available, and all items on the ward had price labels attached.

During the study year, the control unit of 21 beds remained in the customary format of four third-year students, three first-year residents, two second-year residents, and an attending physician who was the physician of record for all patients on the unit.

The program was successful. During that year, the charges per patient on the experimental unit averaged $3,871 per patient compared with a charge of $5,251 on the control unit. The experimental unit was 26 percent below the control unit in charges per discharge. The length-of-stay on the control unit was 8.5 days and on the experimental unit 7.1 days—a difference of almost 20 percent.

The experimental unit accounted for about 10 percent of the medical service admissions during the year of the study. If the entire medical service had achieved similar savings, the charges for its 5,000 admissions would have been reduced by about $7 million—a sizable amount. Two concerns surfaced. First, true cost savings would be much less than the 26 percent reduction in charges, and they would be one-time savings— "trimmed fat." The hospital had also lost the income difference between cost and charges, "profits" that are used to support nonprofitable services necessary for compassionate medical care and high-quality medical education. It is possible, therefore, that these efforts would have ultimately resulted in fewer medical care amenities for the patients. It is hard to give enough emphasis to this often-ignored point. Nonprofit hospitals use the income difference between cost and charges to support nonreimbursable services—pastoral care, "sitters," free telephones or televisions for the indigent, coordination of volunteer services, and all the administrative functions of the hospital.

Second, is $7 million all that much money to a state-supported hospital with a $140 million budget? Who was benefiting? It was probably not the patients, whose bills were paid by insurance companies or their government, and who were subjected to a slightly increased risk by quicker discharge and fewer services. It was certainly not the physicians, who did the work of implementing the cost-containment program but whose reimbursement was decreased because their patients' hospital stays were reduced. And it was certainly not the hospital, which would have to cope with reduced income far in excess of the reduction in costs they experienced.

In other words, the program could actually undermine the economic well-being of the hospital and possibly the patients' welfare, if changes in the provision of services were not planned and synchronous with the change in clinical activities. Some planned reduction in the services offered would have to take place before decreased utilization of the laboratory, x-ray department, or other ancillary services could in fact reduce hospital costs and not just their charges. One final ongoing program is an attempt to do just this—to identify areas within each medical service wherein reduced usage of services might be accompanied by a reduction in the costs of operating the departments offering those services, to generate cost savings commensurate with reductions in charges.

Since 1980, interested members of the Department of Medicine have maintained charge data on all nine medical services at North Carolina Memorial Hospital. Total charges for all medical patients discharged between fiscal year 1980–81 and fiscal year 1984–85 increased by some 59 percent from $19 million to nearly $30 million, with little change in the number of patients discharged. The average charges per patient discharge started at about $3,800 and seemed to plateau at around $6,000 per discharge for the three years 1982–85.

In fiscal year 1984–85, a research project began to do "economic autopsies" on the itemized hospital bill of every patient discharged from the medical services. There was a wide variation of charges among the nine medical services. The average discharge bill for patients on medical services was $5,700, but the variation between services was from a low of $3,400 on one of the general medical services to as high as $17,000 on the medical intensive care unit.

Each individual service was then examined for the average charge per discharge during the period 1980–81 through 1984–85. The national average increase in hospital charges was roughly 15 percent per annum at this time; in comparison, the cardiology service rose almost 40 percent per year, the pulmonary service rose about 25 percent per year, and the coronary care unit some 33 percent per year. The three general medicine services, on the other hand, tended to lag behind the annual increase in charges per discharge. Such data helped to identify areas where the most attention should be focused in planning for reduction in utilization.

Perhaps a better view of utilization of services is offered by charges per patient day by service, because length-of-stay was different on each service. The seven nonintensive care services charged from as little as $484 per patient day to a high of $800. The intensive care unit charges were $1,800 per patient day; in addition, only 30 percent of patients were discharged from the intensive care unit alive. This does not include patients transferred from the unit to other services.

In general for all services, the breakdown of charges was the same— 40 percent for room, 20 percent for laboratory services, 20 percent for pharmacy, and 5 percent for x-ray, with 15 percent for a variety of miscellaneous services. Computerized tomography (CT) scans represented less than 1 percent of medical billings. Patients who had at least some intensive care treatment before being transferred to other units made up 20 percent of the total population but accounted for 46 percent of all hospital charges, and 44 patients with bills greater than $50,000 represented less than 1 percent of total discharges but accounted for 13 percent of all hospital charges on the medical services.

This preliminary analysis led to some difficult ethical decisions before the study could be brought to its conclusion by implementing cost-reducing changes. For example, a major cost savings could result from a coordinated reduction in intensive care unit services. It is important to note, however, that it is not so much the intensive care *unit*, but intensive services that increase charges, although the intellectual atmosphere of the unit certainly does not encourage frugality. Each month, one or two patients with multiple medical problems accrued charges of $50,000 to $100,000; and their survival was at best 90 to 120 days. Not providing intensive care services to such patients would result in greater charge reductions than all of the efforts on the 19-bed cost-awareness unit. Another observation that requires more analysis: patients under the age of 65 who died during their hospitalization incurred average total charges of $14,000, while patients over 65 years old who died had average total charges of above $33,000.

In conclusion, nearly two decades of cost-containment interventions have turned up some unexpected financial and ethical problems that must be faced by physicians and administrators together. A program that allows costs to be reduced through increased efficiency and productivity, as occurred in the ambulatory care study, must be the goal. Reducing charges without reducing costs simply creates a new set of problems that should be avoidable through economic and medical care planning. Reductions in the costs of medical care, as well as a sustained reduction in the rate of increase in the costs of care, may have to come from reductions in intensive care services to the large group of chronically ill, moribund, usually elderly patients who, at least in this analysis, benefited little from rapidly accelerating expenditures.

REFERENCES

Eisenberg, J. M. (1985). "Physician Utilization: The State of Research about Physicians' Practice Habits." *Medical Care* 23: 461–83.
Wennberg, J. E. (1984). "Dealing with Medical Practice Variation: A Proposal for Action." *Health Affairs* 3: 6–32.

SELECTED BIBLIOGRAPHY

Angell, M. "Cost Containment and Physicians." *Journal of the American Medical Association* 254 (1985): 1203–7.
Berkelhamer, J. E. "Charges by Residents and Faculty Physicians in a University Hospital Pediatric Practice." *Journal of Medical Education* 61 (1986): 303–7.
Carel, E. J.; Neuhauser, D.; and Stason, W. B. (eds.). *The Physician and Cost Control.* Cambridge, MA: Oelgeshlager, Gunn & Hain, 1980.
Challah, S.; Wing, A. J.; Bauer, R.; Morris, R. W.; and Schroeder, S. A. "Negative Selection of Patients for Dialysis and Transplantation in the United Kingdom." *British Medical Journal* 288 (1984): 1119–22.
Cohen, D. I.; Breslau, D.; and Porter, D. K. "The Cost Implications of Academic Group Practice: A Randomized Controlled Trial." *New England Journal of Medicine* 314 (1986): 1553–57.

Dans, P. E. "The Great Zebra Hunt: A View of Internal Medicine from the Walk-In Clinic." *Pharos* 41 (1978): 2–6.

Dixon, R. H., and Laszlo, J. "Utilization of Clinical Chemistry Services by Medical House Staff: An Analysis." *Archives of Internal Medicine* 134 (1974): 1064–67.

Eddy, D. M. "Variations in Physician Practice: The Role of Uncertainty." *Health* 3 (1984): 74–89.

Eisenberg, J. M. *Doctors' Decisions and the Cost of Medical Care.* Ann Arbor, MI: Health Administration Press, 1986.

Eisenberg, J. M., and Williams, S. V. "Cost Containment and Changing Physician Behavior. Can the Fox Learn to Guard the Chicken Coop?" *Journal of the American Medical Association* 246 (1981): 2195–2201.

Everett, G. D.; deBlois, C.; Chang, P. F.; et al. "Effect of Cost Education, Cost Audits, and Faculty Chart Review on the Use of Laboratory Services." *Archives of Internal Medicine* 143 (1983): 942–44.

Fineberg, H. C. "Clinical Chemistries: The High Cost of Low Cost Diagnostic Tests." In *Medical Technology: The Culprit Behind Health Care Costs?* ed. S. H. Altman and R. Blendon, 144–65. U.S. Department of Health, Education, and Welfare Publication No. (PHS) 79-3216. Washington, DC: U.S. Government Printing Office, 1979.

Ginzberg, E. "The Destabilization of Health Care." *New England Journal of Medicine* 315 (1986): 757–61.

————. "A Hard Look at Cost Containment." *New England Journal of Medicine* 316 (1987): 1151–54.

Griner, P. F., and Liptzin, B. "Use of the Laboratory in a Teaching Hospital: Implications for Patient Care, Education, and Hospital Costs." *Annals of Internal Medicine* 75 (1971): 157–63.

Himmelstein, D. U., and Woolhandler, S. "Cost without Benefit: Administrative Waste in U.S. Health Care." *New England Journal of Medicine* 314 (1986): 441–45.

Hulka, B. S., and Wheat, J. R. "Patterns of Utilization: The Patient Perspective." *Medical Care* 23 (1985): 438–60.

Lion, J.; Malbon, A.; Henderson, M. G.; et al. "A Comparison of Hospital Outpatient Departments in Private Practice." *Health Care Financing Review* 6 (1985): 69–81.

Lyle, C. B.; Applegate, W. B.; Citron, D. S.; et al. "Practice Habits in a Group of Eight Internists." *Annals of Internal Medicine* 84 (1976): 594–601.

Lyle, C. B.; Bianchi, R. F.; Harris, J. H.; et al: "Teaching Cost Containment to House Officers." *Journal of Medical Education* 54 (1979): 856–62.

Lyle, C. B.; Citron, D. S.; Sugg, W. C.; et al. "Costs of Medical Care in a Practice of Internal Medicine: A Study of a Group of Seven Internists." *Annals of Internal Medicine* 81 (1974): 1–6.

Martin, A. R.; Wolf, M. A.; Thibodeau, L. A.; et al. "A Trial of Two Strategies to Modify the Test Ordering Behavior of Medical Residents." *New England Journal of Medicine* 303 (1980): 1330–36.

May, J. J. "Impact of Diagnosis Related Groups on Medical Practice." *American Journal of Cardiology* 56 (1985): 16c–26c.

McNeil, B. J. "Hospital Response to DRG-Based Prospective Payment." *Medical Decision Making* 5 (1985): 15–21.

McPhee, S. J.; Chapman, S. A.; Myers, L. P.; et al. "Lessons for Teaching Cost Containment." *Journal of Medical Education* 59 (1984): 722–29.

McPhee, S. J.; Myers, L. P.; and Lo, B. "Cost Containment Confronts Physicians." *Annals of Internal Medicine* 100 (1984): 604–6.
McPhee, S. J.; Myers, L. P.; and Schroeder, S. A. "The Cost and Risk of Medical Care: An Annotated Bibliography for Clinicans and Editors." *Western Journal of Medicine* 137 (1982): 145–61.
Myers, L. P.; Chapman, S. A.; McPhee, S. J.; et al. "Unnecessary Service Use at a University Hospital." *Western Journal of Medicine* 143 (1985): 397–98.
Myers, L. P., and Schroeder, S. A. "Physician Use of Services for the Hospitalized Patient: A Review of Implications for Cost Containment." *Milbank Memorial Fund Quarterly* 59 (1981): 481–503.
Pineault, R. "The Effect of Medical Training Factors on Physician Utilization Behavior." *Medical Care* 14 (1977): 51–67.
Schroeder, S. A.; Kenders, K.; Cooper, J. K.; et al. "Use of Laboratory Tests and Pharmaceuticals: Variation among Physicians and Effect of Cost Audit on Subsequent Use." *Journal of the American Medical Association* 225 (1973): 969–73.
Schroeder, S. A.; Myers, L. P.; McPhee, S. J.; et al. "The Failure of Physician Education as a Cost Containment Strategy." *Journal of the American Medical Association* 252 (1984): 225–30.
Scitovsky, A. A. "Change in the Use of Ancillary Services for "Common" Illness. In *Medical Technology: The Culprit Behind Health Care Costs?* ed. S. H. Altman and R. Blendon, 39–56. U.S. Department of Health, Education, and Welfare Publication No. (PHS) 79-3216. Washington, DC: U.S. Government Printing Office, 1979.
Showstack, J. A.; Hughes-Stone, N.; and Schroeder, S. A. "The Role of Changing Clinical Practices and the Rising Costs of Hospital Care." *New England Journal of Medicine* 313 (1985): 1201–7.
Singer, D. E.; Carr, P. C.; Mulley, A. G.; et al. "Rationing Intensive Care: Physician Responses to a Resource Shortage." *New England Journal of Medicine* 309 (1983): 1155–60.
Wertmann, B. G.; Sostrin, S. V.; Pavlova, Z.; et al. "Why Do Physicians Order Laboratory Tests? A Study of Laboratory Test Requests and Use Patterns." *Journal of the American Medical Association* 243 (1980): 2080–82.
White, R. E.; Skipper, B. J.; Applegate, W. B.; et al. "Ordering Decision and Clinic Cost Variation among Resident Physicians." *Western Journal of Medicine* 141 (1984): 117–22.

Chapter 13

A Review of Medical Education Interventions in Cost Containment

J. Dennis Hoban, Charles Hansen, and Jack D. McCue

Editor's Note—Exhortations that we must educate physicians about the importance of cost containment, or encourage frugal clinical decision making by modifying their behavior, frequently ignore the large body of data describing attempts to do so. Hoban et al. review several studies aimed at medical students and resident physicians in graduate medical training, describing their efforts and successes. The studies, overall, are notable for their ingenuity, variety, and ultimately the modesty of the successes. Physicians and administrators who wish to set up cost-containment programs for students, residents, or practitioners can get valuable ideas from this careful review drawn from diverse journals and disciplines.

These studies and the chapter by Lyle et al., however, raise serious questions: Are the countervailing forces that discourage cost containment so strong as to overwhelm educational interventions? Does the effect of behavior modification or education extend beyond the active phase of the intervention study? Is the most common site for these interventions—the acute care hospital, where most medical care money is spent—the best place to work with physicians on cost containment?

More than 550 articles related to cost containment have appeared in the medical literature since 1970. Because the majority of medical care charges are the direct or indirect result of physician decisions, it has been argued that if physicians are made aware of costs and know how to use efficient diagnostic and treatment practices, the will deliver care more cost-effectively (Eisenberg 1986). This review focuses on the cost-containment articles and abstracts (three included) that describe attempts to educate students and physicians-in-training to be more cost-conscious; it investigates the extent to which the scientific literature bears out this hypothesis in the specific case of physicians-in-training. The review analyzes educational interventions only in undergraduate and graduate medical education, and thus excludes other forms of cost-containment intervention strategies and audiences; those interventions have been reviewed by McPhee, Myers, and Schroeder (1982), Hatoum et al. (1986), Eisenberg (1985), Grossman (1983), and Soumerai and Avorn (1984).

The selected articles were also reviewed and analyzed to provide a description of the methods of cost-containment teaching interventions reported during the last 15 years. The decision to include mostly journal articles was based on the assumption that most articles submitted for publication receive peer review and would, therefore, have passed some professional scrutiny by colleagues in the field of study. However, studies may be more likely to be rejected by editorial reviewers if the results do not support the experimental hypothesis; this results in an underrepresentation of studies that showed negative results, and lends our summary a positive bias.

Of the nearly 100 reports relating to cost-containment education that were identified and analyzed for possible inclusion in this review, a total of 31 studies dealt specifically with educational interventions employed in the education of medical students or house officers. We classified articles by the type of outcome each intervention attempted to bring about:

1. Cost Awareness: Interventions to improve knowledge about charges or attitudes toward cost containment.

2. Diagnostic Tests: Interventions to alter ordering of one or more diagnostic tests for cost-related purposes.

3. Treatment: Interventions to alter ordering of treatment modalities that have cost implications.

4. Multiple Service Charges: Interventions to alter behavior to have a global impact on costs/charges.

5. Diagnostic Acumen: Interventions to influence cost by improving the diagnostic process.

OVERVIEW

Most educational interventions have attempted to influence practitioners' uses of "little ticket" services. More than three-fourths of the

TABLE 13.1
Study Audiences, Outcome Measures, and Authors

Educational Measures	Outcome Measures	Author(s)
Medical students	Diagnostic acumen	Smith Spiegel et al.
	Diagnostic tests/charges	Garg et al.
	Knowledge/attitude	Eastaugh Hale et al. Williams et al. Zeleznik and Gonnella

Residents
  Ambulatory
  settings
	Diagnostic tests/charges	Lyle et al.
		Marton et al.
		Neal
		Rhyne and Gehlback

	Knowledge/attitude	Chilton et al. Cummings et al.
	Multiple service charges	Applegate et al. Reid and Lantz
	Treatment modalities	Klein et al.
Inpatient settings	Diagnostic tests/charges	Cohen et al. Dixon and Laszlo Eisenberg et al. Eisenberg Everett et al. Goodspeed et al. Martin et al. Williams and Eisenberg
	Knowledge/attitude	Babington et al.
	Multiple service charges	Forrest et al. Henderson et al. Lyle et al. Schroeder et al.
	Treatment modalities	Johnson et al.

31 studies (24) were aimed at house officers and 23 percent were designed for medical students. Fifteen studies used diagnostic tests as outcome measures; six reported multiple charges (e.g., lab charges, drug charges, and total charges); six studies measured knowledge or attitude; two studies used treatment as an outcome; and two employed measures of diagnostic acumen. Table 13.1 lists the outcome measures used in the studies matched with the populations.

Only eight of the 31 studies randomized their subjects to different interventions, and less than two-thirds of the studies employed a control group. In the vast majority of studies, a simulated intervention or case study approach was used. Given the real world constraints imposed upon most of the reported studies, it is not surprising that experimental intervention was used so infrequently. However, the absence of this intervention weakens the applicability of the results to medical practice. In addition, many of the studies lack the design necessary to establish a cause-and-effect relationship between intervention and outcome.

EDUCATIONAL INTERVENTIONS: MEDICAL STUDENTS

Medical students were the primary audience for seven of the educational interventions: five of the interventions taught cost issues in patient care, and two sought to improve diagnostic reasoning.

In a controlled trial at George Washington University with "after only" measurement, the experimental group received an introductory lecture that presented an analytical framework for making laboratory and other intervention choices. Once during each of the subsequent three weeks, students were given a lecture and a case study based on the lecture material, after which choices of laboratory and other interventions were discussed and critiqued. The average laboratory test charges generated by the experimental third-year student group were half those of the control group, and the experimental group scored significantly higher than the control group in diagnostic acumen; that is, in the ability to determine diagnoses, make patient-management decisions, and choose essential diagnostic procedures (Spiegel et al. 1982).

In a similar study at the University of Pennsylvania, however, Williams et al. (1984) reported that a comprehensive educational program failed to show differences in knowledge about diagnostic test use, attitudes about cost containment, or simulated test-ordering behaviors. The one-month educational program included a 60-minute seminar on "The Economics of Laboratory Use," a simulated patient care exercise with discussion, special student case presentations in which faculty concentrated their teaching on the most appropriate and cost-effective uses of diagnostic tests, ten two-page newsletters describing the appropriate use of diagnostic tests, and feedback of the current bills of patients being cared for by the students' teams to the students.

Smith (1983) studied the effects of a more focused, limited educational intervention. In a community health clerkship at Brown University, half of the students participated in a computerized patient management problem exercise while the rest did not. At the conclusion of the problem, the computer provided feedback to the students on their efficiency, errors of commission and omission, time spent on the problem, the cost of the items selected, and the risk, discomfort, and inconvenience to which they subjected the patient. Pretests and posttests consisted of six patient management problems scored along five dimensions: proficiency, efficiency, errors of omission, errors of commission, and cost. Both groups improved, but there were no statistically significant differences between the experimental and control group on any of the measures.

Hale et al. (1984) found that 26 Dartmouth students on a family medicine rotation that incorporated standardized cost information learning packets had significantly higher levels of cost awareness than 19 controls. The learning packets took advantage of an interpractice medical information system operated by the Primary Care Cooperative Information Project in New England, which could tailor cost data to the practice in which the student was performing a clerkship. Students receiving educational packets were more aware of visit charges and medication costs, and tended to be more confident of their cost estimates.

Thomas Jefferson Medical College used a Student Model Utilization Review Committee as part of a six-week junior clerkship in the Model Family Practice Unit (Zeleznik and Gonnella 1979). During "committee meetings" cases were discussed from a number of perspectives, including those of utilization review coordinators, physicians, and representatives of the local Professional Standards Review Organization (PSRO) and Blue Cross organizations. The intervention group acquired more cost-related knowledge and positive attitudes about utilization review and cost containment.

Eastaugh (1981) described three basic themes underlying a course taught to students at Cornell Medical School. The first theme postulated that physicians must understand the role of cost-benefit analysis in decisions involving policy determinations and expenditure of funds for expensive technological resources. The second theme focused on the physician's need to consider the cost effectiveness of diagnostic tests and procedures. The third theme was professional autonomy. A follow-up attitudinal survey indicated that the course had a positive effect on the participants' attitudes toward the application of decision analysis to medicine and attitudes toward medical economics. Nonparticipants were less mindful of the need for medical cost containment and less conscious of the need for decision analysis applications in medicine than the course takers.

Garg, Gliebe, and Kleinberg (1979), at the Medical College of Toledo, asked medical student clerks to perform retrospective reviews of their peers' laboratory utilization. Students indicated, on the average, that two fewer tests and savings of $24 per patient would have been accrued if the minimum necessary tests had been ordered. The peer review was conducted as part of a quality assurance educational program in a required one-month ambulatory medicine clerkship, which used the patient write-ups from other students on the medicine and pediatric clerkships.

EDUCATIONAL INTERVENTIONS: RESIDENCY TRAINING

Of 23 studies conducted in graduate education programs, three attempted to increase residents' knowledge of cost information, six attempted to influence their practice behavior in ambulatory care practices, and 14 attempted the same in hospitals. We think the distinction between ambulatory care and inpatient care settings may prove important in future studies.

Knowledge of Charges

At the University of Arkansas, Babington, Robinson, and Monson (1983) reported that residents receiving a prescription drugs price booklet did not improve their knowledge on a postintervention questionnaire. A similar study was reported by Chilton et al. (1982) at the New Mexico School of Medicine. No improvement was noted in residents' knowledge of prevailing charges for commonly used clinic services, laboratory and x-ray examinations, and medications after relevant information was provided to the residents by wall posters, discussions with attending physicians, and a catalog of all laboratory, radiologic, and medication charges.

The effects of linking price information to physicians' test-ordering decisions were studied in three family practice centers affiliated with the Wayne State University School of Medicine (Cummings et al. 1982). Residents and faculty were asked to review four case studies, each of which described a patient with ambiguous symptoms. Participants who received test order forms on which the prices of diagnostic tests were printed ordered fewer diagnostic tests than those participants who did not have price information; and the cost of tests ordered per patient was 31 percent less.

Practice Behaviors: Ambulatory Care

At the New Mexico Medical Center, residents' charges in an ambulatory clinic were reviewed after an educational program that included reference materials (a wall poster with charges and a complete catalog of charges), didactic sessions (e.g., decision theory, health economics), resident-faculty interaction, feedback on charges generated by the residents, and faculty review of the cost effectiveness of three of the house officers' clinical encounters per month (Applegate et al. 1983). At the end of each quarter, residents received summaries of their charges compared to the ambulatory clinic as a whole. A statistically significant reduction in laboratory and total charges for all encounters was found, but no long-term follow-up of the residents' test-ordering behavior was done.

Eight of 21 residents in the Primary Care Clinic of the University of Virginia received a quarterly, computer-generated profile derived from each patient encounter (Reid and Lantz 1977). The profile contained the following information: total number of patients seen, average cost of laboratory and x-ray tests ordered, average cost per patient, average patient time in the clinic, compliance rate, and drop-out rate. No effect of distributing the profiles, when compared to the control group, was noted.

At Stanford, residents were randomly assigned to four groups: a control group ($N=14$); a feedback group ($N=14$) which received a computer printout every two weeks indicating the number of patients seen by the resident and the amount of money spent on diagnostic tests; a manual group ($N=15$) which received a reference manual designed to teach principles of cost-effective laboratory use and a 10-minute tutorial on how to use it; and manual-plus-feedback on laboratory use group ($N=14$) (Martin et al. 1980). All intervention groups significantly decreased laboratory use, but the manual-plus-feedback group showed the largest decrease (42 percent) in laboratory charges.

At the Kaiser-Permanente Medical Center at Santa Clara, Neal (1982) reported that for 2½ years attending physicians and house staff received a written brief on indications for radiology procedures developed by respected clinical specialists on the medical staff. The briefs consisted of abbreviated summaries of the literature and recommendations on the use of specific x-ray studies in specific situations. He noted a 28 percent reduction in x-ray utilization per 100 office visits which was sustained for more than three years, compared to the twelve other Kaiser-Permanente Medical Centers in northern California, none of which used the Santa Clara educational approach.

At the Charlotte Memorial Hospital and Medical Center, the clinic attending physician reviewed the costs generated each month by each intern for the first year (Lyle et al. 1979). In subsequent years, the costs were reviewed at a conference at the end of each clinic day. Using the average cost of tests ordered as an indicator of success in this case study, interns in internal medicine had a 28 percent reduction in cost of tests

ordered, compared to interns in family medicine and surgical specialties
who had a 12 percent and 14 percent decrease, respectively.

In the Duke-Watts Family Medicine group practice, two physicians
audited the charts of their patients who had had thyroid function panels
(TFPs) ordered during one six-month period (Rhyne and Gehlback 1979).
A survey, consisting of ten case vignettes, asked the residents to rate the
importance of obtaining a TFP on a five-point scale (essential–unwar-
ranted), the results of which were then presented at a conference. The
conference focused on the process of clinical decision making, using
TFP ordering as an example. The rate of TFP ordering dropped significantly for the first three months after the conference but rose to the
preintervention ordering level during the subsequent three months,
pointing to the need for reinforcement in order to sustain change.

A chart audit at Johns Hopkins' Emergency Room and Walk-in
Clinic revealed that an experimental group receiving a fifteen-minute
tutorial designed to modify misconceptions pertaining to therapy, efficacy, toxicity, and cost of urinary tract infection (UTI) therapy reduced
therapy costs by 44 percent, while the control group did not show a
statistically significant decrease (Klein et al. 1981).

Practice Behaviors: Inpatient

Inpatient studies of cost-containment interventions made up nearly
half of all the studies conducted on physicians-in-training. Nine of these
studies dealt with diagnostic tests and charges as outcomes, and four
measured multiple service outcomes.

At the University of Virginia Medical Center, Forrest et al. (1981)
found that costs incurred by surgical house staff who received cumulative and per diem charges for their cholecystectomy, appendectomy,
breast biopsy, and inguinal hernia repair cases did not differ significantly from their control counterparts who did not receive this information. However, Henderson et al. (1979) found that medicine interns
at the West Virginia University Medical Center who received daily print-
outs of all charges incurred by patients under their care had 29 percent
less total charges per patient than the control group of interns.

The inpatient portion of the study of cost-containment intervention at the Charlotte Memorial Hospital and Medical Center found that
the attending physician's review of the total costs with each resident
reduced the average length-of-stay at that hospital by 21 percent (Lyle
et al. 1979). This case study also claimed that this reduction in length-
of-stay held the rise in cost of an average medical admission to 4.3 percent per year, while the cost of an admission on other services rose 14.5
percent per year.

A research study at the University of California at San Francisco involved 226 medical and surgical house staff; interventions consisted of (1) a one-hour lecture weekly for four weeks, (2) four hour-long sessions of chart audits with feedback, and (3) a combination of the lecture series and chart audit (Schroeder et al. 1984). While certain "little ticket" services showed reduced usage, total charges did not decrease significantly in any of the three intervention groups compared to controls.

Dixon and Laszlo (1974), at the Durham Veterans Administration Hospital, limited the number of total laboratory tests that interns could order to an average of eight per patient per day. Prior to the intervention only 5 percent of the total chemistry determinations altered the care of patients, while afterward, 23 percent altered patient care. Following the limitation in test ordering, the number of tests per patient per day declined from six to two.

At the University of Pennsylvania, an educational program designed to decrease the utilization of prothrombin time determination by house officers included the dissemination of the results of a clinical utility study, a weekly patient management conference devoted to the use of the test, and a memorandum distributed to the house staff urging them to reconsider their use of the test (Eisenberg 1977). Six months after the educational program, the use of the prothrombin time determination as a routine admission test had decreased significantly. Eighteen months after the educational program, the use of this test by the study group had returned to initial levels.

A second study by Eisenberg et al. (1977) involved a computer-based system that detected potential overuse of serum lactose dehydrogenase (LDH) and serum calcium determination. When a review of a patient's chart revealed overutilization of LDH, letters were sent to the responsible resident and attending physician; no letter was sent indicating inappropriate uses of serum calcium determinations. Inappropriate utilization of neither LDH nor serum calcium was influenced by the letters.

A third University of Pennsylvania study included general education about laboratory testing, a nonthreatening letter from the departmental chairman describing an audit process to pick up unnecessary repeat use of a laboratory test, and finally, participation of the residents in planning and conducting the study (Williams and Eisenberg 1986). During the first year there was a significant decrease in the percentage of repeat tests for the experimental group. There were no statistically significant differences, however, among the three intervention groups. In the second year there were no differences among the three groups and the control group. The authors concluded that their educational method was not powerful enough to overcome counteracting influences on the residents' clinical behavior.

An educational study at Brigham and Women's Hospital randomly assigned residents to three groups: (1) four weekly concurrent chart review and discussion sessions, (2) financial incentive, and (3) control (Martin et al. 1980). The financial incentive group was offered $150 worth of medical-educational materials (books or journals) for all study participants, if laboratory tests were reduced by 20 percent and radiologic procedures by 10 percent. If laboratory tests were reduced by 30 percent and radiologic procedures by 15 percent, residents in the incentive group would have received an additional $225 for educational purposes. All groups, including the control, had statistically significant reductions in laboratory testing, but not in the use of radiologic testing. The chart review group had the most dramatic reduction (47 percent) in laboratory testing which was sustained during a four-month follow-up period. The financial incentive group's reduction was not sustained during the follow-up period.

In an interesting study at the Cleveland Metropolitan General Hospital, a "firm" (a group practice of residents and attendings) received a daily report of either the laboratory or x-ray costs for each of their patients (Cohen et al. 1982). The firms that received lab test data reduced test usage during the experimental period, but returned to their pre-experimental usage level after the data feedback was discontinued. The firms receiving only x-ray cost data did not change their use of laboratory testing during the experiment, but an abrupt and significant drop in the use of lab tests by the x-ray firms was noted in the follow-up period. While interviewing the firm team leaders after the experiment, it was determined that the two x-ray firms had leaders who were interested in the study, while the two lab firms had passive leaders.

A study at the University of Connecticut Medical School compared the test-ordering behavior of first-year medical residents in a Probabilistic Reasoning curriculum and a Cost Control curriculum (Goodspeed, Davidoff, and Clive 1985); the authors concluded that a Probabilistic Reasoning curriculum may decrease test-ordering rates more than a Cost Control curriculum.

At the University of Iowa Hospital, medical wards were randomly assigned to either a cost education group, which received a series of cost-containment newsletters and the placement of a charge profile adjacent to the order sheet on the medical charts of the patients; a cost audit intervention group, consisting of weekly computer reports listing tests ordered and the charges incurred per patient day by each first-year resident during the preceding week; or a combined intervention group (Everett et al. 1983). The control group and cost education group had no significant changes, and the cost audit group actually increased the total serum chemistry screening panels (SMA-12s) and complete blood count (CBC) test use during the intervention phase. The combination group significantly reduced the total test use by 9.4 percent and SMA-12 use by 10.8 percent; the total reduction in charges for this group, however, was only 1.2 percent.

In the second Iowa study by the same authors, residents were randomly assigned to a control group or an intervention group consisting of a series of 30-minute, bi-weekly discussions between the attending physician and the residents on appropriate and efficient use of laboratory tests, sensitivity, specificity, and predictive-value measurements. Five randomly chosen charts of patients discharged by the residents provided the basis for discussion. The intervention group ordered significantly fewer total tests and had 9.8 percent less charges than the control group. All of these findings were statistically significant.

Finally, Johnson et al. (1982) reported the results of a cost-containment program directed at medical and surgical residents of the Peter Bent Brigham Hospital. In an attempt to improve the gentamicin prescribing patterns of physicians, an educational program was conducted. The program consisted of: several weekly meetings in which the criteria for acceptable use of gentamicin were discussed in detail, the posting of these criteria at nursing stations, and the dissemination of a monthly hospital publication devoted to the criteria. Results suggest that the educational program improved the acceptable use of gentamicin (78 percent versus 52 percent).

SUMMARY AND CONCLUSIONS

An impressive variety of interventions to encourage more cost awareness and the frugal use of medical resources among students and residents has been reported. Some have involved imaginative and time-consuming educational or behavior-modifying efforts, but results have been inconsistent, regardless of the interventions attempted. The studies involving medical students, as might be expected, investigated ways to help students acquire knowledge, gain positive attitudes toward cost containment, and apply knowledge in a simulated environment. The literature suggests that these goals can, by-and-large, be accomplished. Given undergraduate medical education's emphasis on conformity of knowledge and attitudes, however, these findings are not surprising. In other words, the positive effect on students' awareness of cost issues or knowledge of cost seems relatively independent of the methods used, perhaps indicating that the eagerness of medical students to learn, rather than their perception of the importance of the curriculum content, is responsible for the successful outcomes.

One must seriously ask whether cost containment is a suitable topic for undergraduate medical education. Cost is inextricably part of clinical decision making, and while students must actively learn decision-making skills during their last two years of medical school, it is, nevertheless, hard to justify devoting expensive and scarce teaching time to cost containment. Is that effort not better devoted to improving clinical knowledge, problem definition, and patient-evaluation skills, and to developing humane attitudes? It may be a moot issue, for it is doubtful that cost-related knowledge or attitudes learned during medical school are retained by residents or practitioners. The relearning process that occurs during residency totally reshapes how physicians acquire and process clinical information. Until we can be certain that teaching cost awareness to students makes them better practitioners, our faculty time and resources should be devoted to more traditional educational goals.

Most of the cost-containment educational programs for residents attempted to change practice behaviors in order to reduce costs or charges of medical services. Many of the educational programs appear to have accomplished their goals of changing the behavior of residents, at least for the duration of the experiment. The studies that examined long-term effects, however, usually showed that the newly learned behaviors did not persist when the experimental conditions were removed. After analyzing the results of these studies, it is difficult for us to improve on the conclusions of McPhee et al. (1984), who summarized their experiences at the University of California at San Francisco. Residents pay attention when the purpose of the intervention is improved patient care rather than economy, and when the intervention provides useful cost-related information that is accessible at the time clinical decisions are being made. A single intervention is less likely to be effective than multiple, mutually reinforcing programs. Residents must be given concrete evidence that their clinical decision making needs improvement. Administrative changes that require more awareness of cost and support of educational interventions by influential physicians enormously improve the chance of success. In other words, pleading or reasoning with residents is much less likely to succeed than changing the rules to encourage cost-consciousness (or to penalize cost-unconscious behavior).

The studies involving residents lead to two additional conclusions. If cost containment is important to faculty, they must demonstrate it through personal involvement in the teaching process. The more individual the faculty-resident contact is, the more seriously residents take that interaction and the more likely they are to heed the proffered advice. Personal investment of faculty effort leads to more attention from residents, and in the words of Cohen et al. (1982): "Cost information must, like all data, be perceived by someone whose mind is prepared to use it. . . ."

An unexpected but intuitively correct insight offered by this literature is that it is easier and perhaps more effective to teach cost awareness in ambulatory care settings. Resident-faculty involvement is one-on-one, there are fewer peer pressures for the resident to deal with, and decision making is not surrounded by the sense of urgency and fear of failure that inevitably intrudes on decision making in the inpatient setting. Residents are under great pressures in tertiary care hospitals not to make mistakes, to anticipate needed tests and have them ordered before someone suggests they are needed, to gain a comprehensive understanding of patients quickly, and never to make errors of omission. A corollary of this conclusion, unproved by the literature, is that community hospitals might be a preferable site for teaching frugal, cost-conscious medicine.

It should be apparent that there are strong forces that oppose cost-conscious decision making. It is foolish to assert that residents misuse resources because they are ignorant: when given the knowledge, they tend to use it only when there are behavior-modifying pressures to do so. It should also be clear that a great deal of cost-conscious decision making does go on. Perhaps more attention should be paid to why physicians make good decisions and to using these insights to help them improve their decision-making skills.

A final comment: Teaching cost awareness to residents requires faculty time, resident time, and teaching resources. Considering the meager results indicated by these studies, is this where we should put our time and energies? Schroeder et al. (1984), in pointing out the expense of cost-containment education for such limited results, inspires us to ask: Is teaching cost effectiveness cost-effective?

REFERENCES

Applegate, W. B.; Bennett, M. D.; Chilton, L.; Skipper, B. J.; and White, R. E. (1983). "Impact of a Cost Containment Education Program on Housestaff Ambulatory Clinic Charges." *Medical Care* 21: 286–96.

Babington, M. A.; Robinson, L. A.; and Monson, R. A. (1983). "Effect of Written Information on Physicians' Knowledge of Drug Prices." *Southern Medical Journal* 76: 328–31, 334.

Chilton, L. A.; Applegate, W. B.; Bennett, M. D.; Skipper, B. E.; and White, R. E. (1982). "Evaluation of Educational Methods in a Comprehensive Cost Containment Project in Ambulatory Care." *Southern Medical Journal* 75: 1251–54.

Cohen, D. I.; Jones, P.; Littenberg, B.; and Neuhauser, D. (1982). "Does Cost Information Availability Reduce Physician Test Usage: A Randomized Clinical Trial with Unexpected Findings." *Medical Care* 20: 286–92.

Cummings, K. M.; Frisof, K. B.; Long, M. J.; and Hrynkiewich, G. (1982). "The

Effects of Price Information on Physicians' Test-Ordering Behavior: Ordering of Diagnostic Tests." *Medical Care* 20: 293–301.

Dixon, R. H., and Laszlo, J. (1974). "Utilization of Clinical Chemistry Services
by Medical House Staff: An Analysis." *Archives of Internal Medicine* 134: 1064–
67.

Eastaugh, S. R. (1981). "Teaching the Principles of Cost-Effective Clinical Decisionmaking to Medical Students." *Inquiry* 18: 28–36.

Eisenberg, J. M. (1977). "An Educational Program to Modify Laboratory Use
by House Staff." *Journal of Medical Education* 52: 578–81.

————— (1985). "Physician Utilization: The State of Research about Physician
Patterns." *Medical Care* 23: 461–83.

————— (1986). *Doctors' Decisions and the Cost of Medical Care*. Ann Arbor, MI:
Health Administration Press.

Eisenberg, J. M.; Williams, S. V.; Garner, L.; Viale, R.; and Smits, H. (1977).
"Computer-Based Audit to Detect and Correct Overutilization of Laboratory
Tests." *Medical Care* 15: 915–21.

Everett, G. D.; DeBlois, S.; Chang, P.; and Holets, T. (1983). "Effect of Cost
Education, Cost Audits and Faculty Chart Review on the Use of Laboratory
Services." *Archives of Internal Medicine* 143: 942–44.

Forrest, J. B.; Ritchie, W. P.; Hudson, M.; and Harlan, J. F. (1981). "Cost Containment through Cost Awareness: A Strategy that Failed." *Surgery* 90: 154–
58.

Garg, M. L.; Gliebe, W. A.; and Kleinberg, W. M. (1979). "Student Peer Review
of Diagnostic Tests at the Medical College of Ohio." *Journal of Medical Education* 54: 852–55.

Goodspeed, R.; Davidoff, F.; and Clive, J. (1985). " 'Little Ticket' Laboratory
Tests: Differential Effect of Probabilistic vs. Cost-Control Curriculum on
Ordering Tests." *Clinical Research* 33: 721A.

Grossman, R. M. (1983). "A Review of Physician Cost-Containment Strategies
for Laboratory Testing." *Medical Care* 21: 783–802.

Hale, F. A.; Stone, K. C.; Seibert, D. J.; and Nelson, E. C. (1984). "A Clinical
Cost-Consciousness Learning Packet for Community-Based Clerkships." *Family Medicine* 16: 131–33.

Hatoum, H. T.; Cartizone, C.; Hutchinson, R. A.; and Purohit, A. (1986). "An
Eleven-Year Review of the Literature: Documentation of the Value and Acceptance of Clinical Pharmacy." *Drug Intelligence & Clinical Pharmacy* 20: 33–
48.

Henderson, D.; D'Alessandri, R.; Westfall, B.; Moore, R.; et al. (1979). "Hospital
Cost Containment: A Little Knowledge Helps." *Clinical Research* 27: 279A.

Johnson, M. W.; Mitch, W. E.; Heller, A. H.; and Spector, R. (1982). "The Impact
of an Educational Program on Gentamicin Use in a Teaching Hospital."
American Journal of Medicine 73: 9–14.

Klein, L. E.; Charache, P.; Johannes, R.; et al. (1981). "Effects of Physicians'
Tutorials on Prescribed Patterns of Graduate Physicians." *Journal of Medical
Education* 56: 504–11.

Lyle, C. B.; Bianchi, R. F.; Harris, J. H.; and Wood, Z. L. (1979). "Teaching Cost
Containment to House Officers at Charlotte Memorial Hospital." *Journal of
Medical Education* 54: 856–62.

Martin, A. R.; Wolf, M. A.; Thibodeau, L. A.; Dzau, V.; and Braunwald, E.
(1980). "A Trial of Two Strategies to Modify the Test-Ordering Behavior of
Medical Residents." *New England Journal of Medicine* 303: 1330–36.

Marton, K. I.; Tul, V.; and Sox, H. C. (1985). "Modifying Test Ordering Behavior in the Outpatient Medical Clinic: A Controlled Trial of Two Educational Interventions." *Archives of Internal Medicine* 145: 816–21.

McPhee, S. J.; Chapman, S. A.; Myers, L. P.; Schroeder, S. A.; and Leong, J. K. (1984). "Lessons for Teaching Cost Containment." *Journal of Medical Education* 59: 722–29.

McPhee, S. J.; Myers, L. P.; and Schroeder, S. A. (1982). "The Cost and Risks of Medical Care: An Annotated Bibliography for Clinicians and Educators." *Western Journal of Medicine* 137: 145–61.

Neal, E. A. (1982). "Encouraging Appropriate X-Ray Utilization: A Successful Educational Model." *Clinical Research* 30: 645A.

Reid, R. A., and Lantz, K. H. (1977). "Physician Profiles in Training the Graduate Internist." *Journal of Medical Education* 52: 301–7.

Rhyne, R. L., and Gehlbach, S. H. (1979). "Effects of an Educational Feedback Strategy on Physician Utilization of Thyroid Function Panels." *Journal of Family Practice* 8: 1003–7.

Schroeder, S. A.; Myers, L. P.; McPhee, S. J.; et al. (1984). "The Failure of Physician Education as a Cost Containment Strategy: Report of a Prospective Controlled Trial at a University Hospital." *Journal of the American Medical Association* 252: 225–30.

Smith, S. R. (1983). "An Evaluation of a Computerized Exercise in Teaching Cost Consciousness." *Journal of Medical Education* 58: 146–48.

Soumerai, S. B., and Avorn, J. (1984). "Efficacy and Cost-Containment in Hospital Pharmacotherapy: State of the Art and Future Directions." *Milbank Memorial Fund Quarterly* 62: 447–74.

Spiegel, C. T.; Kemp, B. A.; Newman, M. A.; Birnbaum, P. S.; and Alter, C. L. (1982). "Modification of Decision-Making Behavior of Third Year Medical Students." *Journal of Medical Education* 57: 769–77.

Williams, S. V., and Eisenberg, J. M. (1986). "A Controlled Trial to Decrease the Unnecessary Use of Diagnostic Tests." *Journal of General Internal Medicine* 1: 8–13.

Williams. S. V.; Eisenberg, J. M.; Kitz, D. S.; et al. (1984). "Teaching Cost Effective Diagnostic Test Use to Medical Students." *Medical Care* 22: 535–42.

Zeleznik, C.; and Gonnella, J. S. (1979). "Jefferson Medical College: Student Model Utilization Review Committee." *Journal of Medical Education* 54: 848–51.

Chapter 14

Explicit Rationing of Medical Care: Is It Really Needed?

Jeffrey C. Merrill and Alan B. Cohen

Editor's Note—Rationing is a part of all health care systems: the demand for medical care is nearly unlimited and resources (or, more to the point, the funds we are willing to spend on that care) are limited. Rationing may be implicit: nursing home beds are scarce because public resources required to subsidize their operation are allocated by states to other needs; requiring that patients pay a deductible before their medical care is paid for by Medicare is known to discourage use of medical resources. It may be explicit: the number of nursing home or hospital beds is limited by law in many states, or reimbursement for an expensive new technology such as heart transplant may be restricted to patients under 50 years old.

Explicit rationing, however, is relatively uncommon in the American medical system and is uncomfortable for us to consider openly. As our nation now debates explicitly denying some types of care to some groups of patients, Merrill and Cohen argue that such rationing is not inevitable, that we can decide to afford "first-dollar" equitable care for all. Our national debate, moreover, suffers from a lack of candor. The health care system is an extremely complicated one, and the factors that influence the debate are political, ethical, and social, as well as economic. To have rational, rather than rationed health care, we must face important questions honestly. Do we really spend too much or do we spend it poorly? Do we really believe in equal access to care, and to whom will we be willing to deny care? Is explicit rationing even feasible in our pluralistic health care system?

In the never-ending debate over the future of the American health care system, rationing of care has emerged as a potential policy option for containing health care costs. In fact, some experts have argued that rationing is inevitable. This development is disturbing to many Americans for whom rationing has a pejorative connotation, implying a specific distribution plan that may not treat all individuals equitably. However, equity is often argued to be unattainable in the face of limited resources. This view holds that economic trade-offs are necessary: trade-offs between sectors of the economy, between the young and the old, and between socioeconomic strata within our society (Aaron and Schwartz 1984; Fuchs 1984; Thurow 1984). Implicit in this view is the belief that rationing will be the primary tool by which these trade-offs may be accomplished.

An opposing view holds that attempts to ration care will result in serious negative consequences for many individuals. Although medical care may not deteriorate overall as a consequence of rationing, some populations—particularly the most vulnerable segments (the poor, the elderly, the uninsured)—may experience an erosion of access to appropriate care (Mechanic 1977). This, in turn, could lead to multi-tiered levels of care within the health care system, exacerbating already existing inequities among some population groups.

Why has this debate taken on such significance recently? First, it is significant because it has been brought to our attention by economists and health policy experts such as those noted above.

Second, it is significant because we live in an era when it is again acceptable to acknowledge the existence of inequality in our society. In past eras, such as the New Deal, the New Frontier, and the Great Society, a standard of equity was implicit in the programs that emerged. While equity was not always achieved through these programs, it was assumed to be among the objectives of those efforts. Today, this concept is countered by the assertion that health care is a "privilege" rather than a "right." Thus, rationing has become more palatable in the public policy debate surrounding health care, and it is now acceptable to talk openly about the issue.

Third, there appear to be economic and budgetary imperatives that make rationing a more prominent issue. These include the continued rising cost of health care and its relative share of the gross national product (GNP) that health care represents, as well as concern over how public spending on health care contributes to the large federal budget deficit. While rising costs have been troublesome for many years, many people now perceive that a crisis has been reached both in the general economy and in the federal budget.

These growing concerns, coupled with lessened concern for equity in health care, have fostered an environment in which rationing is actively discussed as a viable public policy option. Whether rationing is in fact a viable option still depends, however, on the answers to three basic questions:

1. Are rising health care expenditures a legitimate concern? Will the increased share of the GNP devoted to health care threaten our economy and our international competitive position?

2. Will American society, with its reverence for human life and almost chauvinistic pride in technology, permit potential restrictions on health care?

3. Even if these first two questions are answered in the affirmative, is rationing an appropriate solution to the problems that we face?

In addressing these questions, we shall define more precisely what we mean by "rationing" and shall discuss the principal factors that are likely to influence rationing decisions. In addition, we shall examine the special case of medical technology and shall conclude with an exploration of the prospects for the future under alternative policy scenarios.

A NEW PROBLEM—OR JUST "OLD WINE IN A NEW BOTTLE"?

Rationing of health care is *not* a new issue; it has always existed in one form or another, and it is currently present in the American health care system. Several authors, most notably Mechanic (1977) and Aaron and Schwartz (1984), have developed frameworks for classifying different forms of rationing. We believe that rationing of care takes either of two forms: implicit or explicit (Merrill and Cohen 1987). The two approaches differ primarily in their intent and in the directness of their effect. Explicit rationing, for instance, may be characterized as a conscious decision to limit the access of a specific population group to a particular medical service, facility, or technology. Barriers to access may be financial, demographic, or geographic in nature (Aday and Andersen 1974). For example, financial barriers may include third-party payer decisions regarding the extent of services covered and the cost-sharing portion to be borne by the consumer. Demographic factors are exemplified by age restrictions that may apply to potential candidates for expensive treatments, such as organ transplants. In some instances, geographic barriers may arise from decisions by providers, especially multi-institutional systems, to locate facilities and services in settings that intentionally favor some population groups and preclude access for others.

Implicit rationing, on the other hand, does not seek to target specific populations or individuals for direct action; rather, it employs global constraints that limit the general availability of resources. Individual institutions, physicians, and patients retain discretion in how those resources may be used. An example of implicit rationing is state-imposed limitations on the total number of magnetic resonance imagers (MRIs) that may be allowed within a defined geographic area. Such limits were implemented to reduce unnecessary duplication and overutilization of services and, in theory, should not pose inequities for specific individuals or populations. However, by virtue of differing personal financial resources, health insurance coverage, or place of residence, these policies can indirectly ration care for segments of the population.

At present, both implicit and explicit forms of rationing operate within the American health care system. Implicit rationing occurs as government agencies attempt to control the diffusion and adoption of new medical technologies through certificate-of-need regulation. Artificially low physician reimbursement rates under many state Medicaid programs serve as an implicit form of rationing for many poor people; although low reimbursement rates are not necessarily overtly set to reduce access, they clearly may have that effect. Explicit rationing is also more common in American health care practices than is commonly recognized, most often in the form of insurance policies under which third-party payers specify the types of covered services and providers, and the settings in which care can be given. However, for programs such as Medicare and Medicaid, the regulatory actions that limit service coverage—and, consequently, costs—are not widely perceived as the explicit rationing mechanisms that they truly are. Rather, they are couched in more euphemistic terms such as cost sharing, coverage restrictions, or, simply, "uncovered" services (Merrill and Cohen 1987).

FACTORS INFLUENCING THE DECISION TO RATION CARE

Thus far, our discussion has explored the controversy surrounding the issue of rationing health care and has attempted to define rationing methods in dichotomous terms. Before we can address the prospects for the future, it is important first to identify and to examine the key factors that influence rationing decisions. Essentially, there are two broad categories: those external to the system, which we may label "environmental" factors, and those intrinsic to the health care system, which we shall term "system" factors.

Environmental Factors

Environmental factors have a profound influence on policy decisions regarding rationing. They may be subdivided into three groups: economic, political and social, and ethical.

The relative importance of *economic* factors in influencing decisions to ration care cannot be underestimated. From the perverse incentives created by cost-based reimbursement systems to the growing competition among health care institutions, economic factors affect the fundamental behaviors of providers and patients alike. Increasing economic pressures in the health care environment are clearly provoking more discussion of rationing. Nevertheless, it is not yet clear how economic factors will ultimately affect access to health care despite the call for action on the part of some (Schwartz 1987).

Political and *social* factors may also play important roles in the rationing debate. They may militate against explicit rationing schemes by tempering efforts to invoke new legislative or regulatory policies that might promote further inequities within the system. In the face of strong economic pressures, however, it remains to be seen whether political and social resistance to implicit and explicit rationing schemes will be able to achieve temporary or partial reprieve for some programs or services.

Lester Thurow (1984) suggests that *ethical* rather than economic considerations are the critical environmental factor. Thurow contends that we actually have a social problem that ultimately will require the American people to learn to say "no" to increased health spending. For example, he believes that "the U.S. cannot maintain its present rate of growth in health care spending while simultaneously restoring productivity growth and increasing international competitiveness." He argues that a shift in standard medical practice is necessary; that is, that physicians must adopt a social ethic and a behavioral practice that help them to decide when the marginal costs of treatment are no longer justified by the marginal benefits accruing to the patient. But the ethical basis of such a decision is generally difficult for many Americans to either acknowledge or comprehend, and we are not really making decisions on the margin in this country (Merrill and Cohen 1987). Nevertheless, we would agree with Thurow that these countervailing forces (i.e, our inability to say "no" and a perceived danger of rising health care costs) are heading toward a collision in the continuing rationing debate.

System Factors

There are two major subgroups of system factors—organizational and professional—and they tend to receive less attention than their environmental counterparts. However, they can also influence decisions to ration care.

Organizational factors can affect both the availability of and access to care for different segments of society. Regionalization of highly specialized services, such as burn units, trauma centers, and neonatal intensive care units, is generally undertaken to achieve economies, but may, in the process, create geographic barriers to care. Moreover, the trend toward corporatization of the health care system—whether it is believed to be good or bad—has implications for access to care, and may ration care for populations considered less profitable to serve. The pluralistic character of our health care system may also make it difficult to adopt any universal rationing scheme, particularly in contrast to England, where there is essentially a single health care financing system.

Professional factors can determine who gets how much access to care. For example, even under the more stringent payment systems, physicians retain enough discretion in medical decision making to produce well-documented variations in clinical practice. In a changing and uncertain environment, fraught with economic and political pressures, some physicians are likely to ration care either by fee or by implicit means (avoiding or queuing, for example, the less desirable or nonpaying patients). Medical decision making at the level of the individual patient may depend, therefore, on the physician's specialty bias, personal inclinations, economic interests, or even social or racial beliefs.

Taken together, system factors and environmental forces are likely to shape the direction of future decisions regarding the rationing of health care.

THE SPECIAL CASE OF MEDICAL TECHNOLOGY

Roger Evans (1983a; 1983b) has argued that resource allocation and resource-rationing decisions will become inevitable, owing to the high cost of rapidly proliferating new medical technology and to the fact that not all individuals with catastrophic or critical illness will be able to benefit from such technology. He distinguishes between "allocation" and "rationing." Allocation refers to aggregate or macro-level decisions applied to health programs, such as determining how much society should invest in one program versus another, whereas rationing pertains to micro-level decisions involving individual patients, such as determining whether or not a given patient should receive a specific treatment, and if so, to what extent.

Couched in terms of the definitions employed in our framework, Evans' notion of interprogram resource allocation approximates our definition of implicit rationing, although we would argue that such rationing could take place in both micro- and macro-level decisions. Evans' concept of rationing at the individual level closely resembles our definition of explicit rationing, but we would not share in his belief that such micro-level rationing decisions are inevitable. He asserts, first, that we currently make these rationing decisions in the arena of medical technology, most notably in the case of organ transplantation; and second, that such decisions will become more commonplace in the future. We would agree with his first point, but would argue the contrary position in the latter. Rather than imposing further limits on who may receive expensive technologies, we believe that other societal imperatives may make some of these technologies even more widely available in the future.

PROSPECTS FOR THE FUTURE

The future rationing of medical care can now be addressed in terms of two opposing arguments: one that states the inevitability of rationing care, and one that does not.

Argument 1: Rationing Is Inevitable

This argument is predicated on the assumption that rationing will not result arbitrarily, but will occur in response to the environmental and system factors discussed earlier. The program would be one of a scarcity of resources: too few physicians, too few hospital or long-term care beds, or too few dollars.

Clearly, an undersupply of physicians and hospitals does not appear to be a problem. While there may be some geographic disparities, we, as a country, may have an oversupply rather than a dearth of these resources. Nursing home beds are not in sufficient supply, but this seems to be, to a great extent, a function of implicit rationing that has already occurred through the certificate-of-need process at the state level, and it is not a new problem. Therefore, the problem seems to stem from inadequate financial resources rather than from insufficient labor or bed supplies.

The question is, will these financial resources continue to be scarce in the future, thereby creating an environment in which rationing becomes inevitable? Federal budget deficits could, for example, dictate greater reductions in public spending for health care. Cutting federal health expenditures, however, may not represent a politically viable option for cutting the deficit. Both Medicare and Medicaid have already undergone major budget reductions, and it is unclear where future cuts might be made.

Most of the spending cuts in health programs have either occurred on the provider side, such as in year-to-year adjustments in the Medicare payment rates and the physician fee freeze under Medicare, or have involved increased premiums to be paid by individuals. Thus, even in this era of concern over federal budget deficits, the actions to date have not reflected any major government move toward rationing.

Argument 2: Rationing Is Not Inevitable

This argument is predicated on the notion that the health care system will continue to expand. Despite some recent claims of victory that health care costs are now under control, the data indicate that the system continues to expand at unprecedented rates. What looks like a slowing in the rate of growth is, in reality, simply the effect of reduced inflation in the economy, and this has little to do with the health care system per se (Merrill and Wasserman 1985). Although some shifting from inpatient to outpatient care has occurred, this is not necessarily a reflection of any form of cost savings or rationing, but may reflect a change in the way that health care is provided. Further, expansion in the system may actually have a salutary, rather than a detrimental, impact on our economy. The health care sector does not exist in isolation, one-sidedly extracting resources from the economy. It is, in fact, an industry like any other that both provides jobs directly and stimulates growth in other sectors of the economy. The concern that 11 percent of the GNP is too much to spend on health care is without empirical basis. Health care is a labor-intensive industry, has a tremendous "multiplier" effect on other segments of the economy, and produces exportable products and services. Thus, one could argue for expanded investment in the health sector rather than for decreasing its relative share through rationing or any other means. The environmental factors discussed earlier may, in fact, militate against rationing in terms of economic considerations.

A second argument against the inevitability of rationing may rest in the underlying ethos of American culture. As a society, we appear unwilling to make the choices that other cultures have consciously made to limit care, particularly for those who are most sick. Early on, we attempted to ration renal dialysis, but we found that choice distasteful and, consequently, established benefits for all, regardless of age, under the Medicare program. Moreover, when we *do* ration, we tend to ration on a first-dollar basis; that is, our public programs are more likely to limit an individual's access to basic services by not paying for the initial costs of care (either because of a lack of coverage for basic services or because of high deductibles and coinsurance), even though more expensive, tertiary care is often covered (Merrill and Cohen 1987). For instance, whereas an indigent Medicare beneficiary with chronic diabetes may be denied coverage for the cost of insulin, that same individual will be afforded every available technological advantage should the illness reach the acute or critical stage! As a society, we have considerable reverence for technology, not just because of its impact on health, but because of an almost chauvinistic belief that improved technology is an American imperative. The last-dollar rationing in Great Britain (where the more expensive tertiary technologies are rationed) may be considered socially impossible in this country, even as denial of coverage for the most basic services continues. Thus, with regard to social considerations, rationing may not be a viable alternative.

MAKING A MORE RATIONAL SYSTEM

As we look to the future, the question is not whether rationing is or is not inevitable. The real question is, how do we make the system more rational? Most observers would agree that rationing should not become a substitute for better management of the health care system, and that equity should not be sacrificed in the process of attaining greater system efficiency. However, a second issue arises when we discuss both rationing and a more rational system: Should we focus solely on rationing, or would it be more appropriate to define a minimum threshold of care to which all people are entitled? Presently, in this country, we seem to be preoccupied with the former.

Even so, when potential schemes for rationing in the United States are discussed, an implicit assumption is made that a minimum level of care is available to everyone. In reality, this is very misleading. In Britain, where the initial, or first-dollar, costs of basic primary care are covered, but access to very high-cost services is impeded, one can argue for or against rationing on the basis of technical efficiency (Merrill and Cohen 1987). In other words, one can weigh the marginal benefit of a given service against its marginal cost precisely because the National Health Service affords a minimum threshold of care for everyone. In the United States, however, where the coverage for basic services is not universal, solutions on the basis of technical efficiency are not realistic and the debate is, indeed, far more complex. Such decisions may well mean trading off one person's organ transplant for another's basic prenatal care.

POLICY QUESTIONS THAT MUST BE ADDRESSED

In order to come to terms with the issue of rationing and its possible future role, we should rely less on the simplistic belief that greater health care spending will inevitably lead to rationing. Rather, we would suggest that the following questions must be thoroughly considered and answered before rationing is posed as a viable public policy alternative:

1. Do we spend too much on health care and do we spend it poorly?

—Is the health care system too big relative to other sectors of the economy? What is an appropriate share of the GNP for health care to absorb, and are we in danger of reaching that level?

—Are federal health dollars being spent appropriately? Can we make better use of these funds? What are our priorities in terms of public dollars spent on health versus other public responsibilities?

—Have we acknowledged the fungibility of health expenditures? When we cut federal expenditures, are we really eliminating them or are we simply shifting those financial responsibilities to other levels of government or to private payers?

2. Can we determine societal expectations within the context of whether or not to ration?

—Do we believe in equity and equal access? Should everyone receive some basic level of services and, if so, should they receive it from the same providers and in the same locations?

—What are we willing to consider as a minimum level of care? Do we consider the status quo an acceptable level? Do we want to reduce that further?

—Are we willing to accept imminent death because of withheld care? If we should decide to make the same choices about rationing that have been made in other countries, are we willing to accept the consequences?

3. If we choose to ration explicitly, how might we accomplish it? Is it as feasible an option as some might imagine?

—Does our pluralistic health care system make it difficult to develop universal rationing schemes?

—Are employers going to ration their health insurance coverage in the same way as the federal government?

—Will rationing in the Medicaid program be uniform across all states?

Given that the current system already relies greatly on personal expenditures for health care, is it more difficult to design and to implement explicit rationing schemes than it would be, for example, in the English system where only about 5 percent of the population has private insurance (Schwartz and Aaron 1984), and most services are completely covered under the National Health Service?

CONCLUSIONS

Rationing as a policy option for cost containment may be a "straw man" in our public debate over the future of our health care financing and delivery system. The forces and principal actors influencing health policy clearly are intrigued by ways of limiting both public and private responsibility for financing health care. Yet, our system is an intricate web of interests that simultaneously coincide and conflict, often operating against continuing cost-containment efforts. For instance, the same corporate executive who is concerned about rising health care insurance premiums may also be a trustee of the local hospital and interested in maximizing that institution's reimbursement levels. Likewise, the member of Congress who is concerned about reducing the federal budget may also be interested in the financial viability of a major private health care concern within his or her district. As with defense, health care permeates society to the extent that major budget reductions or changes that could lead to more rationing may not actually be possible. Instead, the cultural imperatives (i.e., our societal dedication to do everything possible to keep people alive, our reverence for technology, and basic human decency on the part of Americans) may join with the economic imperatives (i.e., those self-interests at the community, corporate, and government levels) to assure a minimum level of care for all Americans. There are indications that this process has already begun, with new coalitions of businessmen, physicians, and other providers, and even the insurance industry seeking new financing mechanisms to address the problems of the uninsured. Rather than viewing rationing as a future inevitability, we must recognize the extent to which it already exists and seek, as a broad spectrum of American leaders already has, solutions to the current problems.

REFERENCES

Aaron, H. J., and Schwartz, W. B. (1984). *The Painful Prescription: Rationing Hospital Care.* Washington, DC: Brookings Institution.

Aday, L. A., and Andersen, R. (1974). "A Framework for the Study of Access to Medical Care." *Health Services Research* 9: 208–20.

Evans, R. W. (1983a). "Health Care Technology and the Inevitability of Resource Allocation and Rationing Decisions. Part I." *Journal of the American Medical Association* 249: 2047–53.

——— (1983b). "Health Care Technology and the Inevitability of Resource Allocation and Rationing Decisions. Part II." *Journal of the American Medical Association* 249: 2208–19.

Fuchs, V. R. (1984). "The Rationing of Medical Care." *New England Journal of Medicine* 311: 1572–73.

Mechanic, D. (1977). "The Growth of Medical Technology and Bureaucracy: Implications for Medical Care." *Milbank Memorial Fund Quarterly* 55: 61–78.

————— (1985). "Cost Containment and the Quality of Medical Care: Rationing Strategies in an Era of Constrained Resources." *Milbank Memorial Fund Quarterly* 63: 453–75.

Merrill, J. C., and Cohen, A. B. (1987). "The Emperor's New Clothes: Unraveling the Myths about Rationing." *Inquiry* 24: 105–9.

Merrill, J. C., and Wasserman, R. J. (1985). "Growth in National Expenditures: Additional Analyses." *Health Affairs* 4: 91–98.

Schwartz, W. B. (1987). "The Inevitable Failure of Current Cost-Containment Strategies." *Journal of the American Medical Association* 257: 220–24.

Schwartz, W. B., and Aaron, H. J. (1984). "Rationing Hospital Care: Lessons from Britain." *New England Journal of Medicine* 310: 52–56.

Thurow, L. C. (1984). "Learning to Say 'No'." *New England Journal of Medicine* 311: 1569–72.

Chapter 15

Cost Containment through Improved Information Systems and Medical Practice Patterns

Anthony L. Komaroff and Thomas H. Lee

Editor's Note—A prospective reimbursement system, such as payment determined by diagnosis-related groups (DRGs), motivates medical providers to economize by eliminating waste. Institutions are paid preset average amounts determined by patients' diagnoses, not according to the resources utilized to provide medical care. Such a system is only as fair and rational, however, as the accuracy of its diagnostic categories. Patient demographics may play an important role in consumption of medical care resources, for example, and unless demographic data are included in diagnostic groupings, they could be clinically accurate but financially incorrect or unfair.

Komaroff and Lee argue that more sophisticated data collection and analysis can refine the DRGs into a more rational list of diagnoses for reimbursement purposes. Their data have led them to conclude, moreover, that such intra- and interhospital analysis is a worthwhile investment for a hospital. It provides them with data to identify cost-inefficient medical practices with precision, to identify the source of wastefulness, to suggest remedies, and to feed back information to administrators and physicians to help them make cost-effective decisions. It may also allow sophisticated financial analysis of technologic innovations that appear expensive, but may reduce the costs of care through shorter or more efficient hospitalizations. In this somewhat technical discussion, actual cases are described in which interventions based on analysis of DRG data led to savings. This study and the preliminary analysis in the chapter by Lyle et al. support the need for prompt ongoing feedback of clinically oriented financial data to practitioners and clinical chiefs.

The organization and financing of health care in the United States is changing in a revolutionary fashion. Traditionally, health care was paid for in a retrospective fashion: doctors and hospitals told insurers how much it had cost to care for a patient, and the insurers paid that cost. Increasingly, however, American health care is being paid for on a prospective basis: the insurers will pay doctors and hospitals according to formulas that take no account of how much it has cost to provide the care. Doctors and hospitals thereby have a strong incentive to deliver care in the most efficient manner possible. If one believes, as we and many others do, that there is currently some waste in the utilization of health care resources, then it is possible to imagine cutting costs without compromising the quality of care.

THE PROSPECTIVE PAYMENT REVOLUTION

The "prospective payment revolution" has many faces: the Medicare diagnosis-related group (DRG) payment system; "caps" on spending by third parties; and the rapid growth of health organizations and financing systems that work primarily on capitated payment of enrolled populations—health maintenance organizations (HMOs), independent practice associations (IPAs), and preferred provider organizations (PPOs).

The "prospective payment revolution" is placing new and often unfamiliar pressures on medical caregivers and medical institutions to examine what we do. Institutions must examine how efficiently they deliver each unit of service which goes into the care of a patient: the cost of each chest x-ray, each dose of a particular medication, and each day of care on a particular patient care unit. Clinicians determine the volume of medical resources—bed days, tests, treatments—used to care for a patient with a particular problem. We are being asked to examine those decisions: Does the patient require hospitalization or surgery? Need the hospitalization be as long for this condition as it traditionally has been? Can the number of tests or treatments be reduced, or can less expensive tests and treatments substitute for more expensive ones?

VARIABILITY IN THE USE OF MEDICAL RESOURCES

For the past 20 years, a growing literature has provided incontrovertible evidence of marked variability among different clinicians caring for patients who appear to have the same clinical problem.[1] The fact that medical practices are so variable is increasingly evident to those concerned with the growing costs of health care. The insurers of health care, and those large organized constituencies that pay the bill (particularly American industry and federal and state government) are asking a simple question of American medicine: If all of you do things so differently, can all of you be doing things correctly?

It has become imperative for clinicians and medical institutions to develop information systems that facilitate an examination of medical practice patterns. This has become particularly true in teaching hospitals, because teaching hospitals typically provide more expensive medical care and typically serve a greater fraction of underinsured patients. In addition, the teaching hospital has always been a laboratory for developing better ways of diagnosing and treating disease, and for teaching about new discoveries and new technologies. The same spirit of examination can be brought to bear on medical practice patterns within a teaching hospital.

The staff at the Brigham and Women's Hospital in Boston have developed systems to help identify and encourage more cost-effective medical care. The initial impetus to do so came from the establishment of a new kind of research and development unit at the hospital, the Center for Cost-Effective Care. Supported initially by grant funding, many of the center's efforts became sufficiently successful and important to be supported by the hospital itself.

DEFINING THE HOSPITAL'S CASE MIX

The center's first task was to define the hospital's case mix: to create groupings of patients with clinically related illnesses who would usually be expected to require similar resources. The definition of such groupings is a tricky business. Every physician recognizes that no two patients with the same illness are necessarily alike. Whereas most industries can define rather precisely a set of products (e.g., Gillette makes a limited number of shaving instruments, and each of these instruments is virtually identical to others of the same type), the hospital "industry" cannot easily define its "products."

DRGs were developed to overcome some of the limitations of traditional diagnostic coding systems, and to identify groups of patients who have the "same" clinical condition and who required reasonably similar resources. It is widely recognized that patients within the same DRG may have variable degrees of illness, and it is argued that teaching hospitals attract sicker patients within the DRGs, because teaching hospitals tend to be the "court of last resort."

The hospital's first task was to adapt DRGs to fit its own needs. There were a number of instances in which, given the kinds of patients seen at the hospital, the DRG system was inadequate. In some cases, because the hospital specialized in a particular medical treatment or surgical procedure, there was great heterogeneity among patients within a DRG. Clinicians and administrators worked together, using computerized analyses of medical practice patterns and resource utilization, to split DRGs into subgroups. Each of these subgroups had a more homogeneous utilization of resources. In other instances, there appeared to be little reason to have several DRGs for a particular condition, since the patients within these DRGs were reasonably similar in their use of resources. In other words, in some cases the DRGs were disaggregated, and in other cases they were lumped together.

AN INFORMATION SYSTEM TO EXAMINE PRACTICE PATTERNS

The hospital's computerized system for analyzing medical practice patterns, the CHASE System, is a data base management system which allows a data base to be created with great flexibility. It also allows the user to ask "what if" questions—questions that could not have been anticipated at the time the system was developed. In other words, the CHASE System not only produces a series of regular reports in a stable format, but can also be used to perform special analyses in response to ad hoc questions.

For each patient, the system combines the information from the hospital discharge abstract and the itemized bill. Every hospitalization since late 1981 is stored in the system, "live" on disc, and can be searched at any time.

The CHASE System groups patients according to any criteria in its data base. It can create groups of patients who share the same DRG, the same doctor, or the same insurer. It also can identify all patients who have had a particular diagnostic technology or form of therapy. Furthermore, this system can find all patients who are characterized by any combination of elements in its data base. For example, it could find all patients within DRG 120, whose care was paid for by Medicare, who were treated on the Medical Service during the month of May, 1985, and whose home address was from a particular zip code.

Having identified groups of patients, the CHASE System can then display any data elements about that group: for example, the average age of the patients, the frequency of a particular complication, or the charges for medications. In so doing, the system automatically performs descriptive statistics and can automatically compare two or more groups of patients using comparative statistics.

The Brigham and Women's Hospital has undertaken a major cost-accounting effort in order to estimate the average cost of each day of care on a particular patient care unit and each diagnostic test and form of treatment. These estimated average costs are maintained within the system and are regularly updated. As a consequence, the system can estimate the average cost of care for any patient, since it knows each of the bed days, and diagnostic and therapeutic resources used for that patient. Because the system can estimate the average costs for any individual patient, it can also estimate the average costs for any group of patients.

The CHASE System can also break down its average cost estimates. For example, the estimated average cost of a bed day on a particular patient care unit is really the total of many component costs: the cost of nursing care on that unit, the cost of house officers, the cost of housekeeping for that unit, the cost of energy for that unit, and indirectly allocated costs such as the institutional cost of general administrative services. The system is built to store estimates for both the fixed and variable costs of each unit of service, and it is able to estimate the marginal cost changes when the volume of a particular unit of service changes.

The CHASE System also includes data to assess the quality of care. Besides storing information about complications of diagnosis and treatment, the system contains special data bases which help assess the quality of care of "tracer" conditions. For example, the Orthopedic Surgery Service uses the system to store information regarding the pre- and postsurgical status of patients undergoing prosthetic joint surgery, including activities of daily living, gait and ambulation status, and so on. As pressures mount to reduce the length-of-stay or the use of resources (e.g., postsurgical physical therapy), the service can follow these outcome parameters to look for evidence that the quality of care is suffering.

PHYSICIAN FEEDBACK

The hospital regularly feeds back information to its physicians and surgeons regarding medical practice patterns in caring for patients with particular clinical problems. These reports include comparisons of the entire service (e.g., medicine, general surgery, orthopedic surgery services) to the service's performance in prior years, and comparisons of individual doctors' use of resources in the care of a particular clinical problem. The CHASE System has also been used to compare the practice patterns of doctors at the hospital with doctors at other teaching hospitals who are caring for patients with the same problem. Data from these other hospitals have been entered into the CHASE System to accomplish these interinstitutional comparisons. Close cooperation between clinicians and administrators is essential, both in the planning of analyses and in the presentation of results as feedback. Interested physicians can serve as liaisons between these two groups who have had an almost adversarial relationship at times in the past. Administrators at the hospital have had little difficulty identifying physicians interested in playing such a role, and clinicians have been included in every stage of virtually every project.

THE CARDIOLOGY SERVICE EXAMPLE

An Examination of DRG 138

In their attempts to define the case mix of the Cardiology Service, cardiologists at Brigham and Women's Hospital were unwilling to accept DRG 138 (Cardiac arrhythmia and conduction disorders, age ≥ 70 and/ or cardiovascular complications) as an adequate case-mix group. They pointed out that there were tremendous clinical differences between an elderly patient with sick sinus syndrome, who might be admitted for monitoring after a presyncopal episode, and another patient who had symptomatic bouts of sustained ventricular tachycardia. In the case of the latter patient, one would not be surprised by hospitalization lasting weeks, as drug after drug was tried. Data lumping such patients together might be valid, but they are of limited use if the clinicians cannot recognize the patients involved.

Accordingly, a small committee of cardiologists and administrators at the hospital subdivided several of the DRGs. DRG 138 was divided into patients with tachyarrhythmias and bradyarrhythmias based on the suspicion that tachyarrhythmias were more likely to be life-threatening and to require prolonged lengths-of-stay. In this case, determining whether these groups actually differ in resource utilization was not especially important, but distinguishing the groups enhanced the physician's interest in and understanding of these data.

Comparison of Recent Versus Historical Performance

Data on changes in resource utilization over time allow analysis of whether clinicians are succeeding in reducing lengths-of-stay and/or test ordering for similar patients. At Brigham and Women's Hospital, length-of-stay fell progressively in patients in DRG 125 (Circulatory disease except acute myocardial infarction; Cardiac catheterization without complex diagnosis). On the other hand, length-of-stay actually increased slightly for patients in DRG 122 (Acute myocardial infarction without complex diagnosis). These findings allowed cardiologists to congratulate themselves on their efficiency with one group of patients while generating interest in investigations of a problem area.

Comparison of Individual Physicians with Their Peers

The system also provides insights into how individual physicians practice in comparison to their peers. For example, patients admitted to one cardiologist had lengths-of-stay that exceeded those in the rest of the cardiology division in almost all DRGs (Table 15.1). While such information is valuable and often intensely interesting to clinicians, differences may be confounded by variability in clinical and socioeconomic considerations. It became apparent (via a retrospective chart review) that the patients admitted by this cardiologist were probably sicker than those in the rest of the cardiology division. His patients were often referred from other cities and communities and had frequently already done poorly with conventional medical therapy. It is not surprising that such patients would have a longer length-of-stay.

Nevertheless, such analyses can help individual physicians recognize areas in which their practice patterns deviate markedly from their peers. Furthermore, they may decrease length-of-stay and resource utilization through a Hawthorne effect alone.

Comparison of Hospitals

An examination of different doctors at the same hospital can be misleading and parochial: physicians at a single hospital may not realize that they all have the same problem. One way to approach this problem is to conduct cooperative analyses of data bases at several hospitals. An analysis of differences in resource utilization, in the care of patients with uncomplicated myocardial infarction, at three Boston teaching hospitals showed that patients at one of these hospitals had significantly shorter total and intensive care unit lengths-of-stay. Furthermore, the patients

TABLE 15.1

Lengths of Hospital Stay for Physician #XXX Compared to
Rest of Division of Cardiology for Several Cardiac Diagnoses, 1983

DRG Number	Abbreviated Diagnosis	MD #XXX	Division
125	No myocardial infarction or catheterization	9.3	4.7
138A	Tachyarrhythmia age >70	11.1	7.2
139A	Tachyarrhythmia age ≤ 70	9.4	5.7
140	Angina	8.8	6.7
All patients		10.7	8.6

at this hospital underwent significantly fewer predischarge tests, suggesting a relationship between test utilization and length-of-stay, and a possible intervention for cardiologists at the other hospitals.

The technical difficulties of such cooperative studies are considerable. Because methods for determining charges and estimating costs vary among institutions, data must usually be analyzed as units of service, such as number of urinalyses or chest x-rays. The analysis will, of course, be as weak as the weakest data base: if one hospital has not collected information on portable versus routine x-rays, no comparison can be made. Steering committees should therefore include a physician and an administrative representative from each hospital. Although it is difficult to plan a study with a large committee, the findings of such analyses can be startling and compelling.

Analysis of the Potential Impact of New Interventions

New technologies and management strategies must be evaluated for their potential economic consequences as well as their medical efficacy. For example, patients admitted from the emergency room with acute chest pain, who were not found to have myocardial infarction, nevertheless had a mean length-of-stay of more than six days, and a mean intensive care unit length-of-stay of two days. These data highlight the importance of increasing the diagnostic accuracy of tests administered to such patients in the emergency room, and the potential impact of triaging patients with a low probability of myocardial infarction to less intensive and less costly levels of care such as intermediate care units (Fineberg, Scadden, and Goldman 1984). Such a unit has just been established at our hospital, based on such analyses.

A more speculative analysis was conducted to determine the potential impact on intensive care unit length-of-stay of using digoxin-specific antibody fragments in digoxin toxicity. Although this drug was developed for treatment of massive overdoses leading to intractable life-threatening arrhythmias, its rapid action and the absence of complications in early testing raise the question of whether it might have a wider application in patients with less severe toxicity. These patients would usually recover with conventional measures, which include monitoring in an intensive care unit, where facilities for arrhythmia treatment or rapid placement of a transvenous pacemaker are available.

The mean intensive care unit length-of-stay in such patients was 3.4 days, suggesting that, since the digoxin-specific antibody fragments can reverse manifestations of digoxin toxicity within 30 minutes, considerable cost savings might be accomplished by using this agent on the first day and reducing intensive care utilization. This drug has not been tested in patients with mild-to-moderate digoxin toxicity, and calculations of potential cost savings are compromised by the difficulty of estimating marginal versus fixed costs. However, this analysis is an example of how such speculation can help direct further, more definitive investigations.

CONCLUSIONS

The prospective payment revolution requires that doctors and medical institutions examine medical practice patterns, and thereby identify and eliminate unnecessary or marginally useful practices. If this is done well, the quality of patient care need not suffer. In order to be successful, the effort requires the development of computerized systems for analysis and, more importantly, working alliances of doctors and hospital administrators.

NOTE

1. The selected bibliography at the end of this chapter lists 21 studies that demonstrate variability in clinical practice.

REFERENCE

Fineberg, H.; Scadden, D.; and Goldman, L. (1984). "Management of Patients with a Low Probability of Acute Myocardial Infarction: Cost-effectiveness of Alternatives to Coronary Care Unit Admission." *New England Journal of Medicine* 310: 1301–7.

SELECTED BIBLIOGRAPHY

Bunker, J. P. "A Comparison of Operations and Surgeons in the United States and in England and Wales." *New England Journal of Medicine* 282 (1970): 135–44.
Daniels, M., and Schroeder, S. A. "Variation among Physicians in Use of Laboratory Tests. II. Relation to Clinical Productivity and Outcomes of Care." *Medical Care* 15 (1977): 482–87.
Dutton, D. B. "Patterns of Ambulatory Health Care in Five Different Delivery Systems." *Medical Care* 17 (1979): 221–43.
Gertman, P. M., and Restuccia, J. D. "The Appropriateness Evaluation Protocol: A Technique for Assessing Unnecessary Days of Hospital Care." *Medical Care* 19 (1981): 855–71.
Griner, P. F., and Liptzin, B. "Use of the Laboratory in a Teaching Hospital: Implications for Patient Care, Education, and Hospital Costs." *Annals of Internal Medicine* 74 (1971): 157–63.

Heasman, M. A. "How Long in Hospital? A Study in Variation in Duration of Stay for Two Common Surgical Conditions." *Lancet* 2 (1964): 539–41.

Lewis, C. E. "Variations in the Incidence of Surgery." *New England Journal of Medicine* 281 (1969): 880–84.

Lovejoy, F. H., Jr.; Carper, J. M.; Janeway, C. A.; and Kosa, J. "Unnecessary and Preventable Hospitalizations: Report on an Internal Audit." *Medical Care* 79 (1971): 868–72.

Lyle, C. B.; Citron, D. S.; and Sugg, W. C. "Cost of Medical Care in a Practice of Internal Medicine: A Study in a Group of Seven Internists." *Annals of Internal Medicine* 81 (1974): 1–6.

MacKintosh, J. M.; McKeown, T.; and Garratt, F. N. "An Examination of the Need for Hospital Admission." *Lancet* 1 (1961): 815–18.

Mushlin, A. I., and Appel, F. A. "Extramedical Factors in the Decision to Hospitalize Medical Patients." *American Journal of Public Health* 66 (1976): 170–72.

Relman, A. S., and Rennie, D. "Treatment of End-Stage Renal Disease: Free but Not Equal." *New England Journal of Medicine* 303 (1980): 996–98.

Restuccia, J. D., and Holloway, D. C. "Barriers to Appropriate Utilization of an Acute Facility." *Medical Care* 14 (1976): 559–73.

Schroeder, S. A.; Kenders, K.; Cooper, J. K.; and Piemme, T. E. "Use of Laboratory Tests and Pharmaceuticals: Variation among Physicians and Effect of Cost Audit on Subsequent Use." *Journal of the American Medical Association* 225 (1973): 969–73.

Schroeder, S. A., and O'Leary, D. S. "Difference in Laboratory Use and Length of Stay between University and Community Hospitals." *Journal of Medical Education* 52 (1977): 418–20.

Schroeder, S. A.; Schliftman, A.; and Piemme, T. E. "Variation among Physicians in Use of Laboratory Tests: Relation to Quality of Care." *Medical Care* 12 (1974): 709–13.

Vayda, E. "A Comparison of Surgical Rates in Canada and in England and Wales." *New England Journal of Medicine* 289 (1973): 1224–29.

Vayda, E., and Anderson, G. D. "Comparison of Provincial Surgical Rates in 1968." *Canadian Journal of Surgery* 18 (1975): 18–26.

Wennberg, J., and Gittelsohn, A. "Health Care Delivery in Maine. I: Patterns of Use of Common Surgical Procedures." *Journal of the Maine Medical Association* 66 (1975): 123–49.

————. "Small Area Variations in Health Care Delivery: A Population-Based Health Information System Can Guide Planning and Regulatory Decision-Making." *Science* 182 (1973): 1102–8.

West, R. R., and Carey, M. J. "Variation in Rates of Hospital Admission for Appendicitis in Wales." *British Medical Journal* 1 (1978): 1662–64.

V

THE MARGINS OF COST CONTAINMENT: CARING FOR THE GROWING ELDERLY POPULATION, ASSURING QUALITY, AND FUTURE RESEARCH

Chapter 16

Geriatric Medicine: Life in the Crucible of the Struggle to Contain Health Care Costs

William R. Hazzard

Editor's Note—The graying of America is a threat of the greatest magnitude to those who are working to reduce medical care costs. The elderly consume a disproportionate amount of medical care resources, and we know that there will continue to be yet more rapidly increasing numbers of older people who live decades longer than had been expected in the 1950s and 1960s. In an insightful analysis of solutions to this socioeconomic threat, Hazzard argues for preventive gerontology, which would improve the health of the elderly by promoting a healthy life-style and reducing disease risk factors. Medical care costs should, therefore, be no greater for the elderly than for younger persons in similar good health.

Aging itself, however, extracts a toll. The elderly have less physiologic reserve, and even the healthy very old may be surviving as a result of delicately maintained homeostasis that could be disrupted by a clinical "trigger"—infection, infarction, trauma, and iatrogenic insults with polypharmacy or invasive procedures. Hence the need for preventive geriatrics—attention to the risks of multiple chronic diseases and to preventing or treating promptly the clinical trigger phenomena that can cause a downward medical spiral resulting in debility or death. With the recognition that fewer problems are reversible, that less may be gained by aggressive intervention, and that the interventions themselves may be trigger phenomena, efficient resource utilization must be one of the skills of the physician who cares for elderly patients.

Of equal significance is an issue that is also raised in several other chapters: the disproportionate use of resources by terminally ill elderly patients. Accurate prediction of the last year or month or week of life is a skill of great economic and humanitarian importance. The medical care system has been designed and refined to care for acutely ill young patients. It is now consumed with the care of chronically ill, debilitated elderly patients. The mismatch between the system and its users leads to the inappropriate waste of resources, often with worse outcomes than if nothing were done—in Hazzard's words, "when less is better."

As the twentieth century nears its end, the "graying of America" cannot be ignored. For health care planners and providers alike, this shift in the population has translated into "the demographic imperative," the need to address the increasing health care needs of an aging American population in an era of diminishing per capita health care resources.

The origin of the demographic shift is familiar to all who have observed the parallel between socioeconomic and cultural development of populations and their increasing median age and longevity. While developing nations (e.g., Mexico) have a population distribution by age resembling that of the United States a century ago (a pyramidal configuration with the greatest proportion in the youngest age group and the smallest in the oldest), fully developed nations (e.g., Sweden and other advanced cultures of northern Europe) have already reached the rectangular configuration representing the steady state.

The United States, by contrast, is a population still in flux, with the bulge of the post–World War II "baby boom" still dominating our culture with a youth-oriented value system. However, as this dominating subpopulation ages, the phenomenon of aging, including the inevitable increase in health care requirements, will become appreciated. As the baby boomers become the elderly, the full rectangularization of the distribution by age will occur (in about 2030). A corollary of those demographic shifts will be an increasing preponderance of surviving women, clearly underscoring the challenge to health care practitioners of the future: the care of the elderly, and specifically of elderly women, will become a dominant force in health care resource allocation in the future, and skill in the management of those resources will become imperative for the successful practitioner.

The association between age and health care resource consumption is exponential, not linear, with increasing age. Moreover, the greatest proportional increase in numbers of the population will be concentrated among the most elderly, those over 75 and even the "oldest old," those over 85. Thus, the health care resource requirements of an aging population are dramatically different from those of one younger: in 1983 the per capita personal health care expenditures of those over 65 (which were increasingly concentrated among those over 75 and 85) were more than four times greater than among those individuals under 65 years of age.

The geriatric health care challenge thus becomes clear. Since:

1. The median age of the population is increasing with an increasing proportion of elderly and a decreasing proportion of younger persons to care for them;
2. The health care needs of "Everyman" increase with age; and
3. Expenditures on health care per capita and as a percent of gross national product appear relatively fixed.

Therefore:

4. The health care of the elderly must become more efficient.

CONTAINING HEALTH CARE RESOURCE EXPENDITURE FOR THE ELDERLY: A TWOFOLD STRATEGY

Two interrelated approaches are necessary to contain such health care costs: gerontology (the study of aging, which begins at conception and ends with death) and geriatrics (the health care of the elderly, including geriatric medicine). It is important to use deliberate program development to control health care costs while extending not only absolute but, more important, functional (including quality-adjusted) longevity.

Preventive Gerontology

Fries (1980) and others have suggested that, by 1980, Americans had achieved 80 percent of the maximum ("ideal") possible increase in average human longevity. This estimate was based on the assumptions of a continuing, inexorable premature attrition from trauma and an absolute upper limit of the human life span of about 110 years. Socioeconomic and cultural development has eliminated much of the vastly premature mortality in children and youth, allowing an ever-increasing proportion of those born in developed nations to achieve nearly their full longevity potential, ultimately succumbing to multisystem frailty in old age ("natural death" in the parlance of Fries).

While this hypothesis, with its average age at death of 85 ± four years (mean ± SD), its exponential rise in death rate in the ninth decade, and its implicit avoidance of a protracted period of preterminal debility, has been widely challenged (Manton 1982; Schneider and Brody 1983), its central truths are nevertheless evident. Chief among these is its logical emphasis upon prevention of adult- and old age–onset chronic diseases through alterations in life-style. Such alterations should attenuate not only the death rate but also, at least hypothetically, the physiological decline in multiple systems which has been shown to accompany increasing age in cross-sectional studies. Hence, one strategy to minimize health care expenditures among an aging population is in the realm of "preventive gerontology." In this conceptualization, the potential for increasing functional longevity is found in the difference between the curve of declining survival or declining physiological competence—which is the resultant of aging of both primary (i.e., genetically determined, inevitable) and secondary (potentially preventable or at least delayable through alterations in life-style) forms of aging—and the curve reflecting the consequences of primary aging alone (by definition quantifiable only after all secondary aging has been eliminated).

Cause for optimism regarding potential in the realm of preventive gerontology was generated by the report of equivalent cardiovascular reserve among men in their eighties (free of ischemic heart disease by thallium scintiscanning) compared with men in their twenties. The subjects were part of the Baltimore Longitudinal Study of Aging, an elite group of health-conscious, highly educated subjects noted for their vigor and good health even at advanced ages (Shock et al. 1984; Weisfeldt, Gerstenblith, and Lakatta 1984). Various health-associated behaviors need to be adopted on a lifelong basis, especially prior to old age, since their impact upon longevity declines with advanced age. Avoidance of health- and accident-associated risks such as cigarette smoking, sedentary life-style, diets high in cholesterol and saturated fats, alcohol and drug abuse, and reckless and hostile behavior are the obvious ploys of a multi-pronged, long-term intervention strategy. Should such a strategy be widely implemented (and recent dramatic, progressive declines in cardiovascular mortality and morbidity suggest that secular, widely adopted population trends are not only possible but are clearly occurring in contemporary American society) (Stern 1979), geriatric medicine of the future may indeed be focused upon those people who are precariously balanced at or near the upper limit of their natural life span.

Two corollaries of successful preventive gerontology must be acknowledged. First, retardation of accelerated disease processes such as atherogenesis may only delay passage of the clinical horizon, and the individual may become equally as disabled in old age as heretofore might have been the case in middle age, but with concomitant debility in multiple other physiological spheres; hence, the need for chronic care of the multiply disabled may conceivably increase rather than decrease as a by-product of successful chronic disease prevention strategies. Second, the prevalence, incidence, and drain on resources of certain disorders that are highly concentrated in old age may increase as a higher proportion of people live to the age of risk (e.g., an "epidemic" of Alzheimer's disease is probably on the horizon).

Another corollary of a successful strategy to delay the onset of time-related disorders is also apparent: whereas the shape of the survival curve of a human population demonstrating senescence may be largely rectangular (in contrast to the semi-logarithmic curve representing the chance survival of radioactive isotopes or, for example, water glasses in a cafeteria), the tail of that human survival curve is semi-logarithmic, suggesting that survival above about 92 years in contemporary American society may be largely a matter of chance. To any health care practitioner who focuses upon the needs of the elderly, the basis of this phenomenon is all too evident: the very old, precariously perched on the edge of a precipice of disaster by virtue of delicately maintained homeostasis in biological, psychological, and social spheres, may be sent over the brink and down the "slippery slope" by seemingly trivial insults (trigger phenomena). While in a younger person such insults would result in short-term disability, in the elderly they may initiate a terminal cascade of complications, decline, and death. Preventive *geriatrics* (prevention in the elderly themselves) differs from preventive *gerontology* in concentrating upon trigger phenomena of proximate importance in avoiding such catastrophes: infections (viral, bacterial, myobacterial); infarctions (myocardial infarction, strokes, and peripheral vascular occlusions); and infirmity (falls and fractures, loss of food and fluid homeostasis, and iatrogenesis, especially polypharmacy).

The ironies implicit from successful preventive gerontology should be appreciated and are, indeed, a new "doctor's dilemma":

1. As they age, people accumulate "life's insults";

2. Most of such diseases and disabilities are only partially reversible;

3. Functional disability in old age may proceed from limitations in several spheres: physical, social, psychological, and economic;

4. As the barrier of the upper limit of the human life span is approached:

   a. the potential reversibility of disability and disease as measured in "person years" is progressively reduced;

   b. the potential risk of complications from any intervention (drugs, diet, diagnostic procedures, surgery, social dislocation) increases;

5. With disease and disability, the elderly and their supporters look increasingly to the physician for aid and comfort at precisely the time when the physician, as conventionally defined, may have the least to offer.

Therefore, the second arm of the twofold strategy to maximize efficiency in health care delivery among the elderly emerges: judgment, multidimensional assessment and thinking, communication, and comfort and compassion are the skills of the effective geriatrician. Resource management becomes a cardinal requirement for such practitioners (and the learning of such skills becomes a primary objective of educational programs for those who will care for the elderly).

Thus, age begins to limit the expected benefits of treatment to the point where treatment may yield risk without benefit as the barrier to immortality is approached among the elderly. Titration of benefits, cost, and risks—especially as measured in terms of the duration and quality of life, potentially prolonged by a given intervention—becomes the quintessential art of the excellent geriatrician. A simple mind's image of the typical elderly patient, a frail old woman clutching a satchel of medications, clearly illustrates the dilemma of caring for the elderly who will increasingly dominate the health care scene in the years to come.

A related phenomenon of particular importance to the issue of health cost containment is the concentration of health care expenditures in the last segments of life, a phenomenon that is particularly evident among the elderly. The vast preponderance of Medicare expenditures in the final year of life are for those in the terminal phases of life (46 percent in the last 60 days), by definition in the dying process. Thus the challenge to research and practice in geriatrics is clear: to define when "doing nothing" is better than "doing something." This will require, first, the identification of the dying patient with a degree of sensitivity and specificity acceptable to the patient, the patient's supporters, and the health care providers involved; and, second, the provision of humane, alternative health care for that dying patient. That such an alternative is possible, acceptable, and appropriate is evident in the widespread acceptance of the hospice movement for those with terminal malignancies. However, it has not yet become possible to predict with sufficient accuracy the death of elderly patients dying of far more common causes, notably cardiovascular disease and multiple system decline. Such identification is therefore an important research topic that will have a major impact on the disposition of health care resources among those who are dying, most of whom will be elderly. Thus a potential, optimistic outcome of increased sophistication in the care of the elderly might be an affirmative answer to the following question: Can less be better in geriatrics?

GERIATRIC MEDICINE: THE HEALTH CARE SYSTEM AS PART OF THE PROBLEM

A source of particular frustration in teaching health care cost containment, given the concentration of health care expenditures among the elderly, is the mismatch between needs and resources that reflects the evolution of the present American health care system. What is wrong?

1. Hospitals dominate.
2. Procedure-oriented practice dominates: cognitive skills are undervalued.
3. Gaps abound in appropriate care for the needs of the chronically disabled.
4. The costs of acute, technology-intensive care are high and compete for expenditures with forms of care more appropriate in the elderly: prevention, social support, and continuing care.
5. The care provided may be inhumane, possibly prolonging the dying process, subjecting the chronically disabled or dying to ineffective, invasive, and painful procedures, and detracting from the comfort and dignity of the patient in the last phase of life.

An obvious organizational answer to this mismatch of needs and resources has been provided by the evolution of health maintenance organizations (HMOs), recently amplified in experimental demonstration projects in the form of social and health maintenance organizations (SHMOs). Given the conservation of resources made possible by avoidance of hospitalization and its associated costly, invasive, and potentially dangerous procedures, the HMO appears especially attractive as a means to meet the health and even social care needs of the elderly. However, only when the continuum of services becomes complete in such HMOs, to include case management and long-term institutional as well as home care, will the efficacy of this organizational structure in meeting the health care needs of the elderly truly be appropriately testable.

Moreover, a perhaps peculiarly American aversion to prepaid health care may inhibit full application of this approach to efficient health resource management. Does health care delivered in HMOs have to be impersonal? Does it have to be bare bones? Does it have to dull the entrepreneurial instincts of its providers? Does it have to blunt the professional instincts of the physician? Will it become inexorably bureaucratic and inflexible? My suspicion is that the answer to these questions is, "probably not." However, the risks of such outcomes are apparent, and protective strategies against such pitfalls should be implemented.

It is difficult to predict the form that health care systems addressing the needs of the elderly will take as the aging of Americans continues over the next four decades. However, conservative estimates can be based upon the following optimistic assumptions:

1. Quality is the first consideration.
2. Flexibility to adapt to changing funding priorities will assure survival of the best geriatric health care systems.
3. Resource management will be a necessary skill to survive economically during the inevitable period of shifting funding patterns to come.
4. Geriatric practitioners and administrators will become skilled in resource management.

How then should academic health care systems prepare to deliver effective geriatric health care and teach it to aspiring practitioners of the future? Fortunately, the following assumptions also pertain:

1. The resources are plentiful to deliver effective and humane care (given the generous support of health care practices in the past).
2. Personal and family resources will continue to predominate in the care of the elderly, and these resources will be ample.
3. People—individually, as families, and as a society—will continue to value quality in the care of the elderly and assign resources accordingly.

If these assumptions are valid, then reallocation of resources toward their more appropriate use will assure excellence in geriatric health care in the decades to come. How then should cost containment (i.e., resource management) in geriatric health care be taught to future practitioners?

The template for developing such programs has been cast by previous successful medical training programs. First, we must develop an appropriate care system with attention to both quality and cost; and second, place the student in the system to learn by managing patients within it, accepting graduated responsibilities appropriate to his or her level of training, experience, and competence.

Selection and, in many cases, development of appropriate health care systems is a necessary antecedent to implementation of teaching programs that emphasize resource management for the elderly. Given that a continuity of health care services constitutes the optimal learning and medical care laboratory, this continuum must stress efficiency. Two models can be compared here: first, one that does not work is a discontinuous system among the various levels of care (hospital, transitional, nursing home, ambulatory, and home-based care), with gaps in physician coverage, nonphysician health providers, and records. One that does work, in contrast, is a closed system emphasizing the role of the same group of physician providers and a linked, multiply accessible record-keeping system among those levels of care and through time. Whereas the nonphysician staff can be different at the various levels of care, the physician or, more commonly, group of physicians assuming ultimate responsibility for patient care must be in close communication, and the records at their disposal must be continuous and readily accessible.

Here, of course, the same challenges facing the teaching of effective health care in the ambulatory sphere will beset the development of appropriate educational programs in the health care continuum. The concentration of resources in the most intensive levels of care and the reimbursement for physician time spent in such intensive care allow education to take place there as an essentially cost-free by-product. However, a decreasing concentration of physicians as one progresses to lesser levels of intensity of care, and the increasing numbers of patients to be cared for (and, to a large extent, the labor-intensive nature of that care), make the cost of focused educational efforts often prohibitive outside the tertiary health care center. Nevertheless, success in teaching resource management where the savings must occur—outside the hospital—is an imperative if health care of the elderly is to become efficient.

Finally, who should teach medical cost containment? Is this a pedagogical dilemma? Does it inherently run counter to the value system and instincts of academic physicians and students (particularly those as yet unjaded by experience in the real world)? Are those faculty in academic medical centers—whose behavior is by definition not primarily driven by material concerns—capable of teaching cost containment?

Failure to consider resource management in the care of the elderly is an abdication of responsibility to the student, to the patient, to the family, and to society. Therefore, to fail to teach effective resource management—including appropriate consideration of the ethical dilemmas—is an abdication of our responsibility as medical educators. In order to teach such skills effectively, however, the imperfections of our approach to health care and health resource management in the elderly must be acknowledged and rectified, requiring vigorous research to improve our knowledge base. We must test drugs in the elderly, in the multiply disabled typical older person. We must assess the efficacy, risk, and cost of all interventions in the elderly. We must formalize decision analysis, as applied specifically to the care of the elderly, and teach it to our students. We must, above all, act as role models for students, attending to details of resource management in our elderly patients, and encouraging our students to learn by example as well as by dictum. The challenge is clear. The need is imperative.

REFERENCES

Fries, J. (1980). "Aging, Natural Death, and the Compression of Morbidity." *New England Journal of Medicine* 303 (3): 130–35.

Manton, K. G. (1982). "Changing Concepts of Morbidity and Mortality in the Elderly Population." *Milbank Memorial Fund Quarterly* 60 (2): 183–245.

Schneider, E. L., and Brody, J. A. (1983). "Aging, Natural Death, and the Compression of Morbidity: Another View." *New England Journal of Medicine* 309: 854–56.

Shock, N. W.; Greulich, R. C.; Andres, R.; Arenberg, D.; Costa, P. T., Jr.; and Tobin, J. D. (1984). *Normal Human Aging: The Baltimore Longitudinal Study of Aging.* U.S. Department of Health and Human Services Publication No. (NIH) 84-2450. Washington, DC: U.S. Government Printing Office.

Stern, M. P. (1979). "The Recent Decline in Ischemic Heart Disease Mortality." *Annals of Internal Medicine* 91: 630–40.

Weisfeldt, M. L.; Gerstenblith, G.; and Lakatta, E. G. (1984). "Alterations in Circulatory Function." In *Principles of Geriatric Medicine,* ed. R. Andres, E. L. Bierman, and W. R. Hazzard, 248–79. New York: McGraw-Hill.

Chapter 17

Quality Assurance: From the Shadows to Center Stage

Peter E. Dans

Editor's Note—Quality assurance (QA) is integral to providing medical care in our complicated world. Multiple providers, high-technology high-risk procedures for which truly informed consent is nearly impossible, and the growth of the health care industry to a size that makes personal and individual attention difficult or impossible, all contribute to the need for conscientious QA. Cost-containment efforts, which inevitably result in restriction or denial of services to patients, make QA more important than ever before, to insure that reductions in services do not substantially imperil patient care.

Dans points out that quality is not an absolute, but that it represents a degree of excellence or conformance to preset standards. QA involves assessment of who provides care and where it is provided (structure), the manner in which care is given (process), and the ultimate results (outcome). The QA process actually measures mortality, complications, efficiency, and satisfaction, all of which are related to or influence the costs of medical care. By prospectively setting standards for high-quality care, QA may save money by reducing unneeded services. It may also help us allocate scarce resources more rationally, in accordance with our desire to maintain those standards.

For decades, hospital quality assurance has been an activity performed in the shadows. Busy practitioners have often regarded attempts to monitor quality to be both unnecessary and bureaucratic. Underlying this feeling has been a sincere belief that they were practicing good medicine. But even the best physicians are subject to error. Furthermore, the potential for miscommunication and misjudgments is heightened by the fact that medical care involves a diverse group of people interacting on numerous occasions over a long time period. When properly done, therefore, QA requires stepping back and taking a broader view than just the analysis of a single encounter.

Quality assurance has been brought out of the shadows by evidence that many impaired and incompetent physicians are not being identified or sanctioned (Feinstein 1985), and that practices vary widely, from community to community and from physician to physician (McPherson et al. 1982). These variations, especially at the extremes, have major implications for both patient care and the use of resources and, not surprisingly, third-party payers are expressing the greatest concern. For example, the disparity in hysterectomy rates of 4:1 for women in different geographic areas needs to be explained. Either some women are being subjected to the procedure unnecessarily or others are not getting it when they should.

Before proceeding further, it is important to dispel the notion that QA is only necessary at the profession's fringe. In 1975, Halsted Holman, a respected physician at Stanford, was highly critical of the self-definition of excellence ("excellence is us and we are excellent") so prevalent at his and other major teaching hospitals (Holman 1976). He recognized that, as great as these institutions are, they are particularly vulnerable to trainee and staff turnover and the inefficiencies associated with size and complexity. His argument is even more persuasive now, as these traditionally Balkanized institutions have been melded into even larger health care conglomerates.

The stress on cost containment as a major consideration in health care delivery has complicated the picture further. Third-party payers and their fiscal intermediaries have entered a territory once thought to be reserved for patients and doctors. Although ostensibly motivated by concerns for better health care, the payers' representatives are measured by the dollars they save. There is a real tension between containing costs and assuring quality (Dans, Weiner, and Otter 1985, 1986). The daily pressures on physicians to limit their use of costly medical technology, to discharge patients from the hospital earlier, and to move surgery and other invasive procedures to outpatient settings increase the potential both for doing harm and for denying beneficial services. This is why quality assurance is assuming such importance. By demanding adherence to high standards of care, QA programs can serve as an early warning system for inappropriate reductions in medical services or for demonstrably poor health care. One of the major benefits of such efforts may be that they force physicians to define an acceptable level of care and to establish standards against which appropriate measurements can be made.

Many see quality assurance as a way of saving money on hospitalization; for example, by eliminating unnecessary procedures or by suggesting improvements in discharge planning to reduce readmissions. However, there are many reasons why QA should not be designed principally as a cost-containment effort. First and foremost, when properly done, QA may lead to the identification of necessary additional services and thereby increase costs. Second, some of the projected "cost savings" are illusory since they may really represent hospital charges which must be covered unless personnel are dismissed or equipment purchases are cancelled (Finkler 1982). Third, quality assurance has its own built-in costs. If inadequately trained or uninterested personnel are assigned to QA activities, or if there is little support from medical and administrative leadership, the costs will clearly outweigh the benefits. On the other hand, if QA is accorded the resources and professional talent it requires, incalculable benefits will result.

There is a final reason to deemphasize cost: the medical ethic. The underlying principles guiding medicine are nonmaleficence ("First, do no harm") and beneficence, which advocates that we do good when we can. When quality assurance is approached from the benefit rather than the cost side of the equation, it commands more respect and attention among physicians. Furthermore, it affirms what should be the unifying desire among patient, physician, and payer to attain the highest quality of care achievable in any given setting.

WHAT IS QUALITY AND CAN IT BE ASSURED?

Much of the skepticism about quality assurance is fueled by the concern that quality is relative and thus "in the eye of the beholder." Quality is usually defined as the degree of excellence or conformation to standards. Thus, patient care can only be measured in relation to what is inherently possible given the current state of the art, the available human and capital resources, and the standards for care set by the community of patients and physicians. Although the ceiling of achievable quality care will be the same worldwide, care at the Massachusetts General Hospital and at a rural hospital in Alaska will always differ. This is no different from wanting to buy a Mercedes but being forced to settle for a less expensive car. Even though you trade off design and performance features, you assume a basic level of safety, comfort, and handling. Similarly, patients should be assured a basic level of care while efforts are directed to closing the gap between that floor and the ceiling of achievable quality care.

Defining and agreeing to assure a reasonable standard of care does not guarantee that care will always meet or exceed this standard. We live in an imperfect world and occasional lapses will occur. Rather, QA must be seen as an ongoing process in which institutions, which change as their personnel do, strive to provide the best care they can. If and when care falls below expectations, the patient as well as the community he or she represents should be guaranteed that corrective action will be instituted immediately to assure that the standard is met once again (Kessner 1978).

A major factor inhibiting the growth of QA has been its threatening nature when done appropriately. Although every attempt should be made in QA programs to accentuate the positive, attention must be focused on defining and correcting problems. None of us likes to have our mistakes highlighted, regardless of whether they are the result of commission or omission. This creates a natural reluctance to shine the light on others for fear that the spotlight will be turned back on us. The specter of malpractice liability reinforces the threatening nature of QA. An adversarial legal system that is intolerant of imperfection has made many physicians concerned about admitting mistakes. Ironically, the society's expectation of perfection may be a direct outgrowth of the profession's overly optimistic claims for "medical advances" as well as the tendency to teach perfection in our training programs (Dubovsky and Schrier 1983).

Another criticism of quality assurance made by some physicians is that the nurses or physicians engaged in it are not their peers and, consequently, are not appropriate judges of their work. Often these same physicians do not involve themselves collaboratively in the peer review process because they "don't have the time." Such a stance is both unfair and untenable. Evidence is mounting that QA is not a frill, but a necessity. The Joint Commission on Accreditation of Healthcare Organizations (JCAHO) is strengthening its supervision of QA activities in the institutions it accredits. Many states are also reviewing their requirements for medical licensure and are considering establishing stricter relicensure procedures. So, either physicians get involved in QA or it will be done for them and, undoubtedly, not as well.

In summary, quality assurance has been unfairly burdened with a poor image. It has been underfunded and, although excellent people have pioneered the field, it has been largely ignored by people of stature in the profession. It has too often involved form rather than substance. The performance of mandated QA activities, such as audits or utilization review, in a half-hearted and perfunctory manner has only served to reinforce this negative stereotype. Ironically, although QA is so integral to the practice of medicine, it is still in its infancy. This concept is difficult for patients to understand because they assume that measuring quality is our primary concern. Now that QA has moved to center stage, that assumption may prove to be true.

WHAT CONSTITUTES QA?

Donabedian has defined three major components to be analyzed in any QA program: (1) structure, (2) process, and (3) outcome (Donabedian 1980). *Structure* refers not only to the facility or setting in which the encounter occurs, but also to components such as equipment and personnel. JCAHO and state licensing boards base their reviews of the structure of care on the culture, the standard of living, and the level of sophistication of the community. These factors may vary considerably from one city or area of the country to another, as well as between countries.

The same type of variability is found among physicians and nurses who carry the same titles but have different capabilities. We tend to ignore this in our training programs when we replace Dr. X with Dr. Y to meet training and scheduling needs. Although credentials such as the type of degree and the stature of the training institution are valuable to know, they do not provide sufficient criteria to predict an individual's success. Furthermore, physicians differ in their personalities and motivations to continue learning. Some are more humble and willing to say "I don't know" (Seegal 1961; Herwig 1986). Some cut corners or have character defects which affect their practice. Others start out well but may develop personal problems such as substance abuse. For this reason, credential reviews now require data on actual physician practice (e.g., the number of times they are mentioned in malpractice suits, their complication rate for specific procedures, and the ratings of their clinical performance by peers).

Process measures usually involve matching actual care to pre-established criteria for appropriate care. For example, in a study of the management of pneumonia, we matched physician management with preset criteria and found many instances of inappropriate antibiotic use and corresponding lower-quality care (Dans et al. 1984). Laboratory and x-ray departments, which more closely resemble industry, have a long tradition of such "quality control" efforts aimed at minimizing the known variability in test performance. As one might expect, the best laboratories monitor themselves and the worst do not. Even so, most laboratory proficiency testing involves mailed specimens and, not surprisingly, laboratories take extra care in handling these test specimens (Goodhart et al. 1981; LaMotte et al. 1977). QA should be concerned with how the laboratory performs routinely (i.e., when it does not know it is being tested).

Finally, more attention is being placed on *outcome* measures. Ironically, although most clinical advances are reported using outcomes (e.g., a five-year survival rate after certain procedures), most health care institutions rarely collect outcome data unless a specific study is being performed. This is because most of us assume that once a procedure is done well, reviews of performance unnecessarily take time away from doing it. Furthermore, careful patient follow-up is difficult in our mobile society. Despite these objections, follow-up data are required of many health care institutions, and many administrators are recognizing the potential utility of such data as a marketing tool.

WHAT SHOULD WE MEASURE?

Mortality and Morbidity

In order to examine specific health care process and outcome measures, it is helpful to draw on an analogy between the quality of health care and the quality of an airplane flight. The first goal of an airplane passenger is to leave the plane alive; the same is true for patients entering a hospital. In the past, we sometimes heard expressions such as "the operation went well but the patient died" or "the patient died in chemical balance." These were small consolations to the patients involved. Fortunately, most patients do leave the hospital alive. For example, the overall mortality at Johns Hopkins Hospital is 2.5 percent. It ranges from 0 percent in psychiatry and ophthalmology, where patients with life-threatening conditions are transferred to other services, to a rate of 9.6 percent in oncology. In order to follow this important measure, we have established a hospital death registry. This allows us to analyze trends in mortality by age, sex, race, payer, diagnosis-related group (DRG), diagnosis, procedure, and physician of record. We have also set up a routine follow-up of survival after cardiopulmonary resuscitation (Dans et al. 1985).

Monitoring mortality trends is only a first step. Because some people who enter the hospital are terminally ill, our major concern is to identify deaths which are unnecessary and untimely (Rutstein et al. 1976; 1980; Roemer, Moustafa, and Hopkins 1968). Traditionally, this has been done at departmental mortality conferences where deaths are reviewed. An autopsy is often required in order to determine whether the death could have been prevented. Unfortunately, autopsy rates have declined at our hospital, from 70 percent in the 1950s to 31 percent in 1987. The decline in autopsy rates has been even greater nationally, from about 50 percent in the 1940s to about 15 percent in the 1980s (McPhee et al. 1986). Many reasons have been given for this decline, including JCAHO's suspension of an autopsy quota for hospital accreditation, failure to reimburse pathologists for the service, and the pervasive feeling that autopsies do not contribute much to our understanding of the cause of death in our high-technology age (Roberts 1978; Lundberg 1984). However, recent studies show that 10 percent or more of patients could have benefited if their autopsy findings had been known before death. That rate is approximately the same as before the technology explosion (Goldman et al. 1983). This is why efforts are now being made to increase the number of autopsies, especially on patients who die under uncertain circumstances (Smith and Zumwalt 1984).

Mortality rates have gained increased prominence as a result of the publication of hospital mortality rates in Medicare patients by the Health Care Financing Administration (HCFA) in 1987 (Health Care Financing Administration 1987). Although such rates cannot be automatically used as proxies for quality because of important patient and institutional variables, their release has generated long-overdue attention to the subject. One of the "dirty little secrets" that has lurked in the shadows of too many hospital corridors is the inadequate performance of some doctors or institutions. This was the concern of Codman in the early 1900s (Codman 1914; Reverby 1981) and later of the National Halothane Study group which surveyed operative mortality in the 1960s (Moses and Mosteller 1968). The power gained by paying for such a large share of hospital costs has enabled the federal government to force the issue to be confronted. In a very practical sense, costs and quality have become entwined.

The next important concern for the airline passenger who arrives alive is to remain in one piece. An analogous measure in the hospital is the rate of morbidity. This involves surveillance of infections and complication rates after procedures such as central line placement or thoracentesis. We have established routine surveillance in potentially high-risk areas, such as the cardiac catheterization laboratory and the endoscopy suite. Comparing trends in complications to reported rates, after adjusting for severity of illness, can help keep this number at an irreducible minimum (Horn 1985; Gonnella, Hornbrook, and Louis 1984; Young, Swinkola, and Zorn 1982). Although our complication rates have been low and well within acceptable levels given our case mix, we still occasionally identify a case or two that lead us to institute corrective action involving either equipment or personnel. This happened recently after two patients developed pneumohydrothoraces in association with the use of a Dobbhoff feeding tube (Woodall, Winfield, and Bissett 1987; Wheeler 1987).

Physicians may be reluctant to report complications because they are seen as "predictable." However, even if the expected rate of complications after a particular procedure is 5 percent, the patient and practitioner both assume the patient will be in the 95 percent group, not the 5 percent group. When things turn out differently, the practitioner's response may be: "Well, I did let the patient know the risk ahead of

time." However, this may underestimate the optimistic tenor of the pre-
procedure discussion during which the patient may have assumed that
he or she would be in the uncomplicated group. Unfortunately, patients
will occasionally sue even though no malpractice has occurred. This
illustrates the link between quality assurance and risk management. The
latter, which is aimed at reducing legal liability, is highly dependent upon
a good QA program to keep adverse events at an irreducible minimum.
Most lawsuits arise when physicians or administrators are unresponsive
to the patient and allow resentment to develop. Thus, physicians must
not only prepare patients adequately, they must also be sensitive to the
patient's or family's appropriate disappointment when predictable complications take place. Our policy has been to urge physicians to report
events which adversely affect care, after taking the necessary steps to
minimize the effects of the complication. This helps alert everyone to
the complication and to any possibility for prevention.

Efficiency, Amenities, and Costs

    After arriving alive and in one piece, the passenger's thoughts turn
to the efficiency of service. Was the plane on time? Were there too many
stops? The analogous measures of health care efficiency for inpatients
are the length of hospital stay related to delays in the admission process,
procedure scheduling, or discharge planning. Monitoring of these variables, known as utilization review (UR), has been the part of QA which
has received the most time and attention. Although useful, UR should
not overshadow other more important components of QA; namely, clinical practice evaluation and physician profiling (Williamson, Hudson,
and Nevins 1982).
    As more and more patient care shifts to ambulatory units, emphasis
is being placed on outpatient QA. Practical measures of ambulatory care
efficiency include no-show rates for appointments and transit time
through the system. In 1980, we studied the obstetrics clinic at our
hospital and identified major delays in patient transit related to late
physician arrival and inappropriate patient scheduling (Dans, Johnson,
and King 1989). Changes were instituted and improvement occurred.
Practicing physicians, who manage their own offices, are very attuned
to these issues since they recognize that "time is money" and that satis-
fied patients are more likely to return. This has not always been the case
in large teaching hospitals, which were, until recently, insulated by serving captive populations. The era of block patient appointments, over-
scheduled or indifferent physicians, and resultant four- to ten-hour transit

times through some clinics and emergency rooms appears to be mercifully passing. This may be one benefit of the "competitive era."

If the flight efficiency has been satisfactory, the passenger may focus on the amenities. Was the experience a pleasant one? Was the flight smooth, the food good, the flight attendant friendly? Similarly, patient satisfaction is extremely important. Many institutions survey patients routinely to identify problems in interpersonal relations, and they are very responsive to complaints in order to assure that service is optimal. Some are even trying to upgrade the food, which has long been the bane of patients well enough to be aware of their surroundings. Unfortunately for the morale of health care workers, this group is dwindling in most hospitals as a result of the pressure for early discharge and for doing procedures on an outpatient basis (Rabkin 1982).

Finally, the passenger does not want to be pauperized by the flight. In the case of airline travel, tickets are purchased ahead of time according to an agreed upon price. Until recently, medical care has been just the opposite, open-ended and charged out after the fact. More and more, however, third-party payers are anticipating patient charges and restricting access to high-cost hospitals and doctors. While such changes are long overdue, an overriding concern about the financial "bottom line" may lead to both covert and overt rationing which can adversely affect quality (Levey and Hesse 1985). In fact, much of the vaunted health care cost savings may be occurring at the expense of family members and patients, as the burden for the extended convalescence of sick patients is shifted to the home. This is occurring even at nonprofit institutions, which are beginning to resemble profit-making ones.

Reports of "patient dumping," the transfer of severely ill patients who do not have health care coverage (Schiff et al. 1986), have resulted in legislation in at least one state (Relman 1986). The allegation that patients are being discharged "sicker and quicker" has led the HCFA to require a review of Medicare patients readmitted to a hospital within seven to fifteen days to assure that they were not inappropriately discharged (Dans and King 1986). In our hospital, in addition to readmission review, we review transfers between nursing units, especially when they involve the intensive care unit.

Attempts are also being made to monitor overall patient care. This is easier to do in prepaid systems and, consequently, HCFA has begun to mandate reviews of health maintenance organizations serving Medicare patients. These reviews may be directed at the wrong group, since most prepaid systems are geared toward lower-risk, generally well patients. Economically disadvantaged patients, who are usually served by less-organized systems, are more vulnerable to cost-quality trade-offs.

Effectiveness

Until now, we have dealt primarily with the adverse aspects of the encounter and have not emphasized the most important aspect; namely, effectiveness, or how much better the patient is for the care (Seegal 1961). This should be the major focus of quality assurance. To return to the airplane flight analogy, some have rightly pointed out that when they board an airplane, they think about why they are going and not about the infrequent morbid complications that may result. This is true for most patients as well and, paradoxically, is why they may appear surprised, even after being forewarned, when adverse events occur. It is here that the analogy between the health care system and the airlines clearly fails. The passenger is on his own after debarking from the plane. Not so for the patient. The physician, because of his covenant with the patient, has a continuing responsibility for the outcome of care.

It is difficult to determine whether the patient is better off for the care. To do so, one must know the patient's functional status on admission and the degree of improvement relative to what might have been expected given the current state of medical treatment and the severity of the patient's condition. Unfortunately, most routine histories and physical examinations do not permit such calculations since they atomize patients into organ systems rather than objectively assess the patient's ability to perform routine activities of daily living (Katz et al. 1983). Nor do medical records usually spell out the likely benefit from any intervention relative to the maximum attainable functional state. The application of already developed and validated measurements of functional status to everyday care is a particularly fruitful area for QA research (Jette 1986; Chambers 1983).

Whereas physicians are oriented to the individual patient or to the individual encounter, most quality assurance studies focus on populations. Although specific problems (so-called tracers or sentinel events) may be important indicators, it usually takes more than one event to measure quality (Kessner, Kalk, and Singer 1973). Gathering data is time consuming and must be done carefully. It involves a basic knowledge of epidemiology and statistics, as well as access to data management systems, and cannot be the sole responsibility of busy practicing physicians and nurses. For this reason, all health care institutions, whether inpatient or outpatient, should have a regular system of self-analysis involving: (1) the review of critical measures of process and outcome; (2) regular feedback to physicians and other caregivers; (3) alteration of practice where necessary; and (4) evaluation of the effectiveness of those corrective actions. It was to that end that our medical school and hospital established a joint Office of Medical Practice Evaluation, a multidisciplinary effort involving medicine, nursing, and administration (Dans and King 1986).

CONCLUSION

Quality assurance means assuring that patient care is not just of high quality but that it is necessary. More is not necessarily better. Although QA can lead to the identification and elimination of unnecessary services, cost reduction is not inevitable. However, because everything we do to and for patients carries some social, medical, or financial costs, QA can serve the purposes of risk and cost reduction, as well as quality enhancement, by requiring us to focus on the cost benefit of medical interventions.

Careful analysis of most "disasters" occurring in hospitals usually reveals a costly cascade of events set into motion by one or more seemingly minor misjudgments or coincidences which act synergistically (Mold and Stein 1986). The same is true of airplane crashes where a few errors compound to erode the margin of safety (Senders 1980). Once the chain of events starts, the patient suffers an inexorable series of complications, too often culminating in death. The outcome is made even more unfortunate when the triggering misjudgment is the decision to perform a test or treatment that appears, in retrospect, to have been unnecessary. The only way to stop such a cascade from occurring is by not starting it in the first place. As with the airlines, cost-cutting may be insidiously harmful. Deregulation of the airlines has led to overloaded airports at peak travel times. In addition, rate wars have led to cuts in personnel and maintenance costs. Similarly, hospitals have eliminated what appears to be "fat" in the system by reducing personnel involved in hands-on care. The added pressure to move patients through the system quickly has increased the potential for error. The need for increased vigilance is obvious.

In conclusion, QA is not an exercise in proving one's superiority and another's inferiority but should be aimed at improving care where possible. It requires analyzing care from both the patient's and the practitioner's perspective. The title Charles Bosk used for his study of how surgeons handle mistakes and errors sounds an appropriate concluding note. The job of anyone involved in QA is to assure that the institution and all those concerned are able to "forgive and remember" (Bosk 1979).

REFERENCES

Bosk, C. L. (1979). *Forgive and Remember: Managing Medical Failure.* Chicago: University of Chicago Press.
Chambers, L. W. (1983). "Physical and Emotional Function of Primary Care

Patients: Scientific Requirements for the Measurement of Functional Health Status" (Editorial). *Journal of the American Medical Association* 249: 3353–55.

Codman, E. A. (1914). "The Product of a Hospital." *Surgery, Gynecology & Obstetrics* 18: 491–96.

Dans, P. E.; Charache, P.; Fahey, M.; and Otter, S. E. (1984). "Management of Pneumonia in the Prospective Payment Era: A Need for More Clinician and Support Service Interaction." *Archives of Internal Medicine* 144: 1392–97.

Dans, P. E.; Johnson, T. R. B.; and King, T. M. (1989). "Improving a University Hospital Obstetrics Clinic: Better But Not Best." *Obstetrics and Gynecology*. In press.

Dans, P. E., and King, T. M. (1986). "An Office of Medical Practice Evaluation: What Is It and Why Have One?" *Quality Review Bulletin* 12: 320–25.

Dans, P. E.; Nevin, K. L.; Seidman, C. E.; McArthur, J. C.; and Kariya, S. T. (1985). "Inhospital CPR 25 Years Later: Why Has Survival Decreased?" *Southern Medical Journal* 78: 1174–78.

Dans, P. E.; Weiner, J. P.; and Otter, S. E. (1985). "Peer Review Organizations: Promises and Potential Pitfalls." *New England Journal of Medicine* 313: 1131–37.

————— (1986). "Peer Review Organizations" (Correspondence). *New England Journal of Medicine* 314: 1121–22.

Donabedian, A. (1980). *The Definition of Quality and Approaches to Its Assessment.* Explorations in Quality Assessment and Monitoring, vol. 1. Ann Arbor, MI: Health Administration Press.

Dubovsky, S. L., and Schrier, R. W. (1983). "The Mystique of Medical Training: Is Teaching Perfection in Medical House-Staff Training a Reasonable Goal or a Precursor of Low Self-Esteem?" *Journal of the American Medical Association* 250: 3057–58.

Feinstein, R. J. (1985). "The Ethics of Professional Regulation." *New England Journal of Medicine* 312: 801–4.

Finkler, S. A. (1982). "The Distinction between Costs and Charges." *Annals of Internal Medicine* 96: 102–9.

Goldman, L.; Sayson, R.; Robbins, S.; Cohn, L.; Bettmann, M.; and Weisberg, M. (1983). "The Value of the Autopsy in Three Medical Eras." *New England Journal of Medicine* 308: 1000–5.

Gonnella, J. S.; Hornbrook, M. C.; and Louis, D. Z. (1984). "Staging of Disease: A Case-Mix Measurement." *Journal of the American Medical Association* 251: 637–46.

Goodhart, G. L.; Brown, S. T.; Zaidi, A. A.; Pope, V.; Larsen, S.; and Barrow, J. E. (1981). "Blinded Proficiency Testing of FTA-ABS Test." *Archives of Internal Medicine* 141: 1045–50.

Health Care Financing Administration (1987). "Medicare Program Selected Performance Information on Hospitals Providing Care to Medicare Beneficiaries." *Federal Register* 52 (August 17): 30,741–45.

Herwig, T. T. (1986). "I Don't Know." *Journal of the American Medical Association* 256: 2348.

Holman, H. R. (1976). "The 'Excellence' Deception in Medicine" (Editorial). *Hospital Practice* 11 (4): 11, 18, 21.

Horn, S. D.; Bulkley, G.; Sharkey, P. D.; Chambers, A. F.; Horn, R. A.; and Schramm, C. J. (1985). "Interhospital Differences in Severity of Illness: Problems for Prospective Payment Based on Diagnosis-Related Groups (DRGs)." *New England Journal of Medicine* 313: 20–24.

Jette, A. M.; Davies, A. R.; Cleary, P. D.; et al. (1986). The Functional Status Questionnaire: Reliability and Validity When Used in Primary Care." *Journal of General Internal Medicine* 1: 143–49.

Katz, S.; Branch, L. G.; Branson, M. H.; Papsidero, J. A.; Beck, J. C.; and Greer, D. S. (1983). "Active Life Expectancy." *New England Journal of Medicine* 309: 1218–24.

Kessner, D. M. (1978). "Quality Assessment and Assurance: Early Signs of Cognitive Dissonance." *New England Journal of Medicine* 298: 381–86.

Kessner, D. M.; Kalk, C. E.; and Singer, J. (1973). "Assessing Health Quality— The Case for Tracers." *New England Journal of Medicine* 288: 189–94.

LaMotte, L. C., Jr.; Cuerrant, G. O.; Lewis, D. S.; and Hall, C. T. (1977). "Comparison of Laboratory Performance with Blind and Mail-Distributed Proficiency Testing Samples." *Public Health Reports* 92: 554–60.

Levey, S., and Hesse, D. D. (1985). "Bottom-Line Health Care?" *New England Journal of Medicine* 312: 644–47.

Lundberg, G. D. (1984). "Medicine without the Autopsy." *Archives of Pathology & Laboratory Medicine* 108: 449–54.

McPhee, S. J.; Bottles, K.; Lo, B.; Saika, G.; and Crommie, D. (1986). "To Redeem Them from Death: Reactions of Family Members to Autopsy." *American Journal of Medicine* 80: 665–71.

McPherson, K.; Wennberg, J. E.; Hovind, O. B.; and Clifford, P. (1982). "Small-Area Variations in the Use of Common Surgical Procedures: An International Comparison of New England, England, and Norway." *New England Journal of Medicine* 307: 1310–14.

Mold, J. W., and Stein, H. F. (1986). "The Cascade Effect in the Clinical Care of Patients." *New England Journal of Medicine* 314: 512–14.

Moses, L. E., and Mosteller, F. (1968). "Institutional Differences in Postoperative Death Rates: Commentary on Some of the Findings of the National Halothane Study." *Journal of the American Medical Association* 203: 150–52.

Rabkin, M. T. (1982). "The SAG Index." *New England Journal of Medicine* 307: 1350–51.

Relman, A. S. (1986). "Texas Eliminates Dumping: A Start Toward Equity in Hospital Care." *New England Journal of Medicine* 314: 578–79.

Reverby, S. (1981). "Stealing the Golden Eggs: Ernest Amory Codman and the Science and Management of Medicine." *Bulletin of the History of Medicine* 55: 156–71.

Roberts, W. C. (1978). "The Autopsy: Its Decline and a Suggestion for Its Revival." *New England Journal of Medicine* 299: 332–38.

Roemer, M. I.; Moustafa, A. T.; and Hopkins, C. E. (1968). "A Proposed Hospital Quality Index: Hospital Death Rates Adjusted for Case Severity." *Health Services Research* 3: 96–118.

Rutstein, D. D.; Berenberg, W.; Chalmers, T. C.; Child, C. G.; Fishman, A. P.; and Perrin, E. B. (1976). "Measuring the Quality of Medical Care: A Clinical Method." *New England Journal of Medicine* 294: 582–88.

——— (1980). "Measuring the Quality of Medical Care: Second Revision of Tables of Indexes" (Correspondence). *New England Journal of Medicine* 302: 1146.

Schiff, R. L.; Ansell, D. A.; Schlosser, J. E.; Idris, A. H.; Morrison, A.; and Whitman, S. (1986). "Transfers to a Public Hospital: A Prospective Study of 467 Patients." *New England Journal of Medicine* 314: 552–57.

Seegal, D. (1961). "Some Symbols of Sound Clinicianship for the Doctor's Bag." *Journal of the American Medical Association* 177: 641–42.

Senders, J. W. (1980). "Is There a Cure for Human Error?" *Psychology Today* 13: 52–62.
Smith, R. D., and Zumwalt, R. E. (1984). "One Department's Experience with Increasing the Autopsy Rate." *Archives of Pathology & Laboratory Medicine* 108: 455–59.
Wheeler, P. S. (1987). "Feeding Tubes that Pierce the Lung: A Case Study in Risk Prevention and Quality Assurance" (Editorial). *Radiology* 165 (3): 861.
Williamson, J. W.; Hudson, J. I.; and Nevins, M. M. (1982). *Principles of Quality Assurance and Cost-Containment in Health Care.* San Francisco, CA: Jossey-Bass.
Woodall, B. H.; Winfield, D. F.; and Bisset, G. S., III. (1987). "Inadvertent Tracheobronchial Placement of Feeding Tubes." *Radiology* 165 (3): 727–29.
Young, W. W.; Swinkola, R. B.; and Zorn, D. M. (1982). "The Measurement of Hospital Case Mix." *Medical Care* 20: 501–12.

Chapter 18

The Future of Health Care Research in Cost Containment

Duncan Neuhauser

Editor's Note—Unfortunately, medical care research tends to follow, rather than lead, public policy changes. By examining the trends in medical care today, Neuhauser identifies cost-related questions that researchers could address to help guide future policymakers. The social support model, rather than the medical model, should be the focus of geriatrics research. A total reworking of the medical-legal liability system is needed, so that injured parties (rather than attorneys) are compensated, and careful practitioners are rewarded (rather than careless ones punished). The incorporation of medical ethics into group medical care financing would encourage recognition that one's culture shapes the cost and value of medical care. To measure the outcome of care economically, one can place a dollar value on life, as is apparent in examples that span more than 1,300 years.

Using ongoing randomization of patients admitted to hospitals can provide quality assurance data that are useful in promoting or marketing a hospital's services; this method also allows piggybacked inexpensive medical care research projects. In addition, cost questions can be an inexpensive piggybacked part of most clinical research projects.

Why do we do research on medical care organization and economics? It is always a good idea to check basic assumptions and beliefs, particularly in this age of "bottom line" medical care. One practical reason for conducting research is because someone wants the answer, and if someone wants an answer, they may even be willing to pay for it. The entrepreneurial medical care researcher needs to spot the changes in health care, to anticipate the questions that will create a demand for new answers.

One measure of the usefulness of applied medical care research is the willingness of delivery systems to pay for it out of operating budgets. This is the case in varying degrees with the Veterans Administration, Kaiser-Permanente, the Hospital Corporation of America, and several large hospitals that have developed and are maintaining in-house applied medical care research activities.

In a 1966 article reviewing medical care research, Odin Anderson concluded that this type of research followed public policy rather than shaped it (Anderson 1966). According to Anderson, politicians or managers would introduce new programs in the belief that it was the right thing to do and, perhaps later, someone would undertake to study its impact. Since then, medical care research has, on occasion, created policy rather than followed it. One notable example is the introduction of diagnosis-related groups (DRGs).

EMERGING RESEARCH CONCERNS

There has been a wave of studies applying the prospective payment concept to medical care other than acute general hospital care, such as psychiatric, ambulatory, rehabilitation, and nursing home care. The next wave of studies looked at the severity of illness measures that undertake to control or explain variance in costs and length-of-stay within DRGs. The third wave is documenting the effect of DRG payment on the delivery of health care. Prior to DRGs, hospital intensive care units (ICUs) were revenue generators, and American hospitals created many more ICUs and ICU beds than countries without a cost-based reimbursement scheme, such as Sweden (Bloom and Jonsson 1978). Under DRG prospective payment, however, ICU care can result in losses for the hospital (Colton et al. 1985), a financial change that may result in a much more rigorous challenge to the appropriate use of ICUs and coronary care units (CCUs) for many patients. This challenge has been long overdue in this country.

Three examples of emerging research interests that are related to cost containment and efficient utilization of resources are as follows:

Geriatrics

Geriatrics and gerontology have become popular medical research topics, and many researchers are becoming involved in this field. However, one approach needs fundamental rethinking: the care of the elderly should not start with the medical model, but rather with a social support model with medical care in a supportive subsidiary role.

An intriguing example of a nonmedical model is the "Beguine." There are two meanings for this word. One refers to a form of music originating in the Caribbean (as in "Begin the Beguine"). The other comes from fourteenth- and fifteenth-century Belgium and Holland, where this word referred to groups of elderly women without families who grouped themselves together around a church to lead devout, but not cloistered, lives in clusters of small houses. They held common beliefs and helped each other. The largest Beguine was in Louvain, Belgium, and the infirmary there is now the faculty dining room of the Catholic University of Louvain (Holmes 1975, 157–61)

Capitation reimbursement schemes and social and health maintenance organizations (SHMOs) provide an opportunity to create a new form of Beguine. The SHMO is perhaps a felicitous word to use for those who remember the Al Capp cartoon "Li'l Abner," in which "schmoos" were perfect little creatures who answered nearly all the needs of the residents of Dog Patch.

Medical-Legal Liability

It is legally possible for a health care delivery system, with appropriate state-enabling legislation and contracts with employee groups, to opt out of the current malpractice nonsystem and to create their own mutually agreed upon compensation system. This creates a great opportunity to improve handling of medical liability problems.

The social psychology literature on behavior change leads one to conclude that malpractice litigation is irrational with respect to improving provider performance. For example, carrots are better than sticks, but the present system uses only a stick, so that although negligence may be punished, good care is not thereby encouraged—only avoidance of negligent care (or of getting caught). In addition, if malpractice litigation is to change behavior, it needs to be a rapid type of feedback, and these decisions now take years. Malpractice litigation, moreover, is wasteful: it is estimated that only about 30 cents on the dollar of malpractice insurance and litigation costs ever gets back to the injured patient, and most harmed patients are probably never compensated. Finally, there are widely different estimates on the costs of defensive medicine, suggesting that we have very little idea of the size of this problem. If the cost is large, there are great potential savings to be achieved by private agreements.

Given this dismal state of affairs, it ought to be possible to create a malpractice insurance program which is a private (perhaps no-fault) system that is much more efficient. A serious effort toward such reform is appropriate for the larger health care delivery systems and should generate much companion research. In the past, there was not the political constituency to change the legal liability system, as exemplified by medical malpractice liability. But when the costs of liability insurance force the closing of the town hockey rink in northern Minnesota, or prevent 10,000 Boy and Girl Scout troops from hiking in the woods, the political constituency for change becomes a potentially overpowering and unstoppable force.

Medical Ethics

Medical ethicists describe different views about how we should allocate scarce resources in medicine, and whether ethical decisions should be based on Catholic, Jewish, or Islamic values, or perhaps based on the ideas of Mill or Rawls. It seems that it should be possible to incorporate different values or philosophies into the financing of medical care. Capitation plans, for example, could be developed to adhere to differing theories of distributive justice, or they could be based on different religious principles, allowing people to choose the medical ethical system they prefer for their medical care.

THE VALUE OF LIFE

When distributive justice, cost containment, and limited resources are the issues, we cannot avoid the central question of how we value human life and the value we assign to the quality of life. Despite its centrality, we try to avoid it. This problem is best addressed head on, with the following working hypotheses: (a) that society *is* willing to place a monetary value on human life and quality of life when they perceive the need to do so; and (b) that doing so can have beneficial social consequences.

Consider the Lex Salica (circa 486–511 AD), a law concerned with valuing life and limb (Lex Salica, n.d.). According to this law, the loss of a hand was worth 4,000 dinarii, the loss of a thumb worth 2,000, and an index finger worth 1,400. To put these figures in perspective, the compensation for stealing a suckling pig was 120 dinarii. The social importance of this law is explained in the Islandic Saga of Burnt Njal (Magnusson and Palsson 1960). The Sagas describe vendettas (blood feuds) during these early centuries that extended over generations. For example, if in a fit of rage, I cut off your finger with my sword, you must do the same to me in order to maintain your social status. But if you miss my finger and cut off my hand, I must respond in kind. If you kill me, my relatives must respond, even if it takes years. One way to stop a vendetta was to pay "wergeld" as compensation for injury, the amount being defined by Salic Law in Belgium, or at the Icelandic Parliament (Althing). One of the important features of wergeld as a money value of life and limb is that to stop the feud, it had to be acceptable to the aggressor (who paid) and the victim (who received), and to their relatives and the community as a whole. If anyone felt the amount to be too much or too little, the balance of vengeance was unstable, and the feud began again. Thus the Salic and other laws that gave a price to life and limb were remarkably humane in their desired result. In Iceland the compensation was fixed at the yearly meeting of the Althing and depended on the social status of the victim (the Sagas do not report a fixed schedule of payment).

The first medically related cost-benefit analysis was apparently carried out by the polymath inventor of political arithmetic, Sir William Petty, on October 7, 1667 (Fein 1971). The medical problem was how to escape death by plague in London during the great epidemic of 1666. Petty proposed that the solution was to get people out of London and into the countryside. He placed a value on human life, and related it to the cost of transporting people. His calculations showed that the removal of people from London would have had benefits greatly in excess of its costs. The rich who could afford to go to their country houses did just that. Petty's analysis suggested that this would have been a socially beneficial policy to adopt for everyone.

The first newspaper published in America was the *Boston News Letter* which started in 1704; a year later it reported a cost-benefit analysis, albeit flawed, for a medically related decision. This weekly paper reported mortality figures by race: 44 slaves died in 1705. At the going market price for slaves, this was a loss of 1,320 pounds, calculated at 30 pounds per person. For only 1,000 pounds, 500 indentured servants could be brought from Europe and would have to work five years for free to pay off their indenture. This would result in 2,500 years of labor. The editor concluded that indenture was the more cost-beneficial choice (Cohen 1982, 88–89). Did New England abandon slavery on the basis of a calculated decision that slavery was not economically justified, rather than on the basis of humanitarian concerns? Regardless, the cost calculations were wrong, because a slave named Onsemus brought knowledge of smallpox innoculation from Africa. This technique was first applied during the Boston smallpox epidemic of 1721 and then during several subsequent epidemics. It resulted in the saving of several thousand New England lives (both black and white) long before the introduction of the Jennarian vaccination for smallpox in 1800 (Hopkins 1983). In February 1777, General Washington required that the American revolutionary troops be inoculated. One could argue that Onsemus' gift of medical technology to America made the American Revolution possible (Hopkins 1983, 261–62).

Lemual Shattuck's 1850 *Report on the Sanitary Condition in Massachusetts* is one of the outstanding documents in America on public health (Shattuck 1948). Shattuck, who was the leader in founding the American Statistical Association, used cost-benefit analysis to justify the need for a state health department. He valued human life by the person's earning capacity, and he put a cost on widowhood related to the state payment to indigent families. He then argued that every dollar spent on a state health department would return a thousand dollars in societal benefits. In spite of this, it took a decade for Massachusetts to start such a department. Although Shattuck was generous in his estimate of the benefits that could be achieved by such a department, history has confirmed his conclusion about the value of public health programs.

On a contemporary, practical note, today our law courts are given the authority to compensate victims for injury. Jury Verdict Research reports that the average award for the loss of one finger was $10,055 and for a hand $192,166 (Jury Verdict Research 1980–81). Such information is used for out-of-court settlements, and for lawyers to explain to their injured clients the expected level of compensation.

These examples that span a millenium show that societies can and do put a price on the value and quality of life. With historical hindsight, we can conclude that such efforts can be humane in their social consequences.

COMPETITION, CAPITATION, DELIVERY SYSTEMS, AND QUALITY OF CARE

With the rapid changes in the structure of the medical care marketplace, there will be a strong concern for demonstrating and documenting quality of care. Primary care capitation plans (HMOs, PPOs, IPA-HMOs) receive fixed monthly amounts of money from enrolled subscribers. In their increasing concern with marketing their services to the public, there will be an interest on the part of such plans and their primary care physicians with "presentation of self," formerly known as the bedside manner. There will probably also be growth in the franchising of physician offices. Franchising organizations must convince people to join their plan. Primary care plans will become more sophisticated in "gatekeeping," "case management," and "block booking" as it relates to the referral of their patients to downstream providers—increasing their concern for both cost and quality of care.

There will be a second group of providers of care, who might be called downstream providers, who will receive their referrals from the primary care plans. Such downstream providers will include tertiary care hospitals, home care programs, and perhaps eventually nursing homes. These downstream providers carry the burden of proof in convincing the primary care groups that their care is of high quality and rendered at low cost. How do downstream providers convince primary care referrers that the cost and quality of the care they offer is the best? In the past, a simple belief in excellence has been sufficient, and there are innumerable large hospitals that have convinced themselves that they are the best. But conviction alone, no matter how persuasively offered, will no longer be adequate. Downstream providers must (and many are beginning to do so) address this question by documenting their operative mortality rates, developing more systematic quality assurance audits, and developing computer-based data systems that not only track cost per patient, but monitor quality of care by comparing expected progress with observed progress.

A most interesting effort by primary providers to assess quality involves the random assignments of patients to more than one downstream provider, allowing controlled comparison of relative performance with respect to cost, outcome, and patient satisfaction. One rehabilitation hospital, for example, encouraged referring HMOs to assign patients randomly to them and any other rehabilitation program. They will measure outcomes of care for comparison if the referrer will ask the same of the other rehabilitation provider, and an outside audit organization would assure comparability of the data collected and inform the HMO of the results. At University Hospitals of Cleveland, contractual agreements with two providers of home care and random assignment of patients could allow the hospital to collect information about the performance of both providers. This approach to evaluating quality, which may provide a quantum leap in the accuracy of quality assessment, may also be used to compare the costs of different downstream providers of medical care.

ONGOING PATIENT RANDOMIZATION

There are several hospitals that use various methods of ongoing randomization as the basis of research and evaluation of medical care (Cohen and Neuhauser 1985). This started at Cleveland Metropolitan General Hospital in 1981, when all new internal medicine patients were randomly assigned to one of four teams of physicians (called "firms"). By 1983, all new house staff were also randomly assigned to one of these firms, allowing the firm system to be used for a series of trials. Since then, ongoing randomization of outpatients has started at University Hospitals of Cleveland, and random assignment of house staff to patients has started at Brook Army Hospital in Fort Houston, Texas. At the St. Louis Veterans Administration Hospital, patients are randomly assigned to two medical school services.

INCLUDING COST IN CLINICAL TRIALS

Future randomized clinical trials in medicine will include cost analysis. This cost analysis should not only consider the economist's definition of social cost, but also net cost to insurer, provider, and patient. The pervasive role of health insurance requires that cost analysis attend to the question of which parties will benefit economically from resultant clinical policy.

Just as we are concerned with efficient medical care, we should be concerned with efficient medical care research. A study by Charles Hershey et al. (1986) worked from an existing computerized data system and the Cleveland Metropolitan General Hospital firm system to carry out a randomized clinical trial for an incremental cost of under a thousand dollars. Not every trial can be so inexpensive, but this trial can stand as a symbol in our efforts to secure low-cost, good-quality medical care research.

DECISION MODELS

The use of the analytic techniques associated with clinical decision analysis, such as decision trees and Markov models, has resulted in a revolution in medical care decision making. Such decision models, however, are reported in printed journals, an inappropriate medium to convey such work. It makes more sense to use microcomputer disks to allow the user to change probabilities and outcome values, so users can perform their own sensitivity analysis, use their preferred values, or modify the decision to fit a unique patient. Unfortunately, more people read journals than use such software; the academic reward system favors the printed page; and many decision analysts are not computer programmers.

CONCLUSION

Today there are many possibilities for innovation in medical care delivery with the associated need for research. The medical care researcher will do well to scan the horizon for such possibilities. The changing environment can lead to changes in the kind of medical research that is acceptable and valuable. Even such things as valuing human life and limb can have socially beneficial uses.

In addition to changes in medical care delivery, changes in research methods should be considered. The randomized clinical trial and the microcomputer are vehicles whose promise has only begun to be exploited. Finally, if one is concerned with medical care cost, one must be concerned with quality of care, and vice versa. These are not, nor should they be, separate issues.

REFERENCES

Anderson, O. W. (1966). "Influence of Social and Economic Research on Public Policy in the Health Field: A Review." *Milbank Memorial Fund Quarterly* 44 (Supplement): 11–51.

Bloom, B., and Jonsson, E. (1978). "Distributing Medical Care Services. Coronary Care Units in the United States and Sweden." *Scandinavian Journal of Social Medicine* 6: 97–104.

Cohen, D., and Neuhauser, D. (1985). "The Metro Firm Trials: An Innovative Approach to Ongoing Randomized Clinical Trials." In *Assessing Medical Technologies*, ed. Institute of Medicine, 529–34. Washington, DC: National Academy Press.

Cohen, P. (1982). *A Calculating People.* Chicago: University of Chicago Press.

Colton, C.; McClish, D.; Doremus, H.; Powell, S.; et al. (1985). "Implications of DRG Payments for Medical Intensive Care." *Medical Care* 23 (8): 977–85.

Fein, R. (1971). "On Measuring Economic Benefits of Health Programs." In *Medical History and Medical Care*, ed. G. McLachlan and T. McKeown. London: Oxford University Press.

Hershey, C. O.; Porter, D. K.; Breslau, D.; and Cohen, D. (1986). "Influence of Simple Computerized Feedback on Prescription Charges in an Ambulatory Clinic." *Medical Care* 24 (6): 472–81.

Holmes, G. (1975). *Europe: Hierarchy and Revolt 1320–1450.* Glasgow: Fontana Collins.

Hopkins, D. (1983). *Princes and Peasants.* Chicago: University of Chicago Press.

Jury Verdict Research Inc. (1980–81). *Personal Injury Valuation Handbooks* (Loose leaf volumes). Cleveland, OH: Jury Verdict Research Inc.

"Lex Salica" (n.d.). In *Leges Barbarorum Fragmenten,* ed. J. Van Ginneken and E. J. J. Van Der Heyden, 1–39. Nymegen-Utrecht, Holland: Nigmeegsche Studie-Teksten.

Magnusson, M., and Palsson, H. (eds.) (1960). *Njal's Saga.* London: Penguin Books.

Shattuck, L. (1948). *Report of the Sanitary Commission of Massachusetts 1850.* Cambridge, MA: Harvard University Press.

Index

Managed delivery networks,
164–66
Managed security organizations. *See* Managed delivery
networks
Maxicare Health Plans, 177
Medicaid: and access to medical
care, 27; budget reductions,
242; cost of, 140–42; cost
sharing, 129, 139; economic
aspects, 139–49; effect on
health services utilization,
144; eligibility, 139–40; and
the Great Society, 32;
"mills," 147; payments, 141,
145–46; and rationing of
health care, 239; recipients,
142–44, 148; reform, 147–
48; reimbursement, 146–47;
services, 139
Medical
—education: in achieving
quality health care, 59;
future methods, 45
—ethics. *See* Ethics
—industrial complex, 169–80;
emergence of, 169–71;
future of, 178–79; legal
power, 179–80; major
companies, 171–77;
physicians in, 179–80. *See
also* Investor-owned medical
institutions
—licensure: and quality
assurance, 274
—schools: and medical politics,
180
—students: in cost-containment
studies, 224–26, 231–32. *See
also* Physicians
—technology: decision making
in use of, 190–95; evaluation
of by AMA, 121; in health
care costs, 31; and increased
health care costs, 121;
international differences,
187; little ticket vs. big

ticket, 186–87, 202–203;
physicians' use of, 185–204;
practice variations in use of,
54–56; rationing of, 241–42;
regional differences, 187;
risks, 195
Medicare: and access to
medical care, 27; budget
reductions, 242; cost sharing
in, 129; DRG prospective
payment system. *See*
Diagnosis-related group
prospective payment system;
and dying patients, 37–39,
83, 266; economic aspects,
128–39; expenditures, 37–
39; fee freezes, 125–26; and
the Great Society, 32; health
insurance (HI), 129–32,
136–38; and investor-owned
companies, 169–70;
legislative cost controls, 130–
33; and nursing home
coverage, 176; participants
in HMOs, 161; and payment
of physicians, 135–36; and
rationing of health care,
239, 243; supplementary
medical insurance (SMI),
129–32, 136, 138–39
Medigap insurance, 130
Mentally retarded: and
Medicaid, 142
Morality: in medical education,
59
Morbidity: in hospitalization,
277–78
Mortality in hospitalization,
276–77
Multihospital system
management, 155–56

N

National Halothane Study of
Operative Mortality, 277
National health insurance: in

Contributors

EDITH E. BRAGDON, M.A. is a research associate for a Kate B. Reynolds Health Care Trust project on cost containment at the University of North Carolina School of Medicine. She received her M.A. in sociology from the University of Virginia.

ALAN B. COHEN, SC.D. is Vice President at the Robert Wood Johnson Foundation. Previously, he served as Associate Director of the Johns Hopkins School of Hygiene and Public Health Center for Hospital Finance and Management. His publications concern a variety of topics, including medical decision making, medical technology assessment, and certificate of need programs. He received his Doctor of Science from the Harvard School of Public Health.

PETER E. DANS, M.D. is Associate Professor of Medicine and Director of the Office of Medical Practice Evaluation at Johns Hopkins. He has written more than 80 papers and chapters on infectious diseases, health policy, quality assurance, ethics, and medical practice evaluation. He received his M.D. from Columbia University and did his internal medicine training at the Johns Hopkins Hospital and Presbyterian Hospital in New York. He did fellowships in infectious diseases at the National Institutes of Health and Boston City Hospital. He was one of the first Robert Wood Johnson Health Policy fellows.

F. DANIEL DUFFY, M.D. is Professor of Medicine and Chairman of Internal Medicine at the University of Oklahoma, Tulsa Medical College. His medical research has been in resident and student education and methods of teaching the medical interview. He received his M.D. degree from Temple University and did his postgraduate training in internal medicine at the University of Oklahoma Health Sciences Center.

JOHN GORDON FREYMANN, M.D. is Professor of Family Medicine at University of Connecticut School of Medicine. Until 1987, he was President of the National Fund for Medical Education. He has been involved in health care policy as a consultant to the Department of Health, Education, and Welfare and has served on many advisory councils and committees. His publications and research have concentrated primarily on health care planning. He received his M.D. from Harvard Medical School and an honorary Doctor of Science degree from the University of Nebraska. He did his internal medicine training at the Massachusetts General Hospital.

THOMAS F. FRIST, SR., M.D. is Chairman, President, and Chief Executive Officer of the Hospital Corporation of America, a major investor-owned health care company. He received his M.D. degree from Washington University School of Medicine and did his surgical internship at Vanderbilt University Medical Center.

CHARLES HANSEN, M.A. is Research Director of the Internal Medicine Training Program at Moses H. Cone Hospital in Greensboro, North Carolina, where he has been actively involved in medical education and medical research. He received his M.A. in sociology from the University of North Carolina at Greensboro.

DONALD M. HAYES, M.D. is Medical Director of the Sara Lee Corporation and Chairman of the Safety and Health Committee of the American Textile Manufacturers Institute. He previously served as Director of Health and Safety at Burlington Industries and was Professor and Chairman of Community Medicine and Associate Dean of Community Health Sciences at the Bowman Gray School of Medicine. He received his M.D. degree from Bowman Gray School of Medicine and trained in internal medicine at the Salt Lake County General Hospital and in psychiatry at the Louisville General Hospital in Kentucky.

WILLIAM R. HAZZARD, M.D. is Professor and Chairman in the Department of Medicine at Bowman Gray School of Medicine of Wake Forest University. He is a coeditor of a major geriatric textbook, *Principles of Geriatric Medicine,* and is also responsible for numerous publications on geriatrics, lipoprotein metabolism, hyperlipidemias, and atherosclerosis. He has served in major faculty positions at the University of Washington and the Johns Hopkins University School of Medicine. He received his M.D. from the Cornell University Medical College and did his internal medicine training at New York Hospital and the University of Washington School of Medicine.

J. DENNIS HOBAN, ED.D. is Director of the Offices of Educational Research and Services and Associate Professor of Medical Education at the Bowman Gray School of Medicine of Wake Forest University. His research and many national presentations have focused on techniques of medical education and curriculum evaluation. He received his Ed.D. at Indiana University.

SAMUEL H. HOWARD, M.A. is founder, President, and Chief Executive Officer of Phoenix Holdings. Formerly, he served as Senior Vice President for Public Affairs for the Hospital Corporation of America. He has received numerous civic and community awards for his public service activities. He received his M.A. in economics from Stanford University.

RICHARD JANEWAY, M.D. is Executive Dean at the Bowman Gray School of Medicine and Vice President for Health Affairs at Wake Forest University. He is a past chairman of the Association of American Medical Colleges and a national spokesman on the economics of medical education.

ANTHONY L. KOMAROFF, M.D. is Associate Professor of Medicine at Harvard Medical School and Director of the Division of General Medicine and Primary Care at Brigham and Women's Hospital. He has been a researcher and national spokesman on the efficient use of technology and management strategies for common illnesses. Cost effectiveness and the use of computers in medical decision making are notable recent research interests. He has served on the editorial boards of *Medical Care* and *Medical Decision Making,* and is the editor of *Journal Watch.* His M.D. was awarded from the University of Washington School of Medicine, and he did his internal medicine training at Cambridge City Hospital and Beth Israel Hospital.

THOMAS H. LEE, M.D. is Assistant Professor of Medicine at Harvard Medical School and Associate Physician at Brigham and Women's Hospital. He has been active in health care and epidemiologic research on cardiovascular topics and in teaching research techniques in these areas. He received an M.S. in epidemiology from the Harvard School of Public Health. He received his M.D. from Cornell University Medical College and did his internal medicine training, cardiology subspecialty, and general internal medicine fellowship at Brigham and Women's Hospital.

CARL B. LYLE, JR., M.D. is Professor of Medicine at the University of North Carolina School of Medicine at Chapel Hill. As a researcher in primary care internal medicine, he is interested in how physician behavior affects economics and productivity of medical care. He received his M.D. degree from Columbia University and did his postgraduate training in internal medicine at the University of California Hospitals, Duke University, and the University of North Carolina at Chapel Hill.

JACK D. McCUE, M.D. is Professor of Medicine at Tufts University School of Medicine, and Vice Chairman of the Department of Medicine and Chief of General Medicine and Geriatrics at Baystate Medical Center, where he directs the internal medicine residency programs. He is the author or editor of six books and an annotated bibliography on medical cost containment. His research and publications reflect his diverse interests in the stresses of medical practice, infectious diseases, and cost containment. He received his M.D. from Case Western Reserve University and did his internal medicine training at Baltimore City Hospitals, the Johns Hopkins Hospital, and Beth Israel Hospital in Boston.

STEPHEN J. McPHEE, M.D. is Associate Professor of Medicine at the University of California in San Francisco and a member of the Institute for Health Policy Studies. He is actively involved in health services research, in which he has published extensively. He received his M.D. from the Johns Hopkins University School of Medicine and completed his internal medicine training at the Johns Hopkins Hospital.

WILLIAM D. MATTERN, M.D. is Associate Dean for Academic Affairs and Professor of Medicine at the University of North Carolina School of Medicine, was cochair of a schoolwide curriculum review, and has been actively involved in the development of new techniques in medical education. He has published extensively in nephrology and medical education. He received his M.D. degree from Columbia Medical School and did his internal medicine training at the New England Medical Center.

DAVID MECHANIC, PH.D. is University Professor and René Dubos Professor of Behavioral Sciences at Rutgers University and Adjunct Professor of Psychiatry at the Robert Wood Johnson Medical School. He is Director of the Institute for Health, Health Care Policy, and Aging Research at Rutgers University. He has held many appointments on federal committees, has served on the editorial boards of major sociology journals, and has published extensively in medical sociology. His research has looked at the effect of cost containment on decision-making processes in medicine and psychiatry and the organization of medical and psychiatric care.

JEFFREY C. MERRILL, M.P.H. is Vice President at the Robert Wood Johnson Foundation. Previous positions include Director of the Center for Health Policy Studies at Georgetown University and Fellow at the Center for Health Policy and Management in the Harvard University Kennedy School of Government. He has worked in the field of human services in both state and federal government. He holds an M.P.H. from Johns Hopkins University and was an Assistant Professor at Georgetown University School of Medicine.

DUNCAN NEUHAUSER, PH.D., M.B.A. is Professor of Epidemiology and Biostatistics at Case Western Reserve University, Professor of Medicine at the Case Western School of Medicine, and Adjunct Professor of Organizational Behavior at the Weatherhead School of Management. He serves as editor of *Health Matrix* and *Medical Care.* He received his Ph.D. and M.B.A. from the University of Chicago and his M.H.A. from the University of Michigan.

STEVEN A. SCHROEDER, M.D., Professor of Medicine and Chief of General Internal Medicine at the University of California at San Francisco, has been a major figure in national general internal medicine activities. He is well known for his innovative research in cost effectiveness and interventions that influence physicians' use of technology, and for his participation on national committees that have examined the use of technology. He was awarded an M.D. from Harvard Medical School and did his internal medicine training at the Boston City Hospital.

M. ROY SCHWARZ, M.D. is Assistant Executive Vice President for Medical Education and Science at the American Medical Association. Formerly, he served as Dean of the University of Colorado and Vice Chancellor for Health Affairs at the University of Colorado Health Sciences Center. The author of more than 150 articles, book chapters, and abstracts, he received his M.D. from the University of Washington School of Medicine.

JONATHAN A. SHOWSTACK, M.P.H. is Associate Adjunct Professor of Health Policy at the University of California at San Francisco. He has researched and published extensively on issues related to medical cost containment. He received his M.P.H. from the University of California at Berkeley.

ALAN L. SORKIN, PH.D. is Professor and Chairman of the Department of Economics at the University of Maryland and Adjunct Professor of the School of Medicine. He is the author or editor of 13 books on economics and has been actively interested in health care economics in developing nations and the economic and social problems of Native Americans. He received his Ph.D. and a master's degree from the Johns Hopkins University.

ROBERT M. VEATCH, PH.D. is Professor of Medical Ethics at the Kennedy Institute of Ethics and Professor of Philosophy and Adjunct Professor in Community and Family Medicine and Obstetrics and Gynecology at the Georgetown University and Georgetown University School of Medicine. He has edited and authored books, monographs, and numerous articles on medical ethics. He holds a master's degree in pharmacology from the University of California Medical Center in San Francisco, and a B.D., M.A., and Ph.D. in religion and society from Harvard University.

STANLEY WOHL, M.D. is Director of Health Services at San Jose State University, San Jose, California. He is actively involved in the study of economics in health care. He has published five books and 26 articles and has consulted for numerous government agencies, both federal and state. He received his M.D. degree from McGill University and did his postgraduate training in surgery at the Montreal General Hospital, Montreal, Canada. He was the 1985 recipient of the American Medical Writers Association book award.